Anopheles Mosquitoes: A Detailed Research

Anopheles Mosquitoes: A Detailed Research

Edited by **Jamie Spooner**

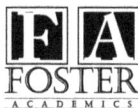

FA
FOSTER
ACADEMICS

New Jersey

Published by Foster Academics,
61 Van Reypen Street,
Jersey City, NJ 07306, USA
www.fosteracademics.com

Anopheles Mosquitoes: A Detailed Research
Edited by Jamie Spooner

International Standard Book Number: 978-1-63242-049-7 (Hardback)

Contents

Preface

This book has been an outcome of determined endeavour from a group of educationists in the field. The primary objective was to involve a broad spectrum of professionals from diverse cultural background involved in the field for developing new researches. The book not only targets students but also scholars pursuing higher research for further enhancement of the theoretical and practical applications of the subject.

Anopheles mosquitoes are the carrier species for transmission of human malaria and its destructive consequences in endemic countries worldwide. In 2010 alone, malaria was the reason for approximately 660,000 deaths. As the study of Anopheles species and populations is an important element for achieving the aim of malaria elimination, a substantial amount of information has been collected over the last century, and together in the last few decades with the advent of new technologies, the acquisition of novel knowledge has accelerated even further. The unique purpose of this book is to present recent compilation on several research, novel concepts, paradigms and innovative approaches for controlling anophelines, using state-of-the-art methodologies and analysis. The content of this book has been compiled from internationally acclaimed experts across 5 continents, covering anopheles mosquito's impact on pathogen transmission and vector control: new approaches and perspectives.

It was an honour to edit such a profound book and also a challenging task to compile and examine all the relevant data for accuracy and originality. I wish to acknowledge the efforts of the contributors for submitting such brilliant and diverse chapters in the field and for endlessly working for the completion of the book. Last, but not the least; I thank my family for being a constant source of support in all my research endeavours.

Editor

Pathogen Transmission and Influencing Factors

Simian Malaria Parasites: Special Emphasis on *Plasmodium knowlesi* and Their *Anopheles* Vectors in Southeast Asia

Indra Vythilingam and Jeffery Hii

Additional information is available at the end of the chapter

1. Introduction

Simian malaria parasites were first reported in Malayan monkeys by Daniels in 1908 [1]. It had been assumed for a long time that transmission of simian malaria to humans would not be possible. However, an accidental infection of scientists in Atlanta, USA by mosquito bites in the laboratory proved that a simian malaria species– *Plasmodium cynomolgi* can be transmitted to humans [2, 3]. In 1965 the first natural infection in human was reported in an American surveyor who was infected in the jungles of Pahang, Malaysia [4]. Fortunately he returned to USA and was detected first as *Plasmodium falciparum* and later revised to *Plasmodium malariae* due to the band form of the parasite. Further examination proved that it was actually *Plasmodium knowlesi* [4].

Plasmodium knowlesi was first found in *Macaca fascicularis* monkeys that were brought to India from Singapore. Drs Knowles and Das Gupta knew that they were dealing with a new malaria parasite but did not provide a binomial nomenclature. It was Sinton and Muligan who formally named the new species as *P. knowlesi* [5] after Dr. Knowles. Studies that were carried out before the first human case was reported unveiled many new simian malaria parasites but no human cases. After the first human case was reported in 1965, blood samples were collected from about 1000 people from surrounding villages in West Malaysia where the case of *P. knowlesi* was found but none were positive for simian malaria [6]. However, a presumptive case was reported from Johore, a southern state in peninsular Malaysia [7].

Mosquito surveys carried out in the area where the first case occurred did not reveal any sporozoite infections in the mosquitoes. However, studies in the coastal areas of Selangor in peninsular Malaysia found *Anopheles hackeri* to be a vector of *P. knowlesi* [8] and this mosquito was attracted only to non-human primates and would not come to bite humans. Thus, at that time it was concluded that simian malaria parasites would not easily affect humans and if it did human malaria cases would occur at very low levels [9]. In 2004 a large focus of knowlesi malaria among humans in Sarawak, Malaysian Borneo was reported [10]. This significant finding stimulated many scientists who were interested in the field of simian malaria in humans and their vectors and hosts. Southeast Asia has now become a focal point for the distribution of *P. knowlesi* in humans. This chapter will describe the simian malaria parasites in non-human primates, the bionomics of vectors involved in transmission, human cases of knowlesi malaria and the challenges in relation to elimination of malaria.

2. Simian malaria parasites and their hosts

In Southeast Asia, there are 13 species of *Plasmodium* affecting non-human primates [11]. Of these *Plasmodium coatneyi, P. cynomolgi, P. fieldi, P. fragile, P. inui, P. knowlesi* and *P. simiovale* are known to occur in macaques and leaf monkeys [12]. However, of the seven species, *P. fragile* has been reported in both India and Sri Lanka while *P. simiovale* is restricted only to Sri Lanka [12]. *Plasmodium eylesi, P. jefferyi, P. youngi* and *P. hylobati* are found in gibbons while *P. pitheci* and *P. silvaticum* are found in orangutans in Borneo. These malaria parasites are found throughout mainland Southeast Asia and associated islands within the Wallace's line [13].

Information is currently available on the non-human primate malaria especially in Malaysia. Thus, so far five species of simian malaria parasites in non-human primates (macaques) have been reported from Malaysia [12, 14]. The simian malaria parasite *P. cynomolgi* is a species that had been experimentally transmitted to humans [3, 15]. *Plasmodium cynomolgi* in monkeys has many of the characteristics seen during infection of humans with *P. vivax* [16]. It was always believed that monkey malaria was specific for monkeys and human malaria was specific for humans. However, in 1960 accidental infections in the laboratory of simian malaria to humans by mosquito bites led to investigative studies to be carried out in Malaysia and this resulted in the description of many new simian malaria parasites [17-20].

Simian malaria parasites have been detected in three main species of non-human primates. They are *Macaca fascicularis, Macaca nemestrina* and *Presbytis melalophos* [19, 20]. In the 1960's studies on malaria parasites of *M. nemestrina* revealed that this non-human primate can harbour the following simian malaria species: *P. cynomolgi, P. inui, P. knowlesi* and *P. fieldi* [19] Of these *P. fieldi* was a new species found in this macaque [17]. Currently, *P. fieldi* has been found as mixed infection in longtailed macaques but less frequently compared to the other simian malaria parasites [14]. Only 4% of the macaques had *P.fieldi* mono-infection in a study in Sarawak, Malaysian Borneo [14]. In Malaysian Borneo the predominant species found in the longtailed macaques was *P. inui* (82%) followed by *P. knowlesi* (78%), *P. coatneyi* (66%) and *P. cynomolgi* (56%) [14]. However, in Singapore *P. knowlesi* was the predominant species among long-tailed macaques (68.2%), followed by *P. cynomolgi* (66.6%), *P. fieldi* (16.7 %), *P. coatneyi* (3%) and *P. inui* (1.5%) [21]. In Selangor, out of the 107 samples of macaque blood tested for malaria, 64.5% were positive for *Plasmodium* of which 23.3 % were positive for *P. knowlesi* [22].

Plasmodium coatneyi was successfully established when sporozoites from *An. hacker* collected from Rantau Panjang Selangor, were inoculated into an uninfected rhesus monkey. The monkey exhibited infection after a prepatent period of 14 days. The young trophozoites were not easily distinguishable from those of *P. falciparum* and demonstrated a tertian cycle thus leading to a new species [23]. This is the first instance of finding a new species of malaria in the vector before it was known from the primate host. Subsequently *P. coatneyi* was also isolated from *M. fascicularis* from the same area and also from the Philippines [24].

The pig-tailed macaque – *Macaca nemestrina* occurs in various sub-species from easternmost India and Bangladesh, through Myanmar and Thailand, Malaysia, Sumatra and Kalimantan [19]. This animal is trained to harvest coconuts from tall trees and is kept as a pet by their owners. They coexist with long-tailed macaques-*M. fascicularis* but are ecologically less diverse in their choice of habitats [19].They are also less commonly seen compared to *M. fascicularis*. The parasites found in the pig-tailed macaques were *P. cynomolgi, P. inui, P. knowlesi, P. fieldi* and Hepatocystis [19].

3. History of natural infection of *P. knowlesi* in human host

Scientists have always been curious as to the possibility of humans being infected with non-human primate malaria. This interest was intensified when two scientists working in the Memphis laboratory were infected with *P. cynomolgi*. They were conducting infection studies in the laboratory and they were dissecting a large number of mosquitoes heavily infected with malaria parasites two weeks prior to coming down with the illness [2]. Following these infections, scientists decided to survey areas in peninsular Malaysia and search for natural transmission of simian malaria in humans. There were also attempts by scientists to probe into the natural transmission of monkey malaria to humans in the northernmost state of peninsular Malaysia [25]. In the first survey they did not come across any human cases but described new species of monkey malaria parasites in macaques [6].

In 1965, an American surveyor working in Bukit Kertau in Pahang, Malaysia came down with malaria. Fortunately he returned to USA where he was diagnosed as *P. knowlesi* [4]. This was the first natural infection reported in humans. The surveyor was apparently working in the forested area at night. American scientists along with the scientists from the Institute for Medical Research carried out extensive surveys in that area where the surveyor was infected. Blood from 1117 persons from 17 villages were examined for malaria parasites by microscopy using Giemsa stained slides. Blood was also inoculated into rhesus monkeys to determine if there were natural infections of simian malaria in humans. Of these only 28 had malaria infection, 11 were *P. falciparum*, 13 *P.vivax* and four were not identifiable. None of the rhesus monkeys developed malaria parasites [6]. Thus it was concluded that simian malaria would not easily infect humans. In 1970's a presumptive case of *P. knowlesi* was reported from Johore, peninsular Malaysia [7].

4. Cases of knowlesi malaria in Southeast Asia

In 2004, a large focus of human knowlesi malaria cases were reported from Sarawak, Malaysian Borneo [10]. In that study it was found that 58% of the patients, admitted at the Sarawak hospital, were found to be infected with knowlesi malaria using molecular tools. These were misidentified by microscopy as *P. malariae*. Early trophozoites of *P. knowlesi* in the erythrocyte resemble that of *P. falciparum* such as double chromatin dots, multiple-infected erythrocytes and appliqué forms [26]. Besides the late and mature trophozoites, schizonts and gametocytes of *P. knowlesi* in human infections were generally indistinguishable from those of *P. malariae*. Moreover, 'band form' trophozoites, which are a characteristic feature for *P. malariae* parasites [27, 28] were observed in more than half of the blood films examined by Lee *et al* [26]. 'Sinton and Mulligan's stippling' in erythrocytes infected with *P. knowlesi* was noted previously in infections in rhesus monkeys [27] and humans [7]. However, in present knowlesi cases only faint stippling was evident in some of the infected erythrocytes with mature trophozoite and schizont stages [10, 26]. Thus, human infections with *P. knowlesi* have been mistaken for *P. falciparum* malaria when the infecting parasites were predominantly at the early trophozoite or ring form developmental stage and as *P. malariae* when in the late trophozoite or band form. Figure 1 shows the different stages of development of *P. knowlesi*.

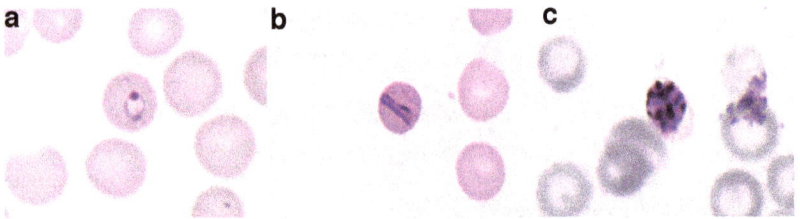

Figure 1. Giemsa stained thin blood film of *P. knowlesi* as seen with 100 x objective. a). trophozoite b) band form of trophozoite, c) schizont

After the publication in 2004 [10], more cases were reported in Malaysia [29-32] and also from other countries in Southeast Asia with the exception of Lao PDR. To date cases have been reported from Thailand [33-35], Philippines [36],Vietnam [37], Indonesia [38], Cambodia [39], Myanmar [40] and Singapore [41]. Malaysia has reported the highest number of cases in the region. *Plasmodium knowlesi* is now considered as the fifth malaria parasite affecting humans [42] and is detected by molecular methods. However, some still believe that it is a simian malaria since human to human transmission has not been proven [13].

A study has shown that *M. fascicularis* experimentally infected with *P. knowlesi* erythrocytic parasites from humans developed pre patent infection on day seven and demonstrated diurnal sub-periodic pattern [43]. It is the only primate malaria with a 24-hour erythrocytic cycle [44] while *P. falciparum* has a 48 hour cycle and *P. malariae* a 72 hour cycle.

Knowlesi malaria has shown to be life threatening and mortality has been reported [29, 31]. From December 2007 to November 2009 six (27%) out of 22 patients with severe knowlesi malaria died in Sabah [31]. Cases of knowlesi malaria are also occurring in areas where human malaria cases have been reduced or in malaria free areas [45]. People can contract malaria either outside their houses in rural settings, in farms where they work or in the forest while hunting or working.

5. Knowlesi malaria associated with travellers to Southeast Asia

Naturally acquired cases of *P. knowlesi* have been reported from travellers visiting this region. A New Zealand pilot working in Sabah and Sarawak north of Bintulu Malaysian Borneo was diagnosed as *P. knowlesi* in New Zealand when he fell ill. The sequence of the parasite had a 100% homology to the Vietnam strain [46]. A lady born in the Philippines and residing in USA for more than 25 years came down with knowlesi malaria after visiting Palawan in the Philippines where she stayed in a log cabin close to the forest edge. She fell ill and on her return to USA was diagnosed as *P. knowlesi* [47]. A Finish traveller spent about 5 days in the jungle on the north-western coast of peninsular Malaysia and fell ill after he returned to Finland. He was diagnosed with *P. knowlesi* parasitaemia by PCR and sequencing showed 100% homology with *P. knowlesi* sequence from Malaysian Borneo and a *Macaca mullata* from Colombia [48]. A Swede who travelled to the Bario Highlands in Malaysian Borneo came down ill on his return to Sweden and was diagnosed as suffering from knowlesi malaria [49]. A Spanish traveller who spent six months travelling around Southeast Asia – in forested areas was diagnosed as knowlesi malaria when he returned to Spain [50]. A French tourist returning from Thailand was diagnosed as *P. knowlesi* [51]. This shows that the knowlesi malaria is currently a serious public health problem and not just single occasional episodes.

6. Bionomics of simian malaria vectors and trapping techniques

6.1. Distribution

The distribution of *P. knowlesi* in the natural monkey hosts and transmission to humans are restricted to mosquito vectors of the *Anopheles* Leucosphyrus Group confined to Southeast Asia [52]. It is currently recognized that under natural forest conditions, most if not all members of the Leucosphyrus Group apparently feed primarily on monkeys in the canopy, transmitting various plasmodia [53]. In Harbach's review [54], the Leucosphyrus Group in the Neomyzomyia Series contains 20 named species [55, 56], one unnamed species (aff. *takasagoensis*) and two geographical forms (Con Son form from island off South Vietnam and Negros form from Negros island in Philippines) [55] divided between the Hackeri, Leucosphyrus and Riparis Subgroups. According to Manguin *et al.* [57] and Sallum *et al.* [56], the Leucosphyrus Subgroup consists of the Dirus and Leucosphyrus complexes, which includes seven and five sibling species, respectively. Species belonging to the Leucosphyrus complex are also important vectors of human malaria and lymphatic filariasis and are distributed in the South and Southeast Asia regions. The current vectorial status and geographical distribution of the Leucosphyrus Group are listed in Table 1 and Figure 2.

Complex	Vector species	Species of *Plasmodium*	Vertebrate hosts	Distribution
Leucosphyrus	*An. leucosphyrus* Donitz (hv)[1]	*Pf, Pv, Pm*[2]	Human	Indonesia, Sumatra
	An. latens Sallum & Peyton (hv, sv, fv)	Pf, Pv, Pm *P. inui* [78] *P. knowlesi, P. inui, P. coatneyi, P. fieldi*[79]	Human *M. fascicularis, M. nemestrina P. melalophos* [19-22]	Indonesia, East Malaysia, West Malaysia, Thailand Sarawak: East Malaysia: Sarawak[45,75] West Malaysia [56]
	An. introlatus Colless (sv)	*P. cynomolgi, P. fieldi* [78]	*M. fascicularis, M. nemestrina P. melalophos* [19-22]	Indonesia West Malaysia, Thailand [56]
	An. balabacensis Colless (hv, sv, fv)	*P. knowlesi* [45]; possibly *P. coatneyi* & *P. inui*[73]	*M. fascicularis* [73]	Brunei, Indonesia, East Malaysia, Philippines [56]
	An. baisasi Colless	Information inadequate		Luzon, Philippines
Dirus	*An. dirus* Peyton & Harrison (hv, sv fv)	*P. knowlesi* [76-77]	Human *M. fascicularis,* [35]	Cambodia, China, Vietnam, Laos, Thailand
	An. cracens Sallum & Peyton (hv, sv, fv)	Probable vector of human malaria [56] *P. knowlesi* [30,72] *P. cynomolgi, P. inui* [80]	*M. fascicularis* [30]	Indonesia, West Malaysia, Thailand
	An. baimaii Sallum & Peyton (hv, fv)	Pf, Pv Pm	Human	Bangladesh, India, Thailand, Myanmar, China
Hackeri	*An. mirans* Sallum & Peyton (sv)	*P. cynomolgi, P. inui* [56] *P. inui shortii; P. fragile* [56]		India, Sri Lanka
	An. hackeri Edwards (sv)	*P. cynomolgi, P. inui, P. fieldi, P. coatneyi, P. knowlesi* [52]	*M. fascicularis*	East and West Malaysia, Philippines, Thailand
	An. pujutensis Colless (sv)?	Probable vector of simian malaria parasites [52]		Indonesia, East and West Malaysia, Thailand

[1] hv,sv and fv indicate human malarial, simian malarial and human lymphatic filarial vectors; sv? Vectorial status awaiting confirmation

Table 1. Simian malaria parasites of Southeast Asia: their Leucosphyrus Group natural vectors, hosts and geographical distribution (modified from Sallum et al [56]

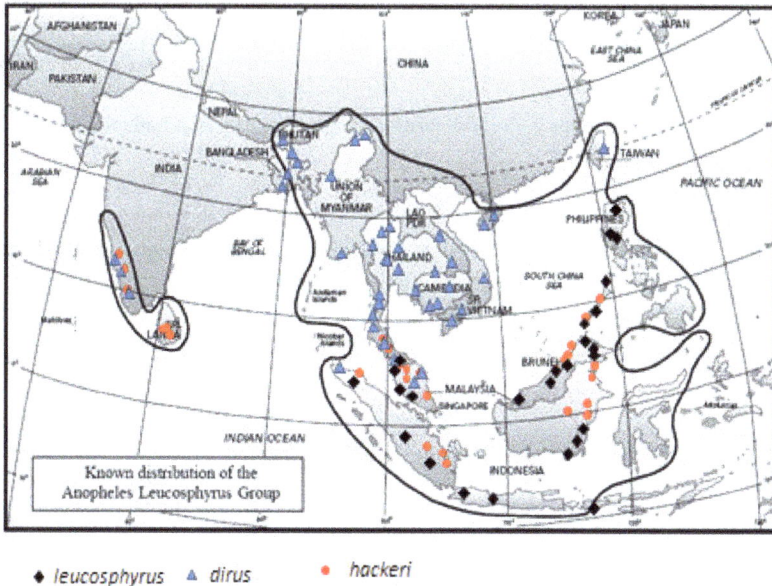

● *leucosphyrus*   ▲ *dirus*   ● *hackeri*

Figure 2. Known limit of the distribution of the *An. leucosphyrus* Group (*An. hackeri* Subgroup, *An, dirus* complex and *An. leucosphyrus* complex) of mosquitoes in South and Southeast Asia adopted from Sallum et al 2005. Only the distribution of those species mentioned in Table 1 are shown

As a member of the Leucosphyrus complex, *An. latens* is widely distributed in Borneo (Kalimantan, Sarawak, Sabah) together with *An. balabacensis* in the forested areas of eastern Borneo (Figure 2). *Anopheles latens* and *An. introlatus* are sympatric with members of the closely related Dirus complex in the Malay Peninsula, including southern Thailand [58, 59] (Figure 2).

The Dirus complex is well known because its species are widespread in forest and forest foothills throughout the Oriental Region from southwestern India eastwards and from 30° north parallel to the Malaysian peninsula [60-62] (Figure2), whereas the Leucosphyrus complex has been investigated to a much lesser degree in Malaysia Borneo and Kalimantan Borneo. *Anopheles cracens* (Dirus complex) was the predominant mosquito species in a recent study and was never reported previously from Pahang, Malaysia [30]. Earlier reports indicate that *An. cracens* was found in Perlis (Northern most state of Peninsular, Malaysia) and in Terengganu (east Coast State of Peninsular Malaysia [56]. Its geographic distribution within peninsular Malaysia is unknown [63].

6.2. Larval biology

Table 2 shows a summary of *Anopheles* larval habitat characteristics adapted from Sinka et al [64]. As forest-dwelling species, the immature stages share an affinity for humid, shaded environments where they make use of transient or temporary larval habitats such as pools and puddles. Like other members of the Leucosphyrus complex, larval habitats of *An. lateens* and *An. balabacensis* are mostly shaded temporary pools and natural containers of clear or turbid water on the ground in forest areas (Table 2). Larvae of *An. latens* are usually found in clear seepage pools in forest swamps in peninsular Malaysia [65] and in pools beside a forest stream and in swampy patches in hilly areas [66]. Habitats occupied by *An. latens* in Thailand include stump ground holes, sand pools, stream margins, seepage-springs, wheel tracks and elephant foot prints [53, 59]. Typical breeding places of *An. balabacensis* are small pools in clay soil containing fairly clean seepage or rainwater, still or slow moving, and under some shade, with the upper altitudinal limit of 4000 ft in Borneo (1220 meters) [66]. Other adventitious and rare breeding sites include swamp edges or in rock pools, bamboo stumps, split bamboos, tins and other artificial containers [66] and wells in Sandakan, Sabah (unpublished report by Dr David Muir, WHO consultant). In inland forest *An. hackeri* was found breeding in split bamboo while in the coastal area it was found breeding in the cavities of leaf bases of nipah palm [8].

Species	Light intensity	Turbidity	Water movement	Small natural water collections	Small man-made water collections
An. latens & leucosphyrus	Heliophobic	Clear, turbid, fresh water Muddy pool (W Malaysia [56])	Still or stagnant	Small streams, seepage streams, pools	Wheel ruts, hoof prints
An. balabacensis	Typical heliophobic	Fresh water	Still or stagnant	Pools; dips in the ground	Wheel ruts, hoof prints
An. dirus	Heliophobic	Clear, turbid, fresh water	Still or stagnant	Small streams, pools, wells, dips in the ground	Borrow pits, wheel ruts, hoof prints
An. hackeri	Heliophobic	Clean non saline water, but found in water containing up to 4% sea-water	Still or stagnant	In split bamboo and cavities at the leaf base of nipa palm	In Thailand, in elephant footprints [56]

Table 2. Larval habitat characteristics of monkey malaria vectors (adapted from Sinka et al [64]) including individual studies reported in the literature.

6.3. Biological characteristics

The important biological charactersitics of the known vectors of simian malaria are shown in Table 3 which has been modified from Meek [67]. Of the known vectors, *An. hackeri* is known to bite only monkeys and rarely comes to bite humans [8]. Although *An. latens* is a vector of human malaria in East Malaysia [68-70], the current studies have shown that the species is more attracted to monkeys compared to humans [71], whilst *An. cracens* is attracted to both monkeys and humans [72]. In Palawan Island, Philippines, *An. balabacensis* was more attracted to a monkey bait trap compared to carabao (water buffalo) and human bait traps [73, 74]. It was also found positive for oocysts and sporozoites but could not be confirmed if it was of monkey origin [73]. However, infection studies carried out by the same authors proved that *An. balabacensis* was the vector of simian malaria in Palawan [73]. So far only the *An.* Leucosphyrus Group (*An. latens, An. cracens, An. balabacensis, An. hackeri* and *An. dirus*) of mosquitoes have been found positive for simian malaria parasites in nature [30, 45, 71, 72, 75-80]. However, *An. dirus* is also a main vector of both human malaria, with sporozoite rates as high as 14% in Myanmar and as low as 2.5% in Lao PDR [61, 81], and *Wuchereria bancrofti* [82].

Species	Peak biting time	Host preference or MBT:HBT	Survivorship	Sporozoite rate/EIR
An. latens	Sarawak: Around midnight in forested areas and soon after dusk in village settlements [68] Forest: 1900-2000 h; farm: 0100-0200 h [69] Monkey biting rate at 6, 3 m above ground and at ground: 6.8:3.2:1.0. HBR highest at forest fringe (6.74%), within the forest (1.85%) and at long house (0.28%) [71]	Similar host preference 1.0 : 1.3 [71]	Sarawak: parous rate 65.8% (farm), 53.7% (forest), 65.8% (longhouse) [71] VC: 2.86 (farm), 0.60 (forest), 0.85 (longhouse) [71]	Sarawak: 1.18% (pooled from forest fringe, forest & longhouse) , 0.7% (farm), 1.4% (forest), all confirmed Pk by PCR; EIR 11.98 (farm), 14.1 (forest) [71]
An. balabacensis	Palawan: In and out; 20.00-03.00 h [73] Sabah: 22:00-02:00 h [85- 86];after midnight [87] Out (76%): 19:00-20:00 h, in(24%): 22:00-23:00 h;[83] Lombok: 19:00-21:00h) [84]	Attracted to humans, monkey & water buffalo; more frequently caught in monkey traps [74]	Sabah: highest in Nov, lowest in July [83]	Kalimantan: 1.3% [88] Palawan: 12.5% sporozoite rate; 29% attracted to monkeys were positive for oocysts [74]
An. dirus	Late or early biting, usually around 22:00 h [60-62]	Highly anthropophilic,	Higher parous rate (76%) & life expectancy during dry season	Human sporozoite rates vary with season and location: from

Species	Peak biting time	Host preference or MBT:HBT	Survivorship	Sporozoite rate/EIR
	9 of 13 *Plasmodium* positive bites occur before 21:00 h (Vietnam) [91]	exophagic as well as endophagic and exophilic [61-62]	compared to wet season (62.4%) in Lao [81]	7.8% in Assam (India) to 14% in Myanmar [61] and 2.5% in Laos [81] 43% of 72 salivary glands were PCR-positive for Pk CSP and Pk 18s rRNA. Mixed infections of Pk with Pv and Pf were common in Vietnam [77]
An. cracens	Thailand: 1900-2100 h [60] West Malaysia: 2000-2100 h; 74% biting before 2100 h; predominantly exophagic (1.11 bites/man-night) in both forest (1.24 bites/man-night) and fruit orchard (4.15 bites/man-night); 60% biting at ground level to 3 m high before 00:00 h; more biting at canopy level (6 m) compared to earlier collections at the same level [72].	West Malaysia: 1: 2.6 [7.2]	West Malaysia: parous rate 65.7% (fruit orchard), 71.5% (forest) VC: 2.46 (fruit orchard), 1.09 (forest) [72]	West Malaysia: 0.60% (fruit orchard), 2.9% (forest) EIR: 0.08 [72]
An. hackeri	Not known since most bite monkeys and rarely found in human bait traps [78]	Most attracted to monkeys at canopy level in mangrove forest does not come to bite humans [78]	No data available	In coastal area of Rantau Panjang West Malaysia 0.7% [78]

[1]VC - vectorial capacity; EIR - entomological inoculation rate; PCR - polymerase chain reaction; HBR - human biting rate; MBT- Monkey bait trap; HBT- human bait trap; CSP - circumsporozoite

Table 3. Biological variations among adults of simian malaria vectors in Southeast Asia (modified from Meek 1995 [67].

The peak biting times of *An. balabacensis* vary from place to place as shown in Table 3. It seems to bite as early as 19:00 h in recent years compared to being late night biters in the previous decades [83-89]. *An. dirus s.s.* tends to bite between 20:00 and 23:00 h [53, 56, 60] and and there is significant biological variability within the Dirus complex, depending on the local circumstances [90]. In Vietnam, sporozoite positive bites from *An. dirus* occur before 21:00 h [91] and co-infections of *P. knowlesi, P. falciparum* and *P. vivax* [76, 77] in mosquitoes are indicative of simultaneous transmission. *Plasmodium knowlesi*-sporozoite infective *An. latens* and *An. cracens* were detected from human landing and monkey bait collections in Sarawak and Pahang, Malaysia, respectively [71, 72] suggesting that *P. knowlesi* is being transmitted to both humans and macaques by these two vector species. Generally the parous rates of the Leucosphyrus Group of mosquitoes where relatively high as shown in Table 3. Overall parous rate of *An. latens* was 59% and those caught in the forest was significantly lower than those caught at the farm or long house (where native people of Sarawak live) [71], while for *An. cracens* the parous rate in the forest was higher than in the farm (Table 3), and on average was above 60% [72]. Heterogeneity in biting rates and parous rates indicates that the vectorial capacities are relatively higher in farms or orchards compared to forests (Table 3), and has significant implications for vector control. Understanding the importance of natural heterogenity in *P. knowlesi* transmission is necessary to elucidate the key variation undermining existing control efforts and to target the vector species for focused interventions [92].

6.4. Laboratory susceptibility studies

In laboratory experiments with *P. knowlesi, An. balabacensis* was found to be a successful vector [93]. However, *An. maculatus* only developed few oocysts and sporozoite infection in salivary glands was of low intensity. Laboratory feeding experiments, *An. maculatus* was susceptible to *P. inui* and was able to transmit the parasite to the non-human primate host after a prepatent period of 11 days [94]. In a series of experiments infectivity conducted in the Institute for Medical Research, with the Gombak strain of *P. cynomolgi*, the following mosquitoes were found with salivary gland infections: *An. maculatus, An. kochi, An. sundaicus* (=*An. epiroticus*), *An. vagus* and *An. introlatus* [16]. However, in field situation it was observed that *An. maculatus* was not attracted to macaques, with only three female mosquitoes entering the monkey bait trap [72]. While *An. kochi* was the second predominant mosquito entering monkey baited trap, none were positive for oocyst or sporozoites [72]. Thus, although species other than the Leucosphyrus Group were able to develop the simian malaria parasites to sporozoites, none were incriminated in nature except the Leucosphyrus Group.

6.5. Trapping techniques

Various trapping methods were tested for the collection of *Anopheles* mosquitoes attracted to non-human primates. Earlier observations indicated that these mosquitoes prefer to feed well above ground level and especially about 6-8 m above ground level. Thus, platforms were built among foliage in the forest or plantations to house the non-human primates for mosquito collections. The following traps that were tested [95] are described hereunder.

Net Traps

This is similar to the human–bait-net trap introduced by Gater [96]. This method provided the best results when tested [95]. The platforms were constructed among the branches of trees to a height of 6 meters. Special metal cages measuring 90 cm x 90 cm x 90 cm and covered by wire mesh were used to house the monkeys on the platform measuring 300 cm X 200 cm. The meshed cages provided a physical barrier to prevent the monkeys from grabbing the collectors and also to prevent the entry of snakes. It is ideal to have two monkeys sharing a cage to increase vector attraction. A mosquito net measuring 190 cm x 180 cm x 150 cm with an opening of about 40 cm lifted on either ends was used to cover the cages with monkeys on each platform. The traps were operated from 18:00 to 06:00 hours and were searched at regular intervals [71, 72]. A collector, upon entering the net, closed the openings and collected all resting mosquitoes with the use of aspirators. Mosquitoes in the aspirator were then transferred to paper cups and were brought to the laboratory for identification and dissection. Platforms were built at various heights, ground level, 3 and 6 meters above ground. Figure 3 shows two different platforms in operation.

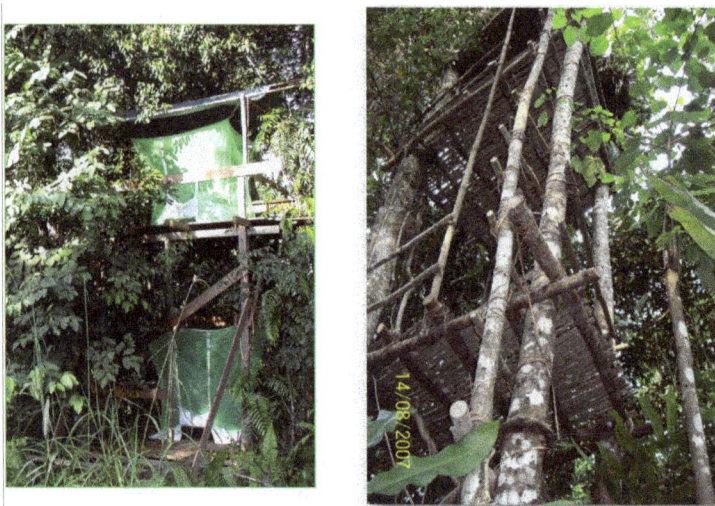

Figure 3. Monkey Baited Net Traps at different levels on platform.

The other traps used were Shannon net trap, drum funnel-trap, Lumsden suction trap and light traps. Detailed descriptions can be found in Wharton [95]. Of all the traps tested, it was found that the monkey- baited traps were superior compared to other types of traps. Although it is a difficult task to collect mosquitoes from the platforms at regular intervals, it is no doubt important to study the behaviour of the mosquitoes. Studies by Wharton [95] demonstrated that 83% of the *An. hackeri* were collected in catches made before midnight, compared to only 62% and 65.8% of *An. latens* and *An. cracens* caught before midnight respectively [71, 72]. Thus, it seems that all night collection is still important despite logistical difficulties, costliness, tediousness and human fatigue.

7. Implications for control

Currently insecticide treated bednets (ITN) and indoor residual spraying (IRS) are the two most important tools for the control of malaria vectors. Scaling up ITN, IRS, artemisinin-based combination therapies and intermittent preventive treatment for infants and pregnant women have contributed to the reported reductions in malaria on a global scale [97]. As part of the Global Malaria Action Plan, the RBM Partnership and World Health Organization has recommended "malaria eradication worldwide by reducing the global incidence to zero through progressive malaria elimination in countries" [98]. However, if human malaria could be eliminated, forests in Southeast Asia provide favourable environments for zoonotic transmission of *P. knowlesi* thus, thwarting efforts to eliminate malaria.

The vectors of *P. knowlesi* malaria have been incriminated only from certain districts or locations in Malaysia [71, 72, 75]. Given that the vectors of monkey malaria show anthropo-phagic, exophagic and exophilic tendencies, it is obvious that the existing front-line vector control tools (IRS, ITN) will not be sufficient to reduce vector density and break the transmission cycle of *P. knowlesi* in the most intensively endemic parts of Southeast Asia. Innovative interventions are needed to control simio-anthropophagic and acrodendrophilic vectors that do not rest and feed indoors. There are two major problems that need to be addressed before considering malaria elimination. It is known that *P. knowlesi* can be life threatening [99] and mortality due to it is increasing [31, 100]. Thus it is important to determine the vectors throughout the country; study the behavior and ecology of the species of mosquitoes and apply the most effective strategy(ies) for control of these vector. To achieve these outcomes, several key areas for strategic investment relevant for malaria elimination have been proposed [101]. Second, there will always be a problem of human population movement (HPM) and thus people moving into the jungle may introduce the parasite which could give rise to new infections if suitable vectors are present and readily establish local transmission. HPM is common among migrants in the Greater Mekong Subregion [102] and in Southeast Asia [103].

In Vietnam, forest malaria caused by *An. dirus* was controlled because workers going into the forest used long lasting insecticide hammocks (LLIH) [104]. The use of LLIH can be encouraged in ecotourism areas where people stay overnight in the community managed guest houses or camps in the forest. However, other types of personal protection methods need to be evaluated for forest workers. A study has demonstrated that military personnel who used permethrin treated uniforms were protected against mosquito bites, thereby reducing malaria transmission [105].

The use of repellents as personal protection measures have been advocated for malaria control. However, this needs to be evaluated in forest settings and large scale implementation will be a public health challenge. Among US Military troops, malaria cases have been reported due to non-compliance of personal protective measures and failure of chemoprophylaxis [106].

Currently in Malaysia people are getting infected when they visit plantations or forests for work or recreational activities as some important vectors do not enter houses [72].

8. Challenges

There is no reason to doubt the possibility and biological capacity of other simian malaria species to infect humans [13, 107]. *An. latens* can develop all the five species of simian malaria [79] and has a biting preference for both humans and macaques, the possibility of humans being infected with *P. cynomologi* or *P. inui* needs to be addressed. As stated by Baird [108], in areas where macaques and vectors are in close proximity to humans and when malaria occurs other species should also be considered and not just the human malarias and *P. knowlesi*.

Currently only three species of mosquitoes have been incriminated as simian malaria vectors in Malaysia (*An. balabacensis, An. cracens* and *An. latens*) [45, 71, 72, 75] and one in Vietnam (*An. dirus*) [76, 77]. However, it is beyond doubt that there would be several more species involved that would feed on both humans and monkeys and establish natural transmission. Before the inception of the malaria eradication program there were many more *Anopheles* species that were vectors [109], but some species were successfully brought down to very low levels due to their endophilic/endophagic behaviours and susceptibility to residual insecticides. Thus the aggressive national control programme has resulted controlling in only three to four important vectors occurring in Malaysia (*An. balabacensis, An. flavirostris, An. latens, An. maculatus*), [110-113].

In Thailand, the main vectors for human malaria are *An. dirus, An. minimus* and *An. maculatus*, mosquitoes [114]. Although *An. dirus* mosquitoes which belong to the Leucosphyrus Group and have been identified as potential vectors for *P. knowlesi* in Vietnam [76, 77], its distribution and abundance have significantly decreased in all major malaria-endemic areas of Thailand during the past decade [34]. Human cases of *P. knowlesi* have been reported from Thailand at a low prevalence (0.57% in 2006-2007), however the vector remains unknown [34].

According to Obsomer et al [61] the mean temperature below 20° C seems to limit the northern distribution of the Dirus complex to just beyond the border of India with Nepal and Bhutan. Rainfall is probably the limiting factor to the west with annual rainfall per year under 800 mm. Thus the lack of information on the distribution and occurrence of *P. knowlesi* cases in large non-forested areas of Thailand, southern Vietnam and central India is probably linked with the lack of suitable habitats [61]. The absence of the complex (besides the newly described species aff. *takasagoensis*) in north of Vietnam is puzzling as this area is still forested and members of the complex occur at the same latitude in neighbouring countries. Laos PDR is the only country in the Greater Mekong Subregion that has not reported the occurrence of *P. knowlesi* malaria. This may be due to the fact that so far investigations have not been carried out for *P. knowlesi*.

Thus it is timely to determine all the vectors of simian malaria throughout the Southeast Asian region. Although old records stating the distribution of the various *Anopheles* species are available, it may not depict the current situation since landscape ecology and vegetation cover have significantly changed over time. The distribution of vectors, in relation to forest areas and human settlements using modern technology such as the GPS, GIS and the behavioral ecology of the vectors, needs to be addressed. These and other key areas identified for specific strategic investment in ecological research [101] should assist to define the target product profiles of completely new control technologies and delivery systems.

9. Conclusion

Since many malaria control programmes in Southeast Asia are moving towards elimination of malaria [115], it is important to determine the prevalence of knowlesi malaria in these countries. In the Greater Mekong Subregion including Bangladesh and India *An. dirus* is one of the primary vector of human malaria and thus it is important to determine if other vectors are involved in knowlesi transmission. Among habitats shared by macaques and vector mosquitoes, it is possible for humans who encroach these areas to be infected. Thus, important issues that need to be determined are as follows: Are other simian malaria parasites affecting humans? Is human to human transmission occurring? What are the other vectors transmitting simian malaria to humans (apart from *An. cracens*, *An. latens*, *An.dirus* and *An. balabacensis*) in the region and what roles do they play in host switching? What innovative technologies or biting prevention are appropriate for the control of these vectors? Thus, knowlesi malaria remains a great challenge for the future.

Acknowledgements

The authors thank Pollie Rueda for his constructive comments. The first author was supported by a grant from University of Malaya UM.C/625/1/HIR/099.J-20011-73822

Author details

Indra Vythilingam[1,3*] and Jeffery Hii[2,3]

*Address all correspondence to: indra.vythilingam@gmail.com

1 Parasitology Department, Faculty of Medicine, University of Malaya, Kuala Lumpur, Malaysia

2 Taman Damai, Jalan Fung Yei Ting, Kota Kinabalu, Sabah, Malaysia

3 Formerly WHO Malaria Scientist, World Health Organization, Philippines

References

[1] Daniels CW. Animal parasites in man and some of the lower animals in Malaya. Studies Institite for Medical Research FMS 1908;3:1-13.

[2] Coatney GR. Simian malaria: Its importance to world wide eradication of malaria. Journal of American Medical Association 1963;184:876-7.

[3] Contacos PG, Elder HA, Coatney GR. Man to man transfer of two strains of *Plasmodium cynomolgi* by mosquito bites. American Journal of Tropical Medicine and Hygiene 1962;11:186-93.

[4] Chin W, Contacos PG, Coatney GR, Kimball HR. A naturally acquired quotidian-type malaria in man transferable to monkeys. Science 1965;149:865.

[5] Sinton JA MH. A critical review of the literature relating to the identification of the malaria parasites recorded from monkeys of the families Cercopithecidae and Colobidae. Rec Malaria Surv India 1932-1933;III:357–443.

[6] Warren MW, Cheong WH, Fredericks HK, Coatney GR. Cycles of jungle malaria in West Malaysia. American Journal of Tropical Medicine and Hygiene 1970;19:383.

[7] Fong YL, Cadigan FC, Coatney GR. A presumptive case of naturally occurring *Plasmodium knowlesi* malaria in man in Malaysia. Transactions of Royal Society of Tropical Medicine and Hygiene 1971;65:839.

[8] Wharton RH, Eyles DE. *Anopheles hackeri*, a vector of *Plasmodium knowlesi* in Malaya. Science 1961;134:279.

[9] Chin W, Contacos PG, Collins WE, Jeter MH, Alpert E. Experimental mosquito-transmission of *Plasmodium knowlesi* to man and monkey. American Journal of Tropical Medicine and Hygiene 1968;17:355-8.

[10] Singh B, Sung LK, Matusop A, Radhakrishnan A, Shamsul SSG, Cox-Singh J, et al. A large focus of naturally acquired *Plasmodium knowlesi* infections in human beings. Lancet 2004;363:1017-24.

[11] Collins WE. Major animal models in malaria research: Simian. In: Wernsdofer WH and McGregor editors. Malaria: Principles and Practice of Malariology. Edinburgh: Churchill Livingstone; 1988. p. 1473-501.

[12] Fodden J. Malaria in Macaques. International Journal of Primatology 1994;15:573-96.

[13] Galinski MR, Barnwell JW. Monkey malaria kills four humans. Trends in Parasitology 2009;25:200-4.

[14] Lee KS, Divis PCS, Zakaria SK, Matusop A, Julin RA, Conway DJ, et al. *Plasmodium knowlesi:* reservoir hosts and tracking the emergence in humans and macaques. PLoS Pathogens 2011;7:e1002015.

[15] Coatney GR, Elder HA, Contacos PG, Getz ME, Greenland R, Rossan RN, et al. Transmission of the M strain of *Plasmodium cynomolgi* to man. The American Journal of Tropical Medicine and Hygiene 1961;10:673-8.

[16] Collins WE, Warren MW, Sullivan JAS, Galland GG, Nace D, Williams A, et al. Studies on two strains of *Plasmodium cynomolgi* in New World and Old World monkeys and mosquitoes. Journal of Parasitology 2005;91:280-3.

[17] Eyles DE, Laing ABG, Fong YL. *Plasmodium fieldi* sp nov, a new species of malaria parasite from the pig-tailed macaque in Malaya. Annals of Tropical Medicine and Parasitology 1962;56:242-7.

[18] Eyles DE. The species of simian malaria: Taxonomy, morphology, life cycle, and geographical distribution of the monkey species. Journal of Parasitology 1963:866-87.

[19] Eyles DE, Laing ABG, Dobrovolny CG. The malaria parasites of the pig-tailed macaque, *Macaca nemestrina* (Linnaeus). Indian Journal of Malariology 1962;16:285-98.

[20] Eyles DE, Laing ABG, Warren M, Sandosham AA. Malaria parasites of the Malayan leaf monkeys of the genus *Presbytis*. Medical Journal of Malay 1962;17:85-6.

[21] Li M. Identification and molecular characterization of simian malaria parasites in wild monkeys of Singapore. Singapore: National University of Singapore; 2011.

[22] Ho G, Lee C, Abie M, Zainuddin Z, Japnin J, Topani R, et al. Prevalance of *Plasmodium* in the Long-tailored Macaque (*Macaca fasicularis*) from Selangor, Malaysia. Proceedings 13th Association of Institutions for Tropical Veterinary Medicine (AITVM) Conference 2010:49.

[23] Eyles DE, Fong, Y.l.,Warren, Mc,W., Guinn,E.,Sabdosham,AA.,Wharton,R.H. *Plasmodium coatneyi*, a new species of primate malaria from Malaya. American Journal of Tropical Medicine and Hygiene 1962;11:597-604.

[24] Eyles DE, Dunn F, Warren McW, Guinn E. *Plasmodium coatneyi* from the Philippines. Journal of Parasitology 1963;49:1038.

[25] Sandosham A. Recent researchers on malaria at the Institute for Medical Research, Kuala Lumpur. Medical Journal of Malaysia 1967;22:145-60.

[26] Lee KS, Cox-Singh J, Singh B. Morphological features and differential counts of *Plasmodium knowlesi* parasites in naturally acquired human infections. Malaria Journal 2009;8:73.

[27] Coatney RG, Collins WE, Warren M, Contacos PG. The Primate Malarias. Washington: U.S. Government Printing Office; 1971.

[28] Sandosham AA. Malariology with special reference to Malaya Singapore. Kuala Lumpur: University of Malaya Press; 1959.

[29] Cox Singh J, Davis TME, Lee KS, Shamsul SSG, Matusop A, Ratnam S, et al. *Plasmodium knowlesi* malaria in humans is widely distributed and potentially life threatening. Clinical Infectious Diseases 2008;46:165-71.

[30] Vythilingam I, NoorAzian YM, Huat TC, Jiram AI, Yusri YM, Azahari AH, et al. *Plasmodium knowlesi* in humans, macaques and mosquitoes in peninsular Malaysia. Parasite Vectors 2008;1:26.

[31] William T, Menon J, Rajahram G, Chan L, Ma G, Donaldson S, et al. Severe *Plasmodium knowlesi* malaria in a tertiary care hospital, Sabah, Malaysia. Emerging Infectious Diseases 2011;17:1248-54.

[32] Barber BE, William T, Jikal M, Jilip J, Dhararaj P, Menon J, et al. *Plasmodium knowlesi* malaria in children. Emerging Infectious Diseases 2011;17:20.

[33] Jongwutiwes S, Putaporntip C, Iwasaki T, Sata T, Kanbara H. Naturally acquired *Plasmodium knowlesi* malaria in human, Thailand. Emerging Infectious Diseases 2004;10:2211-3.

[34] Jongwutiwes S, Buppan P, Kosuvin R, Seethamchai S, Pattanawong U, Sirichaisinthop J, et al. *Plasmodium knowlesi* Malaria in humans and macaques, Thailand. Emerging Infectious Diseases 2011;17:1799-806.

[35] Putaporntip C, Hongsrimuang T, Seethamchai S, Kobasa T, Limkittikul K, Cui L, et al. Differential prevalence of *Plasmodium* infections and cryptic *Plasmodium knowlesi* malaria in humans in Thailand. Journal of Infectious Diseases 2009;199:1143.

[36] Luchavez J, Espino F, Curameng P, Espina R, Bell D, Chiodini P, et al. Human infections with *Plasmodium knowlesi*, the Philippines. Emerging Infectious Diseases 2008;14:811-3.

[37] Eede P, Van H, Van Overmeir C, Vythilingam I, Duc T, Hung L, et al. Human *Plasmodium knowlesi* infections in young children in central Vietnam. Malaria Journal 2009;8:249.

[38] Sulistyaningsih E, Fitri LE, Löscher T, Berens-Riha N. Diagnostic difficulties with *Plasmodium knowlesi* infection in humans. Emerging Infectious Diseases 2010;16:1033.

[39] Khim N, Siv S, Kim S, Mueller T, Fleischmann E, Singh B, et al. *Plasmodium knowlesi* infection in humans, Cambodia, 2007-2010. Emerging Infectious Diseases 2011;17:1900.

[40] Zhu H, Li J, Zheng H. Human natural infection of *Plasmodium knowlesi*. Zhongguo ji sheng chong xue yu ji sheng chong bing za zhi= Chinese Journal Parasitology Parasite Diseases 2006;24:70.

[41] Ng OT, Ooi EE, Lee CC, Lee PJ, Ng LC, Pei SW, et al. Naturally acquired human *Plasmodium knowlesi* infection, Singapore. Emerging Infectious Diseases 2008;14:814.

[42] White N. *Plasmodium knowlesi*: the fifth human malaria parasite. Clinical Infectious Diseases 2008;46:172.

[43] Anderios F, NoorRain A, Vythilingam I. In vivo study of human *Plasmodium knowlesi* in *Macaca fascicularis*. Experimental Parasitology 2010;124:181-9.

[44] Garnham P. Malaria parasites and other haemosporidia. Oxford: Blackwell Scientific Publications; 1966.

[45] Vythilingam I. Review Paper *Plasmodium knowlesi* in humans: a review on the role of its vectors in Malaysia. Tropical Biomedicine 2010;27:1-12.

[46] Hoosen A, Shaw M. *Plasmodium knowlesi* in a traveller returning to New Zealand. Travel Medicine and Infectious Disease 2011;9:144-8.

[47] Mali S, Steele S, Slutsker L, Arguin PM. Malaria surveillance–United states, 2006. MMWR Surveill Summ 2008;57:24-39.

[48] Kantele A, Marti H, Felger I, Muller D, Jokiranta TS. Monkey Malaria in a European Traveler Returning from Malaysia. Emerging Infectious Diseases 2008;14:1434-6.

[49] Bronner U, Divis PCS, Farnert A, Singh B. Swedish traveller with *Plasmodium knowlesi* malaria after visiting Malaysian Borneo: a case report. Malaria Journal 2009;8:15.

[50] Tang TH, Salas A, Ali-Tammam M, Martínez M, Lanza M, Arroyo E, et al. First case of detection of *Plasmodium knowlesi* in Spain by Real Time PCR in a traveller from Southeast Asia. Malaria Journal 2010;9:219.

[51] Berry A, Iriart X, Wilhelm N, Valentin A, Cassaing S, Witkowski B, et al. Imported *Plasmodium knowlesi* malaria in a French tourist returning from Thailand. American Journal of Tropical Medicine and Hygiene 2011;84:535-8.

[52] Warren MW, Wharton RH. The vectors of simian malaria: identity, biology, and geographical distribution. Journal of Parasitology 1963:892-904.

[53] Sallum MAM, Peyton EL, Wilkerson RC. Six new species of the *Anopheles leucosphyrus* group, reinterpretation of *An. elegans* and vector implications. Medical and Veterinary Entomology 2005;19:158-99.

[54] Harbach RE. The classification of genus *Anopheles* (Diptera: Culicidae): a working hypothesis of phylogenetic relationships. Bulletin of Entomological Research 2004;94:537-54.

[55] Peyton E. A new classification for the Leucosphyrus Group of *Anopheles* (*Cellia*). Mosquito Systematics 1989;21:197-205.

[56] Sallum MAM, Peyton EL, Harrison BA, Wilkerson RC. Revision of the Leucosphyrus group of *Anopheles* (*Cellia*)(Diptera, Culicidae). Revista Brasileira de Entomolo 2005;49:01-152.

[57] Manguin S, Garros C, Dusfour I, Harbach RE, Coosemans M. Bionomics, taxonomy, and distribution of the major malaria vector taxa of *Anopheles* subgenus *Cellia* in

Southeast Asia: An updated review. Infection, Genetics and Evolution 2008;8:489-503.

[58] Rattanarithikul R, Harrison BA. An illustrated key to the *Anopheles* larvae of Thailand. United State Army Medical Component, South East Asia Treaty Organization, Bangkok 1973.

[59] Rattanarithikul R, Harrison BA, Harbach RE, Panthusiri P, Coleman RE. Illustrated keys to the mosquitoes of Thailand. IV. *Anopheles*. Southeast Asian Journal of Tropical Medicine Public Health 2006;37 1-128.

[60] Baimai V, Kijchalao U, Sawadwongporn P, Green CA. Geographic distribution and biting behaviour of four species of the *Anopheles dirus* complex (Diptera: Culicidae) in Thailand. Southeast Asian Journal of Tropical Medicine Public Health 1988;19:151-61.

[61] Obsomer V, Defourny P, Coosemans M. The *Anopheles dirus* complex: spatial distribution and environmental drivers. Malaria Journal 2007;6:26.

[62] Trung HD, Bortel WV, Sochantha T, Keokenchanh K, Briët OJT, Coosemans M. Behavioural heterogeneity of *Anopheles* species in ecologically different localities in Southeast Asia: a challenge for vector control. Tropical Medicine & International Health 2005;10:251-62.

[63] Vythilingam I. *Plasmodium knowlesi* and *Wuchereria bancrofti*: their vectors and challenges for the future. Frontiers in Systems Biology 2012;3.

[64] Sinka ME, Bangs MJ, Manguin S, Chareonviriyaphap T, Patil AP, Temperley WH, et al. The dominant *Anopheles* vectors of human malaria in the Asia-Pacific region: occurrence data, distribution maps and bionomic précis. Parasite Vectors 2011;4:1-46.

[65] Reid JA. Anopheline Mosquitoes of Malaya and Borneo. Malaysia: Institute for Medical Research Malaysia; 1968.

[66] Colless D. The *Anopheles leucosphyrus* group. Transactions of Royal Entomological Society London 1956;108:37-116.

[67] Meek S. Vector control in some countries of Southeast Asia: comparing the vectors and the strategies. Annals of Tropical Medicine and Parasitology 1995;89:135-47.

[68] Chang MS, Doraisingam P, Hardin S, Nagum N. Malaria and filariasis transmission in a village/forest setting in Baram District, Sarawak, Malaysia. Journal of Tropical Medicine and Hygiene 1995;98:192.

[69] Colless DH. Observations on Anopheline mosquitoes of the Akah river, 4th Division, Sarawak. Bulletin of Entomological Research 1956;47:115-23.

[70] Zulueta J. Malaria in Sarawak. Bulletin World Health Organisation 1956;15:651-71.

[71] Tan CH, Vythilingam I, Matusop A, Chan ST, Singh B. Bionomics of *Anopheles latens* in Kapit, Sarawak, Malaysian Borneo in relation to the transmission of zoonotic simian malaria parasite *Plasmodium knowlesi*. Malaria Journal 2008;7:52.

[72] Jiram AI, Vythilingam I, NoorAzian YM, Yusof YM, Azahari AH, Fong MY. Entomologic investigation of *Plasmodium knowlesi* vectors in Kuala Lipis, Pahang, Malaysia. Malaria Journal 2012;11:213.

[73] Tsukamoto M, Miyata A, Miyagi I. Surveys on simian malaria parasites and their vector in Palawan Island, the Philippines. Tropical Medicine 1978;20:39-50.

[74] Miyagi I. Studies on malaria vectors in Philippines especially on *Anopheles balabacensis balabacensis* and monkey malaria in Palawan. The Journal of Tropical Medicine 1973;2:163.

[75] Vythilingam I, Tan CH, Asmad M, Chan ST, Lee KS, Singh B. Natural transmission of *Plasmodium knowlesi* to humans by *Anopheles latens* in Sarawak, Malaysia. Transactions Royal Society Tropical Medicine Hygiene 2006;100:1087-8.

[76] Nakazawa S, Marchand RP, Quang NT, Culleton R, Manh ND, Maeno Y. *Anopheles dirus* co-infection with human and monkey malaria parasites in Vietnam. International Journal of Parasitology 2009;39:1533-7.

[77] Marchand RP, Culleton R, Maeno Y, Quang NT, Nakazawa S. Co-infections of *Plasmodium knowlesi, P. falciparum, and P. vivax* among humans and *Anopheles dirus* mosquitoes, southern Vietnam. Emerging Infectious Diseases 2011;17:1232-9.

[78] Wharton RH, Eyles DE, Warren M, Cheong WH. Studies to determine the vectors of monkey malaria in Malaya. Annals of Tropical Medicine and Parasitology 1964;58:56.

[79] Tan CH. Identification of vectors of *Plasmodium knowlesi* and other malaria parasites, and studies on their bionomics in Kapit, Sarawak, Malaysia. MSc Thesis University Malaysia, Sarawak (UNIMAS) 2008.

[80] Cheong WH, Warren MW, Omar AH, Mahadevan S. *Anopheles balabacensis balabacensis* identified as vector of simian malaria in Malaysia. Science 1965;150:1314.

[81] Vythilingam I, Phetsouvanh R, Keokenchanh K, Yengmala V, Vanisaveth V, Phompida S, et al. The prevalence of *Anopheles* (Diptera: Culicidae) mosquitoes in Sekong Province, Lao PDR in relation to malaria transmission. Tropical Medicine International Health 2003;8:525-35.

[82] Pothikasikorn J, Bangs MJ, Boonplueang R, Chareonviriyaphap T. Susceptibility of various mosquitoes of Thailand to nocturnal subperiodic *Wuchereria bancrofti*. Journal of Vector Ecology 2008;33:313-20.

[83] Vythilingam I, Chan ST, Shanmugratnam C, Tanrang H, Chooi KH. The impact of development and malaria control activities on its vectors in the Kinabatangan area of Sabah, East Malaysia. Acta Tropica 2005;96:24-30.

[84] Maekawa Y, Tsuda Y, Dachlan YP, Yotopranoto S, Gerudug IK, Yoshinaga K, et al. Anopheline fauna and incriminatory malaria vectors in malaria endemic areas on Lombok Island, Indonesia. Medical Entomology and Zoology 2009;60:1-11.

[85] Hii J. Evidence for the existence of genetic variability in the tendency of *Anopheles balabacensis* to rest in houses and to bite man. The Southeast Asian Journal of Tropical Medicine and Public Health 1985;16:173.

[86] Rohani A, Lokman Hakim S, Hassan AR, Chan ST, Ong YF, Abdullah AG, Lee HL Bionomics of *Anopheles balabacensis* Baisas, the Principal Malaria Vector in Ranau, Sabah. Tropical Biomedicine 1999;16:31-8.

[87] Chiang G, Cheong W, Samarawickrema W, Mak J, Kan S. Filariasis in Bengkoka Peninsula, Sabah, Malaysia: vector studies in relation to the transmission of filariasis. The Southeast Asian Journal of Tropical Medicine and Public Health 1984;15:179.

[88] Schultz G. Biting activity of mosquitoes (Diptera: Culicidae) at a malarious site in Palawan, Republic of The Philippines. Southeast Asian Journal Tropical Medicine and Public Health 1992;23:464-9.

[89] Harbach RE, Baimai V, Sukowati S. Some observations on sympatric populations of the malaria vectors *Anopheles leucoshpyrus* and *Anopheles balabacensis* in a village forest setting in South Kalimantan. Southeast Asian Journal of Tropical Medicine and Public Health 1987;18:241-7.

[90] Sungvornyothin S, Kongmee M, Muenvorn V, Polsomboon S, Bangs MJ, Prabaripai A, et al. Seasonal abundance and bloodfeeding activity of *Anopheles dirus* sensu lato in western Thailand. Journal of the American Mosquito Control Association 2009;25:425-30.

[91] Van Bortel W, Trung HD, Hoi le X, Van Ham N, Van Chut N, Luu ND, Roelants P, et al. Malaria transmission and vector behaviour in a forested malaria focus in central Vietnam and the implications for vector control. Malaria Journal 2010;9:373.

[92] Lambrechts L, Knox TB, Wong J, Liebman KA, Albright RG, Stoddard ST. Shifting priorities in vector biology to improve control of vector borne disease. Tropical Medicine & International Health 2009;14:1505-14.

[93] Collins WE, Contacos PG, Guinn EG. Studies on the transmission of simian malarias II. Transmission of the H strain of *Plasmodium knowlesi* by *Anopheles balabacensis balabacensis*. Journal of Parasitology 1967:841-4.

[94] Collins WE, Contacos PG, Guinn EG, Held JR. Studies on the transmission of simian malarias, I. Transmission of two strains of *Plasmodium inui* by *Anopheles maculatus* and *A. stephensi*. Journal of Parasitology 1966:664-8.

[95] Wharton RH, Eyles DE, Warren McW. The development of methods for trapping the vectors of monkey malaria. Annals of Tropical Medicine and Parasitology 1963;57:32-46.

[96] Gater BAR. Aids to the identification of anopheline imagines in Malaya. Singapore: Government Printer; 1935.

[97] Takken W, Knols BGJ. Malaria vector control: current and future strategies. Trends in Parasitology 2009;25:101-4.

[98] WHO. The global malaria action plan for a malaria free world. http://wwwrollback-malariaorg/gmap accessed 18Sept 2012. Geneva 2008.

[99] Cox-Singh J, Singh B. Knowlesi malaria: newly emergent and of public health importance? Trends in Parasitology 2008;24:406-10.

[100] Rajahram GS, Barber BE, William T, Menon J, Anstey NM, Yeo TW. Deaths due to *Plasmodium knowlesi* malaria in Sabah, Malaysia: association with reporting as *Plasmodium malariae* and delayed parenteral artesunate. Malaria Journal 2012;11:284.

[101] Ferguson HM DA, Beeche A, Borgemeister C, Gottlieb M, et al. Ecology: A Prerequisite for Malaria Elimination and Eradication. PLoS Medicine 2012;7(8):e1000303. doi: 10.1371/journal.pmed.

[102] Delacollette C, D'Souza C, Christophel E, Thimasarn K, Abdur R, Bell D, et al. Malaria trends and challenges in the Greater Mekong Subregion. Southeast Asian Journal of Tropical Medicine and Public Health 2009;40:674.

[103] Organisation Internationale pour les Migration. Situation report on international migration in East and Southeast Asia. 2008.

[104] Thang ND, Erhart A, Speybroeck N, Xa NX, Thanh NN, Van Ky P, et al. Long-lasting insecticidal hammocks for controlling forest malaria: a community-based trial in a rural area of central Vietnam. PloS One 2009;4:e7369.

[105] Deparis X, Frere B, Lamizana M, N'Guessan R, Leroux F, Lefevre P, et al. Efficacy of permethrin-treated uniforms in combination with DEET topical repellent for protection of French military troops in Cote d'Ivoire. Journal of Medical Entomology 2004;41:914-21.

[106] Wallace MR, Sharp TW, Smoak B, Iriye C, Rozmajzl P, Thornton SA, et al. Malaria among United States troops in Somalia. The American Journal of Medicine 1996;100:49-55.

[107] Collins WE. *Plasmodium knowlesi*: A Malaria Parasite of Monkeys and Humans. Annual Review of Entomology 2012;57.

[108] Baird JK. Malaria zoonoses. Travel Med and Infect Dis 2009;7:269-77.

[109] Sandosham AA, Thomas V. Malariology: with special reference to Malaya: Coronet Books; 1983.

[110] Rahman WA, Che'Rus A, Ahmad AH. Malaria and *Anopheles* mosquitos in Malaysia. Southeast Asian Journal of Tropical Medicine and Public Health 1997;28:599.

[111] Vythilingam I, Foo LC, Chiang GL, Chan ST, Eng KL, Mahadevan S, et al. The impact of permethrin impregnated bednets on the malaria vector *Anopheles maculatus* (Diptera: Culicidae) in aboriginal villages of Pos Betau Pahang, Malaysia. Southeast Asian Journal of Tropical Medicine and Public Health 1995;26:354-8.

[112] Chang MS, Hii J, Buttner P, Mansoor F. Changes in abundance and behaviour of vector mosquitoes induced by land use during the development of an oil palm plantation in Sarawak. Trans Roy Soc Trop Med Hyg 1997;91:382-6.

[113] Hii JLK, Kan S, Vun YS, Chin KF, Lye MS, Mak JW, et al. *Anopheles flavirostris* incriminated as a vector of malaria and Bancroftian filariasis in Banggi Island, Sabah, Malaysia. Transactions of the Royal Society of Tropical Medicine and Hygiene 1985;79:677-80.

[114] Chareonviriyaphap T, Bangs MJ, Ratanatham S. Status of malaria in Thailand. Southeast Asian Journal of Tropical Medicine and Public Health 2000;31:225-37.

[115] APMEN. Vietnam joins Asia Pacific Malaria Elimination Network (APMEN). http://apmenorg/storage/newsmedia/Vietnam assessed 18 Sept 2012.

Chapter 2

The *Anopheles* Mosquito Microbiota and Their Impact on Pathogen Transmission

Mathilde Gendrin and George K. Christophides

Additional information is available at the end of the chapter

1. Introduction

An ecosystem is composed of a biological community and its physical environment. A unique ecosystem is the metazoan digestive tract, which contains and interacts with many microorganisms, e.g. a single human gut contains 10^{13}-10^{14} bacteria belonging to hundreds of species [4, 5]. These microorganisms are important for the host physiology, particularly in shaping the mucosal immune system [6] and protecting the host against infections by colonization resistance [7].

The term microbiota defines the microbial communities that live in contact with the body epithelia. They are composed of bacteria, viruses, yeasts and protists. To date, the bacterial component of the microbiota is the most studied and best characterized. Studies from *Drosophila* to mice have revealed that the microbial flora is tightly regulated by the immune system and that failures in this can have detrimental effects on the host [8, 9]. The microbiota composition and numbers undergo significant changes during a host's lifetime, in particular upon changes of the environment and feeding habits.

Anopheles mosquitoes are of great importance to human health. They transmit pathogens including malaria parasites, filarial worms and arboviruses (arthropod-borne viruses). These pathogens infect the mosquito gut when ingested with a bloodmeal, disseminate through the hemolymph (insect blood) to other tissues and are transmitted to a new human host upon another mosquito bite some days later. The time pathogens spend in mosquitoes is known as extrinsic incubation period. The malaria parasite, *Plasmodium*, undergoes sexual reproduction in the midgut lumen and develops into a motile form that, approximately 24h after infection, traverses the gut epithelium establishing an infection on the basal side that is bathed in the hemolymph [10]. A week to 10 days later, parasites travel to the salivary glands where they become infectious to man. Similarly, after shedding their protective sheath in the mosquito midgut lumen, the elephantiasis nematodes *Wuchereria* and *Brugia* microfilariae migrate through the midgut epithelium to the thoracic muscles where they embark on larval development [11]. Some 10-14 days later, infectious larvae emerge from the mosquito cuticle or the proboscis and infect the human host via a skin wound, such as that caused by the mosquito bite. The O'Nyong Nyong virus (ONNV), the only arbovirus known to be transmitted exclusively by *Anopheles*, mosquitoes infects the muscle bands of the midgut and other visceral tissues after dissemination from infected gut cells [12, 13]. The next steps of the virus migration through the mosquito are not well characterized but it is thought that, as shown for its cousin Chikungunya virus, it infects the salivary glands from where it can be transmitted to the human host. Thus, for all three types of pathogens, the *Anopheles* mosquito midgut is an obligatory gateway to infection and transmission.

The mosquito gut microbiota has recently emerged as an important factor of resistance against pathogens. In particular, midgut bacteria have been shown to have a substantial negative impact on malaria parasite burden through colonization mechanisms involving either direct *Plasmodium*-microbiota interactions or bacteria-mediated induction of the mosquito immune response [1, 2, 14]. Equivalent effects of the microbiota on infection with the Dengue virus and *Brugia* microfilariae are shown in the mosquito *Aedes aegypti* [15-17]. Therefore, the research field of mosquito microbiota has received great attention in the last years and new concepts of microbiota-mediated transmission blocking are currently investigated. These studies face an important challenge: the microbiota of a female mosquito changes considerably as the mosquito shift environments during metamorphosis, from the aqueous developing larva to an air-living adult, and yet during adulthood as its feeding behaviour alternates between flower-nectar feeding and blood feeding [18, 19]. The diversity of the bacterial community is shown to decrease during mosquito development and after the first bloodmeal, whereas bacteria massively proliferate, with a 10 to 900-fold increase registered 24h to 30h after a bloodmeal [18, 20, 21].

In this chapter, we provide an overview on the current knowledge of the composition of the *Anopheles* mosquito microbiota, including important findings from recent high-throughput sequencing studies. We then review studies about the impact of the microbiota on mosquito physiology and infection, focusing in particular on resistance to infection by human pathogens. Finally, we discuss the potential use of this knowledge toward reducing the mosquito vectorial capacity and transmission blocking.

2. The diversity of the *Anopheles* microbiota

The microbiota composition has been studied in several anophelines mainly by culturing or sequencing of the 16S rRNA [14, 18, 20, 22-41]. Together, studies on field-collected or laboratory-reared mosquitoes identified as many as 98 bacterial genera excluding genera of low abundance identified by high-throughput sequencing analyses (Table 1). Of these, 41 genera were found in more than one *Anopheles* species while 9 were reported in at least 7 of these 23 studies and thus appear to be frequently associated with *Anopheles*. *Pseudomonas* was the most frequent of those genera, detected in 16 studies, followed by *Aeromonas, Asaia, Comamonas, Elizabethkingia, Enterobacter, Klebsiella, Pantoea* and *Serratia*, detected in 7-10 studies. No single bacterial genus was found in all the studies, even if culture-dependent studies are not considered – as culturing techniques might be an issue. Thus, there is presumably no obligate symbiont in the *Anopheles* genus, as is the case of some other blood-sucking insects such as the Tsetse fly that hosts *Wigglesworthia spp.*, an obligatory bacterial symbiont important for fly fecundity [42] or the head louse that hosts *Riesia pediculicola* [43]. As the most frequent genera are present in both laboratory and field-collected mosquitoes, it is suggestive that laboratory colonies retain bacterial communities established prior to laboratory colonisation (Table 1 and [18]). There are, however, substantial differences between field-collected and laboratory-reared mosquitoes, as reflected by the loss of microbiota species richness in laboratory-reared mosquitoes [18, 22].

Actinobacteria

Genus	Family	Class	Example	Conditions	stage	Anopheles species	Deep seq	Culture	Non-culture
Agromyces	Microbacteriaceae	Actinobacteria	JX186590	F*	L	gambiae	[17]		
Brevibacterium	Brevibacteriaceae	Actinobacteria	FJ608062	F	L	stephensi			[38]
Corynebacterium	Corynebacteriaceae	Actinobacteria	GQ109703	F, F*	A	funestus, gambiae	[17, 36]		
Janibacter	Intrasporangiaceae	Actinobacteria	NR_043218	F	A	arabiensis		[22]	
Kocuria	Micrococcaceae	Actinobacteria	HQ591424	F	L	stephensi		[23]	
Microbacterium	Microbacteriaceae	Actinobacteria	HQ591431	F, L	A	gambiae, stephensi		[11, 23]	
Micrococcus	Micrococcaceae	Actinobacteria	FJ608230	F, L	A	gambiae, stephensi		[38, 37]	
Propionibacterium	Propionibacteriaceae	Actinobacteria	GQ003306	F, F*	A	funestus, gambiae	[17, 36]		
Rhodococcus	Nocardiaceae	Actinobacteria	AY837749	F	L, A	arabiensis, stephensi		[22, 23]	

Bacteroidetes

Genus	Family	Class	Example	Conditions	stage	Anopheles species	Deep seq	Culture	Non-culture
Chryseobacterium	Flavobacteriaceae	Flavobacteriia	HQ591432	F, F*, L	L, P, A	coustani, funestus, gambiae, stephensi	[17, 36]	[11, 38, 23]	[38]
Dysgonomonas	Porphyromonadaceae	Bacteroidia	FJ608061	F	L	stephensi			[38]
Elizabethkingia	Flavobacteriaceae	Flavobacteriia	EF426434	F*, L	A	gambiae, stephensi	[17, 21]	[22, 37]	[38, 27, 32]
Flavobacterium	Flavobacteriaceae	Flavobacteriia		F, L	A	albimanus, funestus, gambiae, stephensi		[19]	[30]
Flexibacteraceae		Cytophagia	FJ608195	F	A	stephensi			[38]
Myroides	Flavobacteriaceae	Flavobacteriia	HQ832872	F	L, A	stephensi		[23]	
Prevotella	Prevotellaceae	Bacteroidia	JN867317	F*	A	gambiae	[21]		
Sediminibacterium	Chitinophagaceae	Sphingobacteriia	FJ915158	F*	A	gambiae	[21]		
Sphingobacterium	Sphingobacteriaceae	Sphingobacteriia	EF426436	L	P, A	gambiae		[35]	

Firmicutes

Genus	Family	Class	Example	Conditions	stage	Anopheles species	Deep seq	Culture	Non-culture
Bacillus	Bacillaceae	Bacilli	AY837746	F, L	L, A	arabiensis, funestus, gambiae (ss, sl), stephensi		[11, 38, 22, 24]	[38, 27, 30]
Clostridium	Clostridiaceae	Clostridia	JN391577	F*	L	gambiae	[17]		
Enterococcus	Enterococcaceae	Bacilli	HQ591441	F	L, A	funestus, gambiae, stephensi	[36]	[23]	
Exiguobacterium	Bacillales Family XII. Incertae Sedis	Bacilli	HQ591439	F	L	stephensi		[38, 23]	

Lactobacillus	Lactobacillaceae	Bacilli	FJ608053	F, F*	L, A	gambiae, stephensi	[17]		[38]
Lysinibacillus	Bacillaceae	Bacilli	GU204964	F	L	maculipennis, stephensi		[24]	
Paenibacillus	Paenibacillaceae	Bacilli	EF426449	F	A	arabiensis, stephensi			[38, 22]
Staphylococcus	Staphylococcaceae	Bacilli	FJ608067	F, F*, L	L, A	funestus, gambiae, maculipennis, quadrimaculatus, stephensi	[21, 36]	[25, 38, 40]	[38, 26]
Streptococcus	Streptococcaceae	Bacilli	FJ608047	F, F*	L, A	funestus, gambiae, stephensi	[21, 36]		[38]

Proteobacteria

Acetobacter	Acetobacteraceae	Alpha-proteobacteria			L	A	stephensi			[26]
Achromobacter	Alcaligenaceae	Beta-proteobacteria	FJ608301	F		A	stephensi			[38]
Acidovorax	Comamonadaceae	Beta-proteobacteria	AY837725	F		A	arabiensis			[22]
Acinetobacter	Moraxellaceae	Gamma-proteobacteria	FJ608267	F, F*, L	L, A		albimanus, funestus, gambiae, stephensi	[17, 21, 36]	[19, 38]	[38, 26]
Aeromonas	Aeromonadaceae	Gamma-proteobacteria	FJ608130	F, F*, L	L, A		coustani, darlingi, funestus, gambiae, maculipennis, stephensi	[17, 36]	[19, 38, 23, 24]	[22, 33]
Agrobacterium	Comamonadaceae	Beta-proteobacteria	FJ607997	L		A	stephensi		[38]	[38]
Alcaligenes	Alcaligenaceae	Beta-proteobacteria	HQ832875	F		A	funestus, stephensi		[23]	[30]
Anaplasma	Anaplasmataceae	Alpha-proteobacteria	AY837739	F		A	arabiensis			[22]
Aquabacterium	Burkholderiales Genera incertae sedis	Beta-proteobacteria		F		A	gambiae			[26]
Asaia	Acetobacteraceae	Alpha-proteobacteria	FN821398	F, F*, L	L, A		coustani, funestus, gambiae, maculipennis, stephensi	[21, 36]	[11, 26-28, 37]	[26, 28]
Azoarcus	Rhodocyclaceae	Beta-proteobacteria	FJ608071	F		L	stephensi			[38]
Bordetella	Alcaligenaceae	Beta-proteobacteria	HQ832874	F		A	stephensi		[23]	
Bradyrhizobium	Bradyrhizobiaceae	Alpha-proteobacteria	AB740924	F*		A	gambiae	[21]		
Brevundimonas	Caulobacteraceae	Alpha-proteobacteria	GU204962	F		L, A	funestus, stephensi		[24]	[30]
Burkholderia	Burkholderiaceae	Beta-proteobacteria	AY391283	F, F*, L	A		gambiae, stephensi	[21]		[26, 27]
Buttiauxella	Enterobacteriaceae	Gamma-proteobacteria		F		A	darlingi			[33]
Cedecea	Enterobacteriaceae	Gamma-proteobacteria	DQ068869	F, F*, L	A		funestus, gambiae (ss, sl), stephensi	[21]	[19, 29]	[30]
Citrobacter	Enterobacteriaceae	Gamma-proteobacteria	FJ608234	F		A	darlingi, stephensi		[38]	[33]
Comamonas	Comamonadaceae	Beta-proteobacteria	EF426440	F, F*		P, A	dureni, funestus, gambiae, quadrimaculatus, stephensi	[17, 21]	[38, 35, 39, 40]	[30]

Delftia	Comamonadaceae	Beta-proteobacteria	EF426438	L	P	gambiae		[35]	
Ehrlichia	Anaplasmataceae	Alpha-proteobacteria		F	A	arabiensis			[22]
Enterobacter	Enterobacteriaceae	Gamma-proteobacteria	HQ832863	F, F*, L	L, A	albimanus, darlingi, funestus, gambiae (ss, sl), stephensi	[17]	[11, 38, 23, 30, 31]	[38, 23, 26]
Erwinia	Enterobacteriaceae	Gamma-proteobacteria	FJ816023	F, L	A	darlingi, funestus, gambiae		[37]	[30, 33]
Escherichia-Shigella	Enterobacteriaceae	Gamma-proteobacteria	FJ608223	F, F*, L	A	arabiensis, darlingi, funestus, gambiae (ss, sl), stephensi	[21, 36]	[11, 38, 30]	[30, 33]
Ewingella	Enterobacteriaceae	Gamma-proteobacteria		L	A	stephensi		[25]	
Gluconacetobacter	Acetobacteraceae	Alpha-proteobacteria	FN814298	F*, L	A	gambiae	[21]	[27]	
Gluconobacter	Acetobacteraceae	Alpha-proteobacteria		F, L	A	funestus, stephensi			[26, 30]
Herbaspirillum	Oxalobacteraceae	Beta-proteobacteria	FJ608162	F, L	A	gambiae, stephensi		[11]	[38]
Hydrogenophaga	Comamonadaceae	Beta-proteobacteria	FJ608063	F, F*	L	gambiae (ss, sl), stephensi	[17]		[38, 30]
Ignatzschineria	Xanthomonadaceae	Gamma-proteobacteria	FJ608103	F	L	stephensi			[38]
Klebsiella	Enterobacteriaceae	Gamma-proteobacteria	HQ591433	F, F*, L	L, A	darlingi, funestus, gambiae (ss, sl), stephensi	[17]	[23, 30, 37, 39]	[38, 30, 33]
Kluyvera	Enterobacteriaceae	Gamma-proteobacteria		F		funestus, gambiae		[19]	[30]
Leminorella	Enterobacteriaceae	Gamma-proteobacteria	FJ608283	F	A	stephensi			[38]
Leptothrix	Burkholderiales Genera incertae sedis	Beta-proteobacteria	FJ608083	F	L	stephensi			[38]
Morganella	Enterobacteriaceae	Gamma-proteobacteria		F	A	gambiae sl			[30]
Methylobacterium	Methylobacteriaceae	Alpha-proteobacteria	AB673246	F, F*	A	funestus, gambiae	[21, 36]		
Methylophilus	Methylophilaceae	Beta-proteobacteria	FJ517736	F*	P	gambiae	[17]		
Neisseria	Neisseriaceae	Beta-proteobacteria	JX010905	F*	A	gambiae	[21]		
Novosphingobium	Sphingomonadaceae	Alpha-proteobacteria	JX222980	F*	A	gambiae	[17]		
Pantoea	Enterobacteriaceae	Gamma-proteobacteria	JF690934	F, L	L, A	albimanus*, darlingi, funestus, gambiae (*) (ss, sl), stephensi (*)		[11, 19, 24, 35]	[38, 30, 33]
Pelagibacter	SAR11 cluster (no family)	Alpha-proteobacteria	GQ340243	F*	A	gambiae	[17]		
Phenylobacterium	Caulobacteraceae	Alpha-proteobacteria		F	A	gambiae			[26]
Phytobacter	Enterobacteriaceae	Gamma-proteobacteria		L	A	gambiae		[11]	
Porphyrobacter	Erythrobacteraceae	Alpha-proteobacteria	JQ923889	F*	L	gambiae	[17]		

Genus	Family	Class	Example	Conditions	Stage	Species	Deep seq	Culture	Non culture
Pseudomonas	*Pseudomonadaceae*	*Gammaproteobacteria*	EF426444	F, F*, L	L, P, A	*albimanus, darlingi, dureni, funestus, gambiae (ss, sl), maculipennis, quadrimaculatus stephensi*	[17, 21, 36]	[11, 19, 22-24, 29, 35, 38, 39, 40]	[38, 26, 30, 33]
Rahnella	*Enterobacteriaceae*	*Gammaproteobacteria*	GU204974	F	L	*stephensi*		[24]	
Ralstonia	*Burkholderiaceae*	*Betaproteobacteria*	AY191852	F*	A	*gambiae*	[21]		
Raoultella	*Enterobacteriaceae*	*Gammaproteobacteria*	HQ811336	F*	A	*gambiae*	[17]		
Rhizobium	*Rhizobiaceae*	*Alphaproteobacteria*	DQ814410	F*	L	*gambiae*	[17]		
Salmonella	*Enterobacteriaceae*	*Gammaproteobacteria*		F		*funestus, gambiae sl*			[30]
Schlegelella	*Comamonadaceae*	*Betaproteobacteria*	FR774570	F*	A	*gambiae*	[21]		
Serratia	*Enterobacteriaceae*	*Gammaproteobacteria*	FJ608101	F, F*, L	L, A	*albimanus, dureni, gambiae, maculipennis, quadrimaculatus, stephensi*	[17, 21]	[11, 19, 25, 31, 37-40]	[38]
Shewanella	*Shewanellaceae*	*Gammaproteobacteria*	HQ591421	F	L	*stephensi*		[23]	
Sphingobium	*Sphingomonadaceae*	*Alphaproteobacteria*	GU940735	F*	A	*gambiae*	[17]		
Sphingomonas	*Sphingomonadaceae*	*Alphaproteobacteria*	GU204960	F, F*, L	L, A	*funestus, gambiae, stephensi*	[21, 36]	[11, 24]	[26]
Stenotrophomonas	*Xanthomonadaceae*	*Gammaproteobacteria*	EF426435	F, F*		*arabiensis, funestus, gambiae*	[17, 21]	[35]	[22, 30]
Thorsellia	*Enterobacteriaceae*	*Gammaproteobacteria*	NR_043217	F, F*	L, A	*gambiae, stephensi*	[17]	[38, 22]	[38, 34]
Vibrio	*Vibrio*	*Gammaproteobacteria*	FJ608116	F	L, A	*arabiensis*		[38, 22]	
Xenorhabdus	*Enterobacteriaceae*	*Gammaproteobacteria*	FJ608329	F	A	*stephensi*			[38]
Yersinia	*Enterobacteriaceae*	*Gammaproteobacteria*		F	A	*darlingi*			[33]
Zymobacter	*Halomonadaceae*	*Gammaproteobacteria*	FR851711	F	A	*funestus, gambiae*	[36]		
Others									
Bacillariophyta (Eukaryota: Diatom)			JQ727029	F*	L	*gambiae*	[17]		
Chlorophyta (green algae)			EF114678	F*	L	*gambiae*	[17]		
Calothrix	*Rivulariaceae*	(no data)	FJ608095	F	L	*stephensi*			[38]
Deinococcus	*Deinococcaceae*	*Deinococci*	FJ608089	F	L	*stephensi*		[38]	[38]
Mycoplasma	*Mycoplasmataceae*	*Mollicutes*	AY837724	F	A	*arabiensis*			[22]
Spiroplasma	*Spiroplasmataceae*	*Mollicutes*	AY837733	F	A	*funestus*			[22]
Cyanobacteria-GpI			HM573452	F*	P	*gambiae*	[17]		
Cyanobacteria-GpIIa			JQ305084	F*	L	*gambiae*	[17]		
Cyanobacteria-GpV			AB245143	F*	L	*gambiae*	[17]		
Fusobacterium	*Fusobacteriaceae*	*Fusobacteriia*	JX548360	F*	A	*gambiae*	[17, 21]		

Table 1. List of bacterial genera associated with *Anopheles* mosquitoes reported in the following studies: [11, 17, 19, and 21-40]. For high-throughput sequencing studies; only genera found to represent at least 1% of the total population in at least one study/condition are listed. Genera are classified by phyla, which are indicated in bold. In column "Conditions", F, F* and L indicate field, semi-natural and laboratory conditions, respectively. In column "Stage", L, P and A indicate larvae, pupae and adults, respectively. Column "Example" shows NCBI accession number of a sequence example for each genus (first hit after BLAST). Columns "Deep seq", "Culture", "Non culture" list studies based on 16S rRNA gene deep sequencing, culture-dependent methods, conventional sequencing (including 16S rRNA gene libraries and DGGE) and gas chromatography, respectively. In the line "*Pantoea*", * refers to what was identified in [19] as *Enterobacter agglomerans*, since then renamed *Pantoea agglomerans*.

Three metagenomics studies were recently carried out using 16S RNA from bacteria found in the *Anopheles* gut [18, 22, 37]. Wang and co-workers examined the microbiota composition throughout the mosquito life cycle, using a laboratory colony of *A. gambiae* mosquitoes (the main vector of malaria in sub-Saharan Africa) reared in semi-natural microcosms in Kenya [18]. The microcosms contained local rainwater and topsoil and were kept outside to allow microbial colonization. Boissière and co-workers investigated the microbiota of adult *A. gambiae* mosquitoes in Cameroon and how these microbiota may be related to *Plasmodium* infection [22]. They collected larvae from the field, reared them to adulthood in the laboratory and monitored the microbiota composition of individual mosquitoes 8 days after infection with *Plasmodium falciparum* sampled directly from gametocytemic patients. Finally, Osei-Poku and co-workers collected adult mosquitoes in Kenya and analysed the microbiota of individual mosquitoes of 8 different species, including 3 species of *Anopheles* (*A. coustani*, *A. funestus* and *A. gambiae*) [37].

These studies led to 5 main observations. First, the microbiota diversity is high: when defining species as $OTU_{97\%, V1\text{-}V3}$[1], Wang et al. detected more than 2,000 species in a pool of 30 adult *A. gambiae* [18]. The highest diversity was registered in larvae and pupae, with an estimate of 4,000-8,000 species in a pool of 30 individuals of each stage. Diversity decreased during adulthood to 2,000-4,000 species upon emergence and dropped further to 600-900 species after a bloodmeal. As all of these high-throughput sequencing studies used bacterial DNA, which is a very stable molecule, an important question is whether these results genuinely reflect the *Anopheles* gut communities or include environmental contaminants. By direct sampling of the larval aquatic environment, Wang et al. indeed showed that the microbial communities differed from those in the larvae, suggesting that – at least in this study – bacteria were able to persist in, if not colonise, the mosquito host (Figure 1A).

Second, this diversity is partially explained by significant diversity within a single mosquito [22, 37], varying from 5 to 71 $OTUs_{97\%, V3}$ per individual (median: 42 $OTUs_{97\%, V3}$) [37]. Diversity is higher than what observed by metagenomics studies in other insects such as the honeybee which hosts 8 dominant species ($OTU_{97\%, V6\text{-}V8}$), the estimated species richness within a colony being 9-10 [44], and *Drosophila* where 31 $OTUs_{97\%, V2}$ were observed in a pool of 50 females [45]. Nevertheless, a single $OTU_{97\%, V3}$ represents on average 67% of a mosquito bacterial community and the median mosquito gut species richness is only 17% to that of humans, where an individual hosts 150-300 $OTUs_{99\%, whole\ 16S}$ [4, 37].

Third, another component of the observed biodiversity lies within the high variability in microbial communities between individuals. This is quantified by calculating the UniFrac distance between mosquitoes. UniFrac varies from 0 when two mosquitoes have exactly the same microbiota to 1 when there is no phylogenetic overlap between the microbiota of two mosquitoes. The mean UniFrac distance between individuals is high, 0.72 and 0.74 in *A. funestus* and *A. gambiae*, respectively [37]. This variability is almost as high between *Anopheles* individuals of the same species as between mosquitoes of different species and/or genera [37].

---

1 As not all the studies were based on the same region of 16S or the same threshold of differences, we refer here to OTU97%, V1-V3 as the operational taxonomic unit with more than 97% identity in the V1-V3 regions of 16S rRNA gene sequences.

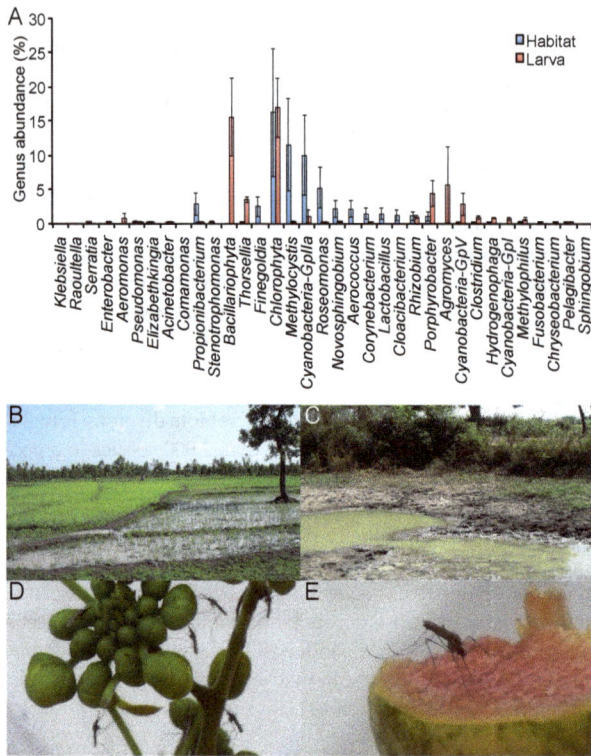

Figure 1. *Anopheles* microbiota and environment. A: Abundance of bacterial genera

Figure 1. Anopheles microbiota and environment. A: Abundance of bacterial genera in larval habitat and in larvae found in [17]. B, C: Natural habitat of A. gambiae. Permanent habitats such as rice fields (B) are colonized with M molecular form of A. gambiae and temporary water ponds (C) with S plus M forms (mostly S). D, E: Mosquitoes feeding on Senna siamea flowers (D) and papaya fruit-Carica papaya (E).

Fourth, the microbiota composition partly reflects the larval origin but bacteria acquired during adulthood may affect the microbiota composition to the extent that the geographic origin cannot be traced. Osei-Poku and co-workers did not observe any correlation between geographic location and microbiota composition in their Kenyan adult collections [37]. This is in sharp contrast to the Boissière et al. observations that microbiota were more similar between adults derived from larvae breading in the same pond than between adults derived from larvae of different geographic origins [22]. These results are, however, not contradictory if we consider differences in experimental designs of these studies. The latter study focused almost exclusively on bacteria transmitted from larvae to adults since larvae from the field were sampled and adults where fed with sterile sugar upon emergence, while the former study additionally sampled bacteria acquired during adulthood, and related to presumably diverse adult life histories. Together, these studies suggest that the acquisition of new strains of bacteria during adulthood can potentially increase the inter-individual diversity and mask similarities linked to the larval origin. However, this hypothesis requires further investigation, as mosquitoes from the two geographical origins reported in the Boissière et al. study belonged to the M and S molecular forms of *A. gambiae*, respectively, which are thought to be emerging species breading in different types of aquatic environments, i.e. permanent and temporary (rain-dependent) water pools, respectively (see Figures 1B, C) [22]. These environments are likely to contain different microbiota that largely determine the mosquito enterotype. Additionally, genetic differences between the two molecular forms may also partly account for the observed differences in microbiota composition.

Fifth, when considering the *Plasmodium* infection status, Boissière and co-workers found that the abundance of bacteria of the *Enterobacteriaceae* family was higher in *P. falciparum*-infected mosquitoes than in non-infected mosquitoes fed with the same infectious bloodmeal. This observation may indicate that *Enterobacteriaceae* favour *P. falciparum* infection or, conversely, that *P. falciparum* infection influences the composition of microbiota to the benefit of *Enterobacteriaceae* [22].

3. Bacterial colonization of mosquitoes

In addition to metagenomics studies, factors determining the composition of the adult mosquito microbiota were also investigated by conventional methods. Evidence that mosquitoes are colonized by bacteria both found in the environment and transmitted between individuals or developmental stages was revealed, but the relative contribution of these transmission routes to the microbiota diversity remains largely unknown. Laboratory studies investigated the vertical (from parent to progeny), transstadial (between developmental stages) and horizontal (between individuals of the same stage) transmission of specific bacterial strains. In particular, horizontal transfer of *Asaia sp.* is found to occur both by feeding and by mating (from male to female), but it is yet unclear whether vertical transmission occurs via egg spreading or by contamination of the environment during egg-laying [27]. Transstadial transmission of *Pantoea stewartii* is shown to occur from larvae to pupae but not from pupae to adults [36]. This is likely due to gut sterilization during metamorphosis; bacterial counts are high in the gut of fourth instar larvae, decrease after final larval defecation, increase again during pupal development and are very low or null in newly emerged adults [46].

Two mechanisms are thought to be involved in gut sterilization during adult emergence [46]. Firstly, bacteria are enclosed in the degenerated larval midgut, the meconium, enveloped by 2 meconial peritrophic matrixes and egested during molting. Secondly, during emergence, adults ingest exuvial liquid that has bactericidal properties. Nevertheless, sterilisation is thought to be incomplete, thus allowing some direct transmission from pupae to adults [46] and being responsible for the contribution of the larval/pupal breading sites to the adult microbiota, as mentioned earlier [22]. Moreover, emerging adults have been reported to ingest water and uptake bacteria during or shortly after emergence, with colonization efficiencies depending on the bacterial strains, e.g. *Elizabethkingia anophelis* (previously thought to be *E.*

meningoseptica) is more successful than *Pantoea stewartii* [33, 36]. During adulthood, mosquitoes take sugar-meals of floral and extra-floral nectar, sap, ripe fruit and honeydew (Figure 1D, E) [47-49]. These meals potentially provide new bacterial species and are likely to affect the relative growth of existing species or strains depending on their properties, such as the concentration of each sugar type, typically glucose, fructose or gulose [50]. This might well be the case for *Asaia* and *Gluconacetobacter*, two genera usually found in flowers, and which have been identified as part of the adult *Anopheles* microbiota [22, 27].

The *Anopheles* tissue specificity of *Asaia sp.* was studied using a bacterial strain expressing GFP (green fluorescent protein) [27]. *Asaia* was found in the female gut and salivary glands, two tissues of particular interest to vector biology, but also in the male reproductive tract and the larval gut, which are potentially important tissues for the bacterial spread [27]. The microbiome of *Anopheles* other tissues than the gut has not yet been characterized. Interestingly, *Wolbachia sp.*, a maternally transmitted intracellular bacterium able to colonize multiple tissues in other insects, has not yet been found in any *Anopheles* species. This is of particular interest, as this endosymbiont colonizes around half of the insect species including several *Culex* and *Aedes* mosquito species [51]. Reasons for the apparent incompatibility between *Anopheles* and *Wolbachia* are unknown, but the generation of *Wolbachia*-infected *Anopheles* colonies is currently being pursued. Laboratory infection has been achieved for *Ae. aegypti* [52, 53], where *Wolbachia* is a promising candidate for reducing the vector competence (see below). To our knowledge, no endosymbiont has been described in *Anopheles* to date.

Non-bacterial members of the *Anopheles* microbiota are poorly understood. Such studies are of special interest, as these microorganisms can potentially interact directly with the bacterial microbiota as well as the human pathogens and are likely to affect the mosquito physiology. An initial study, based on sequencing a 18S-library, identified 6 fungal clones related to *Candida sp.*, *Hanseniaspora uvarum*, *Pichia sp.*, *Wallemia sebi*, *Wickerhamomyces anomalus* and uncultured fungi in laboratory-reared *A. stephensi* [54]. *W. anomalus* is also found in wild and laboratory-reared *A. gambiae* [55]. TEM observation of mosquito tissues revealed the presence of yeasts in the female midgut and of actively dividing yeasts in the male gonoduct of *A. stephensi* [54, 55].

4. Impact of microbiota on *Anopheles* physiology and pathogen transmission

The studies reviewed above suggest that *Anopheles* mosquitoes do not host any particular obligate symbiont. However, bacteria as a whole appear to be essential for mosquito physiology. In particular, it has not been possible to date to maintain *Anopheles* colonies on conventional laboratory diet in axenic conditions. In addition, *A. stephensi* larval development is slowed down in the presence of antibiotics and putatively blocked at the 3rd or 4th instar, but an antibiotic-resistant strain of *Asaia* is sufficient to revert this effect [56]. Although the mechanism involved in this dependence is unknown, several lines of experimental evidence point to the important nutritional role of gut commensals. First, the development of aseptic

A. stephensi mosquitoes was achieved from sterilized eggs to adults in a custom aseptic medium [57], although no mention is made about adult fertility under these conditions. Second, a delay in the development was also observed in *Drosophila melanogaster* raised in axenic conditions under protein deprivation, which was rescued by the addition of live *Lactobacillus plantarum* in the fly medium [58]. *L. plantarum* was shown to promote larval growth under poor dietary conditions by enhancing nutrient sensing in a TOR-dependent manner, thus acting on ecdysone and insulin-like-peptide pathways [58]. Third, larval mortality was reported in the clothing louse deprived of its bacterial symbionts and can be avoided by supplementing the blood with B-vitamins (ß-biotin, pantothenate and nicotinic acid) [59]. The *Anopheles* microbiota may also participate in metabolism, as adult mosquitoes fed with radiolabelled-Glycine *Pseudomonas* displayed radioactive signal throughout their body [40]. Interestingly, *Plasmodium* oocysts and sporozoites developing in these mosquitoes also contained radioactive compounds, suggesting that bacteria also participate in parasite nutrition [40].

Anopheles females appear to also sense bacterial presence in the water, which influences oviposition in a bacterial strain dependent manner [60]. The underlying stimuli are not known but they are likely semiochemicals, i.e. messenger molecules produced by bacteria [60]. A principal component analysis of volatiles emitted by 17 bacterial strains, including 6 oviposition-inducing strains, failed to identify compounds shared between all oviposition-inducing bacterial strains, suggesting that such semiochemicals are acting as cocktails [60].

An aspect of the *Anopheles* microbiota that received great interest recently is the colonisation resistance effect towards *Plasmodium* infection, as depicted in Figure 2. First, bacterial growth after a bloodmeal is reported to trigger an immune response via the Immune-deficiency (Imd) pathway, which causes synthesis of antimicrobial peptides and other immune effectors [2]. These effectors target bacterial populations in the mosquito midgut and exert antiparasitic effects. Second, an *Enterobacter* strain (*EspZ*) isolated from wild *A. arabiensis* mosquitoes is shown to directly affect *Plasmodium* development in the mosquito gut via elevated synthesis of ROS (reactive oxygen species) [1]. Third, microbiota-dependent immune priming is reported upon *Plasmodium* infection. This effect protects mosquitoes from subsequent *Plasmodium* infections and is likely to be mediated by hemocyte differentiation [3].

As mentioned above, *Anopheles* mosquitoes are also vectors of filarial worms and ONNV (anophelines are also secondary vectors of West Nile virus). The effect of gut microbiota on infection with these pathogens has not been thoroughly investigated to date, but feeding *A. quadriannulatus* with an antibiotic/antimycotic mixture is shown to increase *Brugia malayi* infection [61]. In *Ae. aegypti*, antibiotic treatment increases the susceptibility of mosquitoes to Dengue virus via a decrease in antimicrobial gene transcription [53]. This can be reverted by addition of bacterial strains such as *Proteus sp.* and *Paenibacillus sp.* [62]. The role of *Anopheles* microbiota upon viral infections is still unclear, but our unpublished observations suggest that antibiotic treatment of *A. gambiae* increases significantly the prevalence of infection with ONNV.

Vertically-transmitted *Wolbachia* endosymbionts are under special focus as promising candidates to stop pathogen transmission. Research in this field has advanced in *Ae. aegypti*, where stable infections of *Wolbachia* strains have been established in laboratory colonies [52, 53]. The

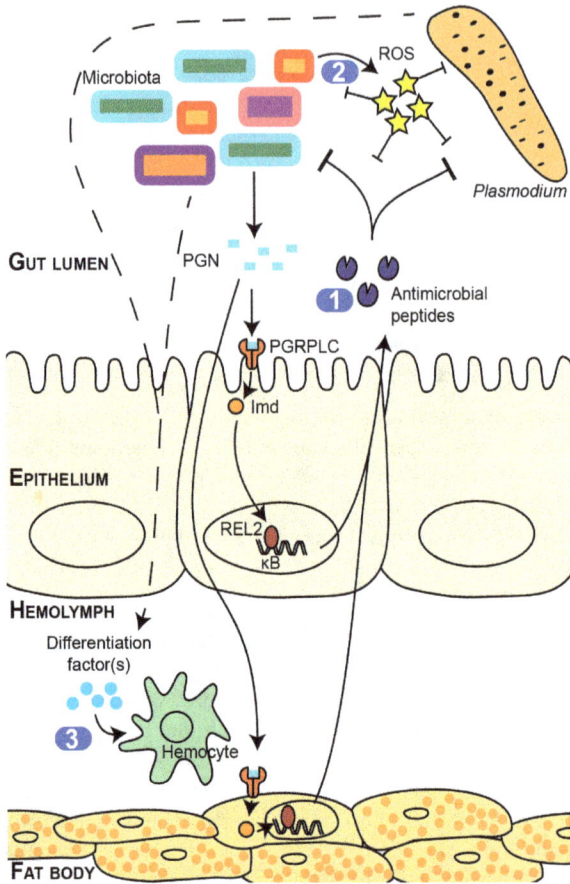

Figure 2. Mechanisms of colonization resistance conferred by *Anopheles* microbiota against *Plasmodium* infection. 1 — Direct effect via synthesis of ROS by the *Enterobacter EspZ* strain [1]. 2 — Indirect effect via induction of NF-κB antibacterial responses that have antiparasitic effects [2]. This is likely to be the most general mechanism. 3 — Induction of hemocyte differentiation by unknown soluble hemolymph factors during *Plasmodium* infection, which has a priming effect against asubsequent *Plasmodium* infection [3].

fast growing wMelPop strain of *Wolbachia* halves the mosquito lifespan, thus potentially affecting the capacity of mosquitoes to transmit pathogens with long extrinsic incubation periods [52]. It also induces a constitutively elevated immune response that negatively impacts on the infection prevalence and intensity of *Brugia pahangi* microfilariae, Chikungunya and Dengue viruses and the avian parasite *Plasmodium gallinaceum* [15, 17]. wAlbB and wMel, which naturally infect the Asian tiger mosquito *Aedes albopictus* and *D. melanogaster*, respectively, also render *Aedes* mosquitoes resistant to Dengue virus when introduced into laboratory populations [16, 63, 64]. Moreover, wMel is shown to successfully spread into wild *Ae. aegypti* populations in North-Eastern Australia [65] and is a strong candidate for Dengue biocontrol. When injected into *Anopheles* mosquitoes, *Wolbachia* seems to positively or negatively impact on *Plasmodium* infection depending on the *Wolbachia/Plasmodium* strain/species combination [66-68].

The immune system of *Anopheles* is known to control the microbiota population, by both resistance and tolerance mechanisms. On the one hand, the Imd pathway is shown to control the midgut bacterial numbers, especially after a bloodmeal [2], together with the production of ROS [21]. The melanization reaction might also contribute to limiting the bacterial numbers, as shown in the hindgut of the silkworm *Bombyx mori* [69]. On the other hand, induction of the Duox-IMPer (Dual oxidase - Immunomodulatory peroxidase) pathway after a bloodmeal leads to the formation of a dityrosine-linked mucus layer in the space between the peritrophic membrane and the midgut epithelium that reduces the permeability to immune elicitors. This tolerance mechanism leads to increased bacterial and *Plasmodium* loads [21]. Interestingly, such protection from oxidative stress is also identified in *Ae. aegypti*, where blood heme induces a protein kinase C-dependent mechanism leading to decreased ROS production and bacterial proliferation [70]. In *Drosophila*, several negative regulators of the Imd pathway are involved in tolerance to gut bacteria, but equivalent tolerance mechanisms have not yet been described in *Anopheles*. In particular, PGRP-LB and PGRP-SC1A/B degrade peptidoglycan into non-immunogenic fragments and Pirk downregulates the activity of the PGRP-LC and PGRP-LE receptors [71-76]. Orthologs of these regulators PGRPs, but not of Pirk, are present in *Anopheles* [77, 78].

In several insect species, microbiota are shown to also impact on host behavior. Notably, *Drosophila* mating preference is influenced by the microbiota composition [79]. *Klebsiella oxytoca* is proposed as a probiotic able to rescue the loss of copulatory performance that follows male sterilization by irradiation in medfly (*Ceratitis capitata*), by restoring the *Klebsiella/ Pseudomonas* ratio to its normal levels [80]. In termites, a Rifampicin treatment is shown to reduce the queen oviposition rate and to decrease longevity and fecundity of termite reproductives [81]. As *Anopheles* mosquitoes are able to sense the presence of bacteria in water as well as on human skin and modulate their oviposition rate and feeding behavior accordingly [60, 82], the microbiota composition could also influence the mosquito social and/or reproductive behavior and feeding preference. This may prove to be of particular importance to vector control.

5. Potential exploitations to reduce *Anopheles* vector competence

Reduction of the *Anopheles* competence to transmit human pathogens, especially malaria, will have great implications on public health. Any perspective of reducing vector competence should affect at least one of the parameters of the Ross-McDonald model of disease transmission [83]. These parameters include the mosquito-to-man ratio, the mosquito biting rate, the probability of successful man-to-mosquito and mosquito-to-man transmission, the mosquito daily survival probability, the days needed for the parasite in the mosquito to become infective and the daily rate at which humans become non-infectious to mosquitoes. From studies carried out to date and reviewed in preceding sections, it is evident that the mosquito microbiota can potentially affect most of these parameters except those referring only to disease progression in the vertebrate host. The most important of these parameters are mosquito longevity, feeding behavior and capacity to support pathogen development and/or replication.

A direct way to reduce vector competence using our current knowledge of the *Anopheles* microbiota would be to use bacterial strains that are naturally incompatible with pathogen development and/or replication. Potential candidates are either natural microbiota such as the EspZ strain of *Enterobacter* that causes resistance to *Plasmodium* [1] or artificially introduced bacteria such as *Wolbachia*, which apparently induce a wide spectrum of resistance to human pathogens [15]. The great advantage of the latter is its ability to spread into populations by manipulating insect reproduction in several ways. In particular, *Wolbachia* induces death of young embryos laid by *Wolbachia*-free females mated with infected males; *Wolbachia*-infected females are always fertile independently of the male infection status [84]. This so-called cytoplasmic incompatibility confers a reproductive benefit to *Wolbachia*-infected females and leads to propagation of *Wolbachia* even if it bears small fitness cost to the host, including reduced fecundity (discussed in [85, 86]). The challenge of this approach is the fact that *Wolbachia* and *Anopheles* seem to be incompatible in nature and introduction of the endosymbiont in laboratory colonies of *Anopheles* has not yet been achieved. Screening of *Wolbachia* strains able to infect the *Anopheles* reproductive tissues, when cultured *ex vivo*, has been reported [87]. Alternatively, preadaptation of *Wolbachia* strains by long-term culturing in mosquito cell lines has been suggested as a strategy to infect new hosts, as shown successfully for *Aedes* [52, 88]. As previously reported in *Aedes* [15-17], *Wolbachia* might impact both on mosquito longevity and successful development and/or replication of all three taxa of *Anopheles*-borne pathogens, i.e. *Plasmodium*, viruses and nematodes.

An alternative approach is paratransgenesis, the introduction of genetically modified bacteria into the vector, which would confer resistance to pathogens. *Pantoea agglomerans*, a natural *Anopheles* symbiont, is a candidate for this approach and has been successfully engineered to express and secrete proteins that either inhibit midgut invasion by *Plasmodium*, such as [EPIP]$_4$ (*Plasmodium* enolase-plasminogen interaction peptide) that competes with *Plasmodium* EPIP for plasminogen binding, or by directly targeting the parasite, such as the scorpion-derived antiplasmodial scorpine [89, 90]. Green fluorescent protein (GFP)-tagged *P. agglomerans* persists and grows in the *Anopheles* gut, while transgenic *P. agglomerans* confers resistance against *P. falciparum* infection in both *A. stephensi* and *A. gambiae* without affecting the mosquito lifespan [90]. Applicability to more than one mosquito species is particularly advantageous for a transmission blocking approach. *Asaia* has also been proposed as a candidate for paratransgenesis, as it is quite frequent in *Anopheles* microbiota and can be successfully transformed [27]. Interestingly, this genus has been found in all of the 30 individuals assessed in the metagenomics study of Boissière et al. suggesting that it can easily spread into field populations [22]. *Asaia* can be transmitted both horizontally and vertically presenting an additional advantage for the spread of a transgenic strain into mosquito populations [27]. The introduction of such microbiota into mosquito populations could be achieved by using baiting stations, i.e. clay jars containing cotton balls soaked with sugar and bacteria, around malaria endemic villages, but this approach requires further investigation [90].

Finally, transmission-blocking interventions could involve drugs or other interventions that would impact on the microbiota, thus affecting mosquito homeostasis and efficiency of pathogen development. For example, the effects of antibiotics in the human blood could significantly impact the mosquito microbiota upon blood feeding, indirectly influencing mosquito physiology and infection with pathogens. Depending on its spectrum, an antibiotic could influence the microbiota composition and thus have a positive or negative impact on pathogen development and/or replication.

6. Conclusion

Recent high-throughput sequencing studies of the *Anopheles* microbiota have revealed the extent of the microbiota diversity, mostly in field or semi-natural conditions. A diverse range of bacteria is able to colonize the *Anopheles* gut, and there is a vast diversity of microbiota between mosquitoes. To some extent, this diversity needs to be considered at the bacterial strain level, as different strains of one species may have diverse effects on the mosquito physiology and other microbes of the gut ecosystem. Although bacteria may be the most abundant and important members of the gut microbiota, characterization of the viral, fungal and protist communities could prove insightful into the understanding of the homeostasis of this complex biological system (e.g. phage predation is thought to regulate bacterial popula- tions [91]) and its effects on pathogen transmission. An important question that may arise from further studies is whether variability and/or discrepancies in experimental findings about the interactions between mosquitoes and pathogens could be attributed to differences in the microbiota between laboratories. Toward exploiting the knowledge on *Anopheles* microbiota to reduce vector competence, research is currently at its infancy, but some bacteria such as *Pantoea* and *Asaia* already emerge as promising candidates of paratransgenesis. The use of *Wolbachia* to reduce *Aedes* vectorial capacity and fitness may be of particular importance, if this technology can be effectively transferred to *Anopheles*. Finally, the possibility to use drugs such as antibiotics to target specific mosquito microbiota and affect vector competence or fitness is a new concept that merits further investigation.

Acknowledgements

We thank Jiannong Xu, Jewelna Osei-Poku, Anne Boissière and Isabelle Morlais for providing example sequences of some of the bacterial genera shown in Table 1 and Thierry Lefèvre for helping with mosquito pictures presented in Figure 1.

Author details

Mathilde Gendrin and George K. Christophides*

*Address all correspondence to: g.christophides@imperial.ac.uk

Department of Life Sciences, Imperial College London, UK

References

[1] Cirimotich CM, Dong Y, Clayton AM, Sandiford SL, Souza-Neto JA, Mulenga M, et al. Natural microbe-mediated refractoriness to *Plasmodium* infection in *Anopheles gambiae*. Science. 2011 May 13;332(6031):855-8.

[2] Meister S, Agianian B, Turlure F, Relogio A, Morlais I, Kafatos FC, et al. *Anopheles gambiae* PGRPLC-mediated defense against bacteria modulates infections with malaria parasites. PLoS pathogens. 2009 Aug;5(8):e1000542. DOI: 10.1371/journal.ppat. 1000542.g006

[3] Rodrigues J, Brayner FA, Alves LC, Dixit R, Barillas-Mury C. Hemocyte differentiation mediates innate immune memory in *Anopheles gambiae* mosquitoes. Science. 2010 Sep 10;329(5997):1353-5.

[4] Eckburg PB, Bik EM, Bernstein CN, Purdom E, Dethlefsen L, Sargent M, et al. Diversity of the human intestinal microbial flora. Science. 2005 Jun 10;308(5728):1635-8.

[5] Dethlefsen L, McFall-Ngai M, Relman DA. An ecological and evolutionary perspective on human-microbe mutualism and disease. Nature. 2007 Oct 18;449(7164):811-8.

[6] Bouskra D, Brezillon C, Berard M, Werts C, Varona R, Boneca IG, et al. Lymphoid tissue genesis induced by commensals through NOD1 regulates intestinal homeostasis. Nature. 2008 Nov 27;456(7221):507-10.

[7] Stecher B, Hardt WD. Mechanisms controlling pathogen colonization of the gut. Current opinion in microbiology. 2011 Feb;14(1):82-91.

[8] Ryu JH, Kim SH, Lee HY, Bai JY, Nam YD, Bae JW, et al. Innate immune homeostasis by the homeobox gene caudal and commensal-gut mutualism in *Drosophila*. Science. 2008 Feb 8;319(5864):777-82.

[9] Saha S, Jing X, Park SY, Wang S, Li X, Gupta D, et al. Peptidoglycan recognition proteins protect mice from experimental colitis by promoting normal gut flora and preventing induction of interferon-gamma. Cell host & microbe. 2010 Aug 19;8(2): 147-62.

[10] Yassine H, Osta MA. *Anopheles gambiae* innate immunity. Cell Microbiol. 2010 Jan; 12(1):1-9.

[11] Manguin S, Bangs MJ, Pothikasikorn J, Chareonviriyaphap T. Review on global co-transmission of human *Plasmodium* species and *Wuchereria bancrofti* by *Anopheles* mosquitoes. Infection, genetics and evolution : journal of molecular epidemiology and evolutionary genetics in infectious diseases. 2010 Mar;10(2):159-77.

[12] Brault AC, Foy BD, Myles KM, Kelly CL, Higgs S, Weaver SC, et al. Infection patterns of O'nyong nyong virus in the malaria-transmitting mosquito, *Anopheles gambiae*. Insect Mol Biol. 2004 Dec;13(6):625-35.

[13] Waldock J, Olson KE, Christophides GK. *Anopheles gambiae* antiviral immune response to systemic O'nyong-nyong infection. PLoS neglected tropical diseases. 2012;6(3):e1565. DOI: 10.1371/journal.pntd.0001565.

[14] Dong Y, Manfredini F, Dimopoulos G. Implication of the mosquito midgut microbiota in the defense against malaria parasites. PLoS pathogens. 2009 May;5(5):e1000423. DOI: 10.1371/journal.ppat.1000423.

[15] Moreira LA, Iturbe-Ormaetxe I, Jeffery JA, Lu G, Pyke AT, Hedges LM, et al. A *Wolbachia* symbiont in *Aedes aegypti* limits infection with dengue, Chikungunya, and *Plasmodium*. Cell. 2009 Dec 24;139(7):1268-78.

[16] Bian G, Xu Y, Lu P, Xie Y, Xi Z. The endosymbiotic bacterium *Wolbachia* induces resistance to dengue virus in *Aedes aegypti*. PLoS pathogens. 2010;6(4):e1000833. DOI: 10.1371/journal.ppat.1000833.g006.

[17] Kambris Z, Cook PE, Phuc HK, Sinkins SP. Immune activation by life-shortening *Wolbachia* and reduced filarial competence in mosquitoes. Science. 2009 Oct 2;326(5949):134-6.

[18] Wang Y, Gilbreath TM, 3rd, Kukutla P, Yan G, Xu J. Dynamic gut microbiome across life history of the malaria mosquito *Anopheles gambiae* in Kenya. PloS one. 2011;6(9):e24767. DOI: 10.1371/journal.pone.0024767.

[19] Muller GC, Beier JC, Traore SF, Toure MB, Traore MM, Bah S, et al. Field experiments of *Anopheles gambiae* attraction to local fruits/seedpods and flowering plants in Mali to optimize strategies for malaria vector control in Africa using attractive toxic sugar bait methods. Malaria journal. 2010;9:262.

[20] Pumpuni CB, Demaio J, Kent M, Davis JR, Beier JC. Bacterial population dynamics in three anopheline species: the impact on *Plasmodium* sporogonic development. The American journal of tropical medicine and hygiene. 1996 Feb;54(2):214-8.

[21] Kumar S, Molina-Cruz A, Gupta L, Rodrigues J, Barillas-Mury C. A peroxidase/dual oxidase system modulates midgut epithelial immunity in *Anopheles gambiae*. Science. 2010 Mar 26;327(5973):1644-8.

[22] Boissiere A, Tchioffo MT, Bachar D, Abate L, Marie A, Nsango SE, et al. Midgut microbiota of the malaria mosquito vector *Anopheles gambiae* and interactions with *Plasmodium falciparum* infection. PLoS pathogens. 2012 May;8(5):e1002742. DOI: 10.1371/journal.ppat.1002742.

[23] Lindh JM, Terenius O, Faye I. 16S rRNA gene-based identification of midgut bacteria from field-caught *Anopheles gambiae sensu lato* and *A. funestus* mosquitoes reveals new species related to known insect symbionts. Applied and environmental microbiology. 2005 Nov;71(11):7217-23.

[24] Chavshin AR, Oshaghi MA, Vatandoost H, Pourmand MR, Raeisi A, Enayati AA, et al. Identification of bacterial microflora in the midgut of the larvae and adult of wild caught *Anopheles stephensi*: a step toward finding suitable paratransgenesis candidates. Acta tropica. 2012 Feb;121(2):129-34.

[25] Dinparast Djadid N, Jazayeri H, Raz A, Favia G, Ricci I, Zakeri S. Identification of the midgut microbiota of *An. stephensi* and *An. maculipennis* for their application as a paratransgenic tool against malaria. PloS one. 2011;6(12):e28484. DOI: 10.1371/journal.pone.0028484.

[26] Pumpuni CB, Beier MS, Nataro JP, Guers LD, Davis JR. *Plasmodium falciparum*: inhibition of sporogonic development in *Anopheles stephensi* by gram-negative bacteria. Experimental parasitology. 1993 Sep;77(2):195-9.

[27] Favia G, Ricci I, Damiani C, Raddadi N, Crotti E, Marzorati M, et al. Bacteria of the genus *Asaia* stably associate with *Anopheles stephensi*, an Asian malarial mosquito vector. Proceedings of the National Academy of Sciences of the United States of America. 2007 May 22;104(21):9047-51.

[28] Chouaia B, Rossi P, Montagna M, Ricci I, Crotti E, Damiani C, et al. Molecular evidence for multiple infections as revealed by typing of *Asaia* bacterial symbionts of four mosquito species. Applied and environmental microbiology. 2010 Nov;76(22): 7444-50.

[29] Damiani C, Ricci I, Crotti E, Rossi P, Rizzi A, Scuppa P, et al. Mosquito-bacteria symbiosis: the case of *Anopheles gambiae* and *Asaia*. Microbial ecology. 2010 Oct;60(3): 644-54.

[30] Noden BH, Vaughan JA, Pumpuni CB, Beier JC. Mosquito ingestion of antibodies against mosquito midgut microbiota improves conversion of ookinetes to oocysts for *Plasmodium falciparum*, but not *P. yoelii*. Parasitology international. 2011 Dec;60(4): 440-6.

[31] Straif SC, Mbogo CN, Toure AM, Walker ED, Kaufman M, Toure YT, et al. Midgut bacteria in *Anopheles gambiae* and *An. funestus* (*Diptera: Culicidae*) from Kenya and Mali. Journal of medical entomology. 1998 May;35(3):222-6.

[32] Gonzalez-Ceron L, Santillan F, Rodriguez MH, Mendez D, Hernandez-Avila JE. Bacteria in midguts of field-collected *Anopheles albimanus* block *Plasmodium vivax* sporogonic development. Journal of medical entomology. 2003 May;40(3):371-4.

[33] Kampfer P, Matthews H, Glaeser SP, Martin K, Lodders N, Faye I. *Elizabethkingia anophelis sp. nov.*, isolated from the midgut of the mosquito *Anopheles gambiae*. Int J Syst Evol Microbiol. 2011 Nov;61(Pt 11):2670-5.

[34] Terenius O, de Oliveira CD, Pinheiro WD, Tadei WP, James AA, Marinotti O. 16S rRNA gene sequences from bacteria associated with adult *Anopheles darlingi* (*Diptera: Culicidae*) mosquitoes. Journal of medical entomology. 2008 Jan;45(1):172-5.

[35] Briones AM, Shililu J, Githure J, Novak R, Raskin L. *Thorsellia anophelis* is the dominant bacterium in a Kenyan population of adult *Anopheles gambiae* mosquitoes. The ISME journal. 2008 Jan;2(1):74-82.

[36] Lindh JM, Borg-Karlson AK, Faye I. Transstadial and horizontal transfer of bacteria within a colony of *Anopheles gambiae* (Diptera: Culicidae) and oviposition response to bacteria-containing water. Acta tropica. 008 Sep;107(3):242-50.

[37] Osei-Poku J, Mbogo CM, Palmer WJ, Jiggins FM. Deep sequencing reveals extensive variation in the gut microbiota of wild mosquitoes from Kenya. Molecular ecology. 2012 Sep 18. DOI: 10.1111/j.1365-294X.2012.05759.x.

[38] Kajla MK, Andreeva O, Gilbreath TM, 3rd, Paskewitz SM. Characterization of expression, activity and role in antibacterial immunity of *Anopheles gambiae* lysozyme c-1. Comparative biochemistry and physiology Part B, Biochemistry & molecular biology. 2010 Feb;155(2):201-9.

[39] Rani A, Sharma A, Rajagopal R, Adak T, Bhatnagar RK. Bacterial diversity analysis of larvae and adult midgut microflora using culture-dependent and culture-independent methods in lab-reared and field-collected *Anopheles stephensi*-an Asian malarial vector. BMC Microbiol. 2009;9:96.

[40] Jadin J. [Role of bacteria in the digestive tube of insects, vectors of plasmodidae and trypanosomidae]. Annales des sociétés belges de médecine tropicale, de parasitologie, et de mycologie. 1967;47(4):331-42.

[41] Jadin J, Vincke IH, Dunjic A, Delville JP, Wery M, Bafort J, et al. [Role of *Pseudomonas* in the sporogenesis of the hematozoon of malaria in the mosquito]. Bulletin de la Société de pathologie exotique et de ses filiales. 1966 Jul-Aug;59(4):514-25.

[42] Aksoy S. *Wigglesworthia gen. nov.* and *Wigglesworthia glossinidia sp. nov.*, taxa consisting of the mycetocyte-associated, primary endosymbionts of tsetse flies. International journal of systematic bacteriology. 1995 Oct;45(4):848-51.

[43] Kirkness EF, Haas BJ, Sun W, Braig HR, Perotti MA, Clark JM, et al. Genome sequences of the human body louse and its primary endosymbiont provide insights into the

permanent parasitic lifestyle. Proceedings of the National Academy of Sciences of the United States of America. 2010 Jul 6;107(27):12168-73.

[44] Moran NA, Hansen AK, Powell JE, Sabree ZL. Distinctive gut microbiota of honey bees assessed using deep sampling from individual worker bees. PloS one. 2012;7(4):e36393. DOI: 10.1371/journal.pone.0036393.

[45] Wong CN, Ng P, Douglas AE. Low-diversity bacterial community in the gut of the fruitfly Drosophila melanogaster. Environmental microbiology. 2011 Jul;13(7):1889-900.

[46] Moll RM, Romoser WS, Modrzakowski MC, Moncayo AC, Lerdthusnee K. Meconial peritrophic membranes and the fate of midgut bacteria during mosquito (Diptera: Culicidae) metamorphosis. Journal of medical entomology. 2001 Jan;38(1):29-32.

[47] Gary RE, Jr., Foster WA. Anopheles gambiae feeding and survival on honeydew and extra-floral nectar of peridomestic plants. Medical and veterinary entomology. 2004 Jun;18(2):102-7.

[48] Muller G, Schlein Y. Plant tissues: the frugal diet of mosquitoes in adverse conditions. Medical and veterinary entomology. 2005 Dec;19(4):413-22.

[49] Gouagna LC, Poueme RS, Dabire KR, Ouedraogo JB, Fontenille D, Simard F. Patterns of sugar feeding and host plant preferences in adult males of An. gambiae (Diptera: Culicidae). Journal of vector ecology : journal of the Society for Vector Ecology. 2010 Dec;35(2):267-76.

[50] Manda H, Gouagna LC, Foster WA, Jackson RR, Beier JC, Githure JI, et al. Effect of discriminative plant-sugar feeding on the survival and fecundity of Anopheles gambiae. Malaria journal. 2007;6:113.

[51] Wiwatanaratanabutr I. Geographic distribution of Wolbachia infection in mosquitoes from Thailand. Journal of invertebrate pathology. 2012 May 23. DOI: 10.1016/j.jip. 2012.04.010.

[52] McMeniman CJ, Lane RV, Cass BN, Fong AW, Sidhu M, Wang YF, et al. Stable introduction of a life-shortening Wolbachia infection into the mosquito Aedes aegypti. Science. 2009 Jan 2;323(5910):141-4.

[53] Xi Z, Ramirez JL, Dimopoulos G. The Aedes aegypti toll pathway controls dengue virus infection. PLoS pathogens. 2008 Jul;4(7):e1000098. http://www.ncbi.nlm.nih.gov/entrez/query.fcgi?cmd=Retrieve&db=PubMed&dopt=Citation&list_uids=18604274.

[54] Ricci I, Damiani C, Scuppa P, Mosca M, Crotti E, Rossi P, et al. The yeast Wickerhamomyces anomalus (Pichia anomala) inhabits the midgut and reproductive system of the Asian malaria vector Anopheles stephensi. Environmental microbiology. 2011 Apr; 13(4):911-21.

[55] Ricci I, Mosca M, Valzano M, Damiani C, Scuppa P, Rossi P, et al. Different mosquito species host *Wickerhamomyces anomalus* (*Pichia anomala*): perspectives on vector-borne diseases symbiotic control. Antonie van Leeuwenhoek. 2011 Jan;99(1):43-50.

[56] Chouaia B, Rossi P, Epis S, Mosca M, Ricci I, Damiani C, et al. Delayed larval development in *Anopheles* mosquitoes deprived of *Asaia* bacterial symbionts. BMC Microbiol. 2012 Jan 18;12 Suppl 1:S2.

[57] Lyke KE, Laurens M, Adams M, Billingsley PF, Richman A, Loyevsky M, et al. *Plasmodium falciparum* malaria challenge by the bite of aseptic *Anopheles stephensi* mosquitoes: results of a randomized infectivity trial. PloS one. 2010;5(10):e13490. DOI: 10.1371/journal.pone.0013490.

[58] Storelli G, Defaye A, Erkosar B, Hols P, Royet J, Leulier F. *Lactobacillus plantarum* promotes *Drosophila* systemic growth by modulating hormonal signals through TOR-dependent nutrient sensing. Cell metabolism. 2011 Sep 7;14(3):403-14.

[59] Puchta O. Experimentelle Untersuchungen ueber die Symbiose der Kleiderlaus *Pediculus vestimenti* Burm. Die Naturwissenschaften. 1954 1954;41(3):71-2.

[60] Lindh JM, Kannaste A, Knols BG, Faye I, Borg-Karlson AK. Oviposition responses of *Anopheles gambiae s.s.* (Diptera: Culicidae) and identification of volatiles from bacteria-containing solutions. Journal of medical entomology. 2008 Nov;45(6):1039-49.

[61] Nayar JK, Knight JW. Nutritional factors and antimicrobials on development of infective larvae of subperiodic *Brugia malayi* (Nematoda: Filarioidea) in *Anopheles quadrimaculatus* and *Aedes aegypti* (Diptera: Culicidae). Journal of medical entomology. 1991 Mar;28(2):275-9.

[62] Ramirez JL, Souza-Neto J, Torres Cosme R, Rovira J, Ortiz A, Pascale JM, et al. Reciprocal tripartite interactions between the *Aedes aegypti* midgut microbiota, innate immune system and dengue virus influences vector competence. PLoS neglected tropical diseases. 2012;6(3):e1561. DOI: 10.1371/journal.pntd.0001561.

[63] Blagrove MS, Arias-Goeta C, Failloux AB, Sinkins SP. *Wolbachia* strain *w*Mel induces cytoplasmic incompatibility and blocks dengue transmission in *Aedes albopictus*. Proceedings of the National Academy of Sciences of the United States of America. 2012 Jan 3;109(1):255-60.

[64] Walker T, Johnson PH, Moreira LA, Iturbe-Ormaetxe I, Frentiu FD, McMeniman CJ, et al. The *w*Mel *Wolbachia* strain blocks dengue and invades caged *Aedes aegypti* populations. Nature. 2011 Aug 25;476(7361):450-3.

[65] Hoffmann AA, Montgomery BL, Popovici J, Iturbe-Ormaetxe I, Johnson PH, Muzzi F, et al. Successful establishment of *Wolbachia* in *Aedes* populations to suppress dengue transmission. Nature. 2011 Aug 25;476(7361):454-7.

[66] Hughes GL, Koga R, Xue P, Fukatsu T, Rasgon JL. *Wolbachia* infections are virulent and inhibit the human malaria parasite *Plasmodium falciparum* in *Anopheles gambiae*. PLoS pathogens. 2011 May;7(5):e1002043. DOI: 10.1371/journal.ppat.1002043.

[67] Hughes GL, Vega-Rodriguez J, Xue P, Rasgon JL. *Wolbachia* strain *wAlbB* enhances infection by the rodent malaria parasite *Plasmodium berghei* in *Anopheles gambiae* mosquitoes. Applied and environmental microbiology. 2012 Mar;78(5):1491-5.

[68] Kambris Z, Blagborough AM, Pinto SB, Blagrove MS, Godfray HC, Sinden RE, et al. *Wolbachia* stimulates immune gene expression and inhibits *Plasmodium* development in *Anopheles gambiae*. PLoS pathogens. 2010;6(10):e1001143. DOI: 10.1371/journal.ppat.1001143.

[69] Shao Q, Yang B, Xu Q, Li X, Lu Z, Wang C, et al. Hindgut innate immunity and regulation of fecal microbiota through melanization in insects. The Journal of biological chemistry. 2012 Apr 20;287(17):14270-9.

[70] Oliveira JH, Goncalves RL, Lara FA, Dias FA, Gandara AC, Menna-Barreto RF, et al. Blood meal-derived heme decreases ROS levels in the midgut of *Aedes aegypti* and allows proliferation of intestinal microbiota. PLoS pathogens. 2011 Mar;7(3):e1001320. DOI: 10.1371/journal.ppat.1001320.

[71] Bischoff V, Vignal C, Duvic B, Boneca IG, Hoffmann JA, Royet J. Downregulation of the *Drosophila* Immune Response by Peptidoglycan-Recognition Proteins SC1 and SC2. PLoS pathogens. 2006 Feb;2(2):e14. DOI: 10.1371/journal.ppat.0020014.sg002.

[72] Zaidman-Remy A, Herve M, Poidevin M, Pili-Floury S, Kim MS, Blanot D, et al. The *Drosophila* amidase PGRP-LB modulates the immune response to bacterial infection. Immunity. 2006 Apr;24(4):463-73.

[73] Paredes JC, Welchman DP, Poidevin M, Lemaitre B. Negative regulation by amidase PGRPs shapes the *Drosophila* antibacterial response and protects the fly from innocuous infection. Immunity. 2011 Nov 23;35(5):770-9.

[74] Aggarwal K, Rus F, Vriesema-Magnuson C, Erturk-Hasdemir D, Paquette N, Silverman N. Rudra interrupts receptor signaling complexes to negatively regulate the IMD pathway. PLoS pathogens. 2008;4(8):e1000120. DOI: 10.1371/journal.ppat.1000120.t001.

[75] Kleino A, Myllymaki H, Kallio J, Vanha-aho LM, Oksanen K, Ulvila J, et al. Pirk is a negative regulator of the *Drosophila* Imd pathway. J Immunol. 2008 Apr 15;180(8):5413-22.

[76] Lhocine N, Ribeiro PS, Buchon N, Wepf A, Wilson R, Tenev T, et al. PIMS modulates immune tolerance by negatively regulating *Drosophila* innate immune signaling. Cell host & microbe. 2008 Aug 14;4(2):147-58.

[77] Waterhouse RM, Kriventseva EV, Meister S, Xi Z, Alvarez KS, Bartholomay LC, et al. Evolutionary dynamics of immune-related genes and pathways in disease-vector mosquitoes. Science. 2007 Jun 22;316(5832):1738-43.

[78] Waterhouse RM, Zdobnov EM, Tegenfeldt F, Li J, Kriventseva EV. OrthoDB: the hierarchical catalog of eukaryotic orthologs in 2011. Nucleic acids research. 2011 Jan; 39(Database issue):D283-8.

[79] Sharon G, Segal D, Ringo JM, Hefetz A, Zilber-Rosenberg I, Rosenberg E. Commensal bacteria play a role in mating preference of *Drosophila melanogaster*. Proceedings of the National Academy of Sciences of the United States of America. 2010 Nov 16;107(46):20051-6.

[80] Ben Ami E, Yuval B, Jurkevitch E. Manipulation of the microbiota of mass-reared Mediterranean fruit flies *Ceratitis capitata* (Diptera: Tephritidae) improves sterile male sexual performance. The ISME journal. 2010 Jan;4(1):28-37.

[81] Rosengaus RB, Zecher CN, Schultheis KF, Brucker RM, Bordenstein SR. Disruption of the termite gut microbiota and its prolonged consequences for fitness. Applied and environmental microbiology. 2011 Jul;77(13):4303-12.

[82] Verhulst NO, Beijleveld H, Knols BG, Takken W, Schraa G, Bouwmeester HJ, et al. Cultured skin microbiota attracts malaria mosquitoes. Malaria journal. 2009;8:302.

[83] Smith DL, Battle KE, Hay SI, Barker CM, Scott TW, McKenzie FE. Ross, macdonald, and a theory for the dynamics and control of mosquito-transmitted pathogens. PLoS pathogens. 2012;8(4):e1002588. DOI: 10.1371/journal.ppat.1002588.

[84] Engelstadter J, Telschow A. Cytoplasmic incompatibility and host population structure. Heredity. 2009 Sep;103(3):196-207.

[85] Douglas AE. The microbial dimension in insect nutritional ecology. Funct Ecol. 2009 Feb;23(1):38-47.

[86] Walker T, Moreira LA. Can *Wolbachia* be used to control malaria? Mem I Oswaldo Cruz. 2011 Aug;106:212-7.

[87] Hughes GL, Pike AD, Xue P, Rasgon JL. Invasion of *Wolbachia* into *Anopheles* and other insect germlines in an ex vivo organ culture system. PloS one. 2012;7(4):e36277. DOI: 10.1371/journal.pone.0036277.

[88] McMeniman CJ, Lane AM, Fong AW, Voronin DA, Iturbe-Ormaetxe I, Yamada R, et al. Host adaptation of a *Wolbachia* strain after long-term serial passage in mosquito cell lines. Applied and environmental microbiology. 2008 Nov;74(22):6963-9.

[89] Bisi DC, Lampe DJ. Secretion of anti-*Plasmodium* effector proteins from a natural *Pantoea agglomerans* isolate by using PelB and HlyA secretion signals. Applied and environmental microbiology. 2011 Jul;77(13):4669-75.

[90] Wang S, Ghosh AK, Bongio N, Stebbings KA, Lampe DJ, Jacobs-Lorena M. Fighting malaria with engineered symbiotic bacteria from vector mosquitoes. Proceedings of the National Academy of Sciences of the United States of America. 2012 Jul 31;109(31):12734-9.

[91] Rohwer F, Prangishvili D, Lindell D. Roles of viruses in the environment. Environmental microbiology. 2009 Nov;11(11):2771-4.

Chapter 3

Thermal Stress and Thermoregulation During Feeding in Mosquitoes

Chloé Lahondère and Claudio R. Lazzari

Additional information is available at the end of the chapter

1. Introduction

Many arthropods have acquired the ability to use the blood of endothermic vertebrates as their main or even unique food. Among insects, haematophagy has evolved independently in different groups [1], which have converged to this way of life under strong selective pressures that modelled many morphological, physiological and behavioural traits.

Blood is a rich source of nutrients and, except for the possible presence of parasites, otherwise sterile. However, being haematophagous is a risky task, as the food circulates inside vessels hidden beneath the skin of mobile hosts, able to defend themselves from biting or even predate on blood-sucking species. Thus, in order to minimize the contact with the host, blood-sucking insects need to pierce the host-skin without being noticed and gather blood in relatively high amounts and as quick as possible. Large blood-meals produce a strong osmotic misbalance at its ingestion and toxic metabolites as by products of its digestion. In addition, the rapid ingestion of a fluid which temperature can exceed that of the insects by 20°C or more and account for many times the insect's own body weight also implies a rapid transfer of heat into the insect's body. Thus, the inner temperature of the insect could exceed the physiological limits of certain functions, causing deleterious effects [2]. Numerous studies report the impact of temperature on different behavioural [3] and physiological processes such as development [4-6], metabolism [7, 8], blood-feeding and reproduction [9] of mosquitoes and insects in general.

Thermal stress may not only affect the insect itself but also its symbiotic flora [10-12] and the parasites that it transmits with an important impact on vector infectivity [13-15]. Finally, heat constitutes a main cue to find a food source (*i.e.* a warm-blooded vertebrate). Consequently, a recently fed insect could be exposed to cannibalism if its body temperature is higher than that of the surrounding environment, facilitating the horizontal transmission of parasites between vectors [16-17].

Provided their ectothermic nature, as well as their ability to colonize all kind of habitats, insects must cope with highly variable temperatures. Therefore, many insect species have developed particular physiological and behavioural mechanisms and strategies to avoid the risk to be submitted to thermal stress [18, 19]. To avoid the effect of environmental heat, insects can seek for fresher environments or adjust their water loss to increase evaporation. In the case of haematophagous insects such as mosquitoes, they must in addition confront the exposition to thermal stress at each feeding event.

The problem of heat transfer between hosts and blood-sucking insects during blood feeding remained largely overlooked until recently, when unexpected physiological mechanisms against thermal stress were unravelled in mosquitoes. We present in this chapter a brief account of these findings and the perspectives that they open in both, fundamental and applied research.

2. Thermal stress and protective strategies in *Anopheles*

The first evidences of thermal stress during feeding in haematophagous insects were obtained only recently [20]. The variation of the temperature of the body during the feeding process was measured in different species of blood-sucking insects, including two mosquitoes, *Aedes aegypti* and *Anopheles gambiae* using thermocouples. As soon as feeding begins, a steady increase of the body temperature occurs, reaching peak values of up to +10°C a few minutes later. After feeding, the temperature decreases gradually to come back similar to the environmental one. Depending on the values of environmental temperature, which is the initial temperature of the insect, and that of the blood, the amplitude and dynamics of heating and cooling vary.

Physiological responses of insects to heat include molecular changes, as is a rapid increase in the level of heat shock proteins (Hsps), which have a role as molecular chaperones that preserve the function of enzymes and other critical proteins [20]. More than a dozen Hsps are synthetized after exposure to high temperature, being the Hsp70 the most widely recognised as associated to thermal and other stresses. As in many other organisms, mosquito Hsp70s have been shown to increase during environmental stress [21, 22].

Benoit and co-workers [20] showed that, correlated with feeding and the associated elevation of the body temperature, a synthesis of heat-shock proteins occurs in *Aedes aegypti* in the few hours following a blood meal, in particular of Hsp70. In this species, the Hsp70 synthesis peaks 1 hour after feeding, reaching maximal expression in the mosquito midgut, where the relative amount of Hsp70 increases about 7 times after feeding. Similar increases in Hsp70 were showed immediately after blood feeding in *Culex pipiens* and in *Anopheles gambiae*, as well as in the bed bug *Cimex lectularius*. Nevertheless this increase, measured as the relative increase of mRNA by Northern blot, is not identical in the three mosquito species. Whereas in *Aedes aegypti* and

Culex pipiens the relative level increases between nine and ten times, in *Anopheles gambiae* only three times. This last result is particularly interesting, since it is probable that the last named species would be less submitted to thermal stress, as we will discuss in the following sections.

3. Heterothermy during feeding in *Anopheles*

To better understand to what extent mosquitoes are exposed to thermal stress during feeding, we recently conducted a real-time infrared thermographic analysis of the evolution of the body temperature of *Anopheles stephensi* during feeding on live hosts at different skin temperatures and using an artificial feeder [23].

Thermal imaging analysis has first revealed that during feeding, the different regions of the mosquito's body exhibited different temperatures. When *Anopheles stephensi* fed on mice or human volunteers, their head temperature remained close to that of the ingested blood while the abdomen temperature stayed closer to that of the ambient temperature (Figure 1). The thermal profile along a mosquito's body during feeding, notwithstanding the exact temperature of the host skin, can be summarized as in this: $T°_{head} > T°_{thorax} > T°_{abdomen}$. The fact of maintaining different temperatures in different regions of the body by an animal is named "regional heterothermy" and it is common in vertebrates living in cold aquatic or terrestrial environments. When the body temperature changes with time, this condition is called "temporal heterothermy". A combination of both types of heterothemy is frequently found in insects that perform pre-heating of flight muscles before taking off. By means of simultaneous isometric contractions of antagonist muscles, insects like bumble-bees and moths heat their thorax up to reach the optimal temperature for muscular work [18].

In the case of *Anopheles stephensi*, an average difference of 3.3° C between $T°_{head}$ and $T°_{abdomen}$ was measured when the $T°_{host}$ was 34° C and 2.2° C when T_{host} was 28° C. At the end of feeding, when mouthparts are retracted from the skin, the mosquito temperature returns rapidly to environmental temperature (ectothermy).

Infrared thermography revealed a quite different pattern of body temperature in *Aedes aegypti*. In this species, the abdominal temperature during feeding remains close to that of the host, rather than to that of the environment as in *Anopheles stephensi* [23]. On the other hand, when the two species fed on sugar solution, despite the muscular activity of the ingestion pump, no heterothermy occurs: the temperature of the whole body remained that of the environment. As a consequence males, which don't feed on blood, exhibit a typically ectothermic thermal profile even when resting on a warm host, demonstrating that heating is only due to blood ingestion and not to the proximity of the host [23].

4. Prediuresis and drop-keeping

During blood feeding, most haematophagous species excrete drops of fluid, a process referred in mosquitoes as "prediuresis". The physiological function of prediuresis has been related to

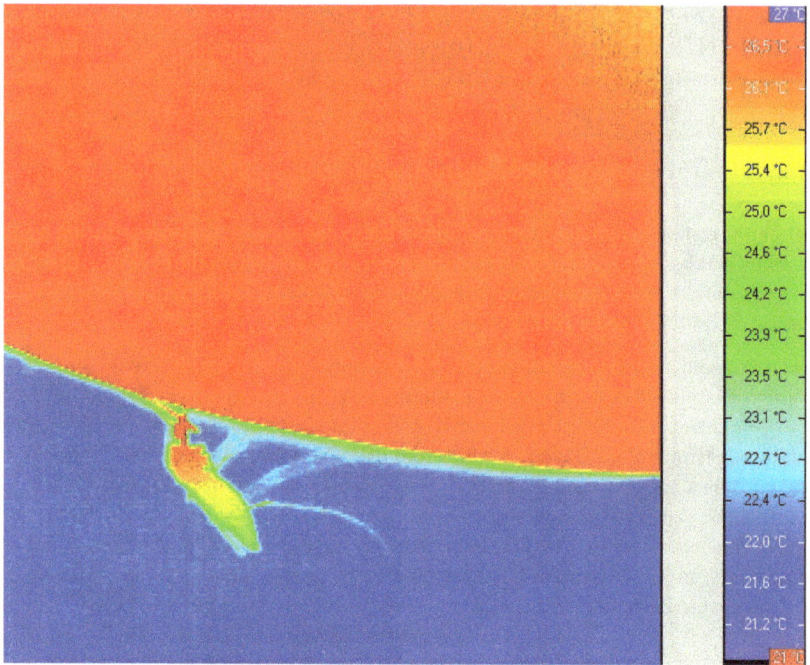

Figure 1. Thermographic image of an *Anopheles stephensi* female at the beginning of feeding on an anesthetized mouse (T°_{host} = 28° C, $T^\circ_{environment}$ = 22° C). The temperature of the head is very close to the mouse one and a temperature gradient along the mosquito body can be observed (i.e., heterothermy).

erythrocytes concentration and elimination of water excess. The eliminated fluid is in most insects composed of urine, but in some blood-sucking species, such as mosquitoes and sandflies, it also contains fresh ingested blood that gives to the drop a bright red appearance. In mosquitoes, which feed not only on vertebrate blood, but also on nectar, prediuresis occurs during blood-feeding but it is rare or absent when they take a sugar meal.

In *Anopheles stephensi*, notwithstanding the nature of the host, blood-feeding almost always proceeds in a similar way: drops of fluid start being excreted during the first or second minute after the insect begins to feed. Frequently, a drop remains attached to the end of the abdomen for several minutes, increasing its size during feeding. Eventually the drop felt, and a new one is emitted and retained at the abdomen's end. The number of drops produced until complete gorging may vary.

Real-time thermography revealed that when *Anopheles stephensi* performs prediuresis and keeps a drop attached to its anus, a transient fall of 2° C or more of the abdominal temperature occurs and the characteristic heterothermy along its body becomes even more pronounced (Figure 2). The same phenomenon was observed in females of this species feeding in mice, human volunteers or using an artificial feeder [23]. Besides, when ingesting blood at the same temperature, the abdominal temperature of drop-keepers is significantly lower than that of mosquitoes that just perform prediuresis but that do not keep drops. These results demonstrate the existence of a physical cooling process in *Anopheles stephensi*. Conversely, drop-keeping was never observed to occur in *Aedes aegypti* among the individuals producing pre-urine while feeding, even if the frequency of prediuresis is the same in both mosquito species [23].

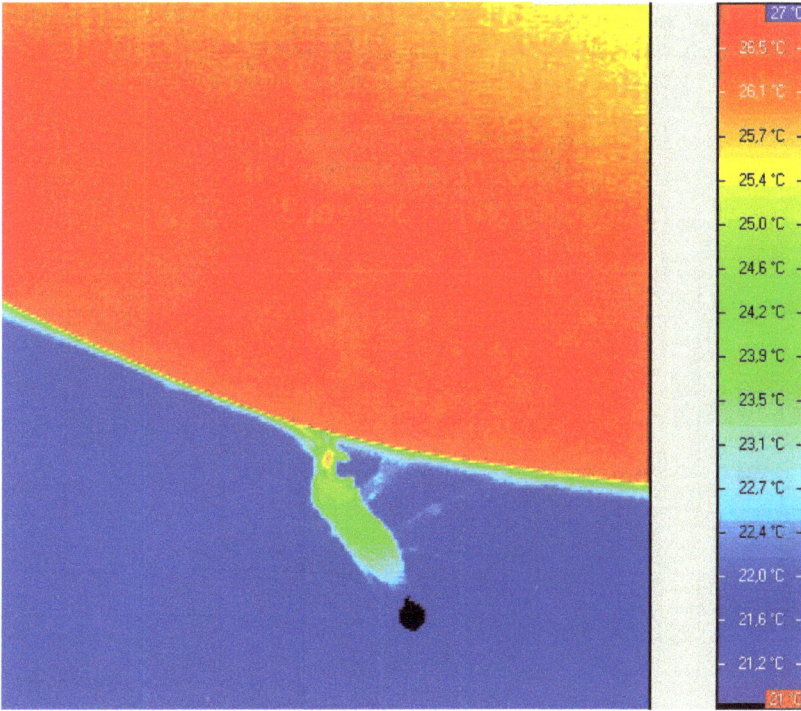

Figure 2. Thermographic image of the same *Anopheles stephensi* female as Figure 1, but during prediuresis. The mosquito performs evaporative cooling. The retention of the fluid drop attached to the abdomen end leads to a fall of the abdomen temperature causing a clear temperature gradient along the mosquito body. The colour of the droplet does not reflect the real temperature, because of the difference in the emissivity between the cuticle of the mosquito and the drop surface.

5. Thermoregulation in *Anopheles*

Many insects, in particular those having easy access to water, produce and retain drops of fluid, such as nectar, honey-dew, water or urine, depending on species, which evaporates in contact with the air, causing heat loss by evaporative cooling and the consequent decrease of the temperature of the insect body. Evaporative cooling constitutes an adaptive and effective response to risks associated to high temperature and has been observed in different groups of insects [24, 25].

This decrease of temperature helps them to avoid the deleterious physiological consequences of thermal stress. Some insects such as honeybees and bumblebees produce heat with their thoracic muscles while flying (endothermy) and regurgitate a droplet of nectar through their mouthparts to cool down their head, thus keeping the brain safe from overheating [26, 27]. Moths emit fluid, which is retained on the proboscis to refresh their head whereas others, like aphids, excrete honey-dew through their anus that consequently refresh their abdomen. The recorded loss of temperature is between 2 and 8° C depending on species [28].

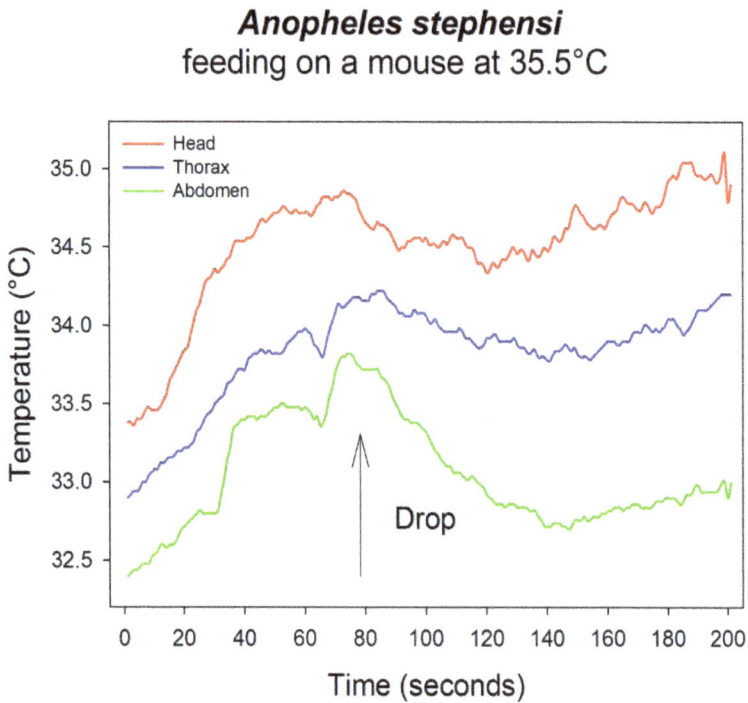

Figure 3. Evolution of the body temperatures of *Anopheles stephensi* during feeding on an anesthetized mouse. The arrow indicates the excretion of a droplet. ($T°_{host}$ = 35.5° C, $T°_{environment}$ = 28° C)

In *Anopheles* mosquitoes, the abdominal temperature of drop-keepers decreases of about 2° C during drop retention. For mosquitoes and in general for all haematophagous insects that need to manage an excess of water into their body during feeding and keep a well-adjusted water balance, evaporative cooling represents an efficient protective mechanism against overheating.

To what extent prediuresis and drop-keeping occurs is variable and it is known that the rate of production and the size of the droplets excreted in mosquitoes during prediuresis differ not only between species but also within the same species, as also differs the amount of erythrocytes from the ingested blood [29].

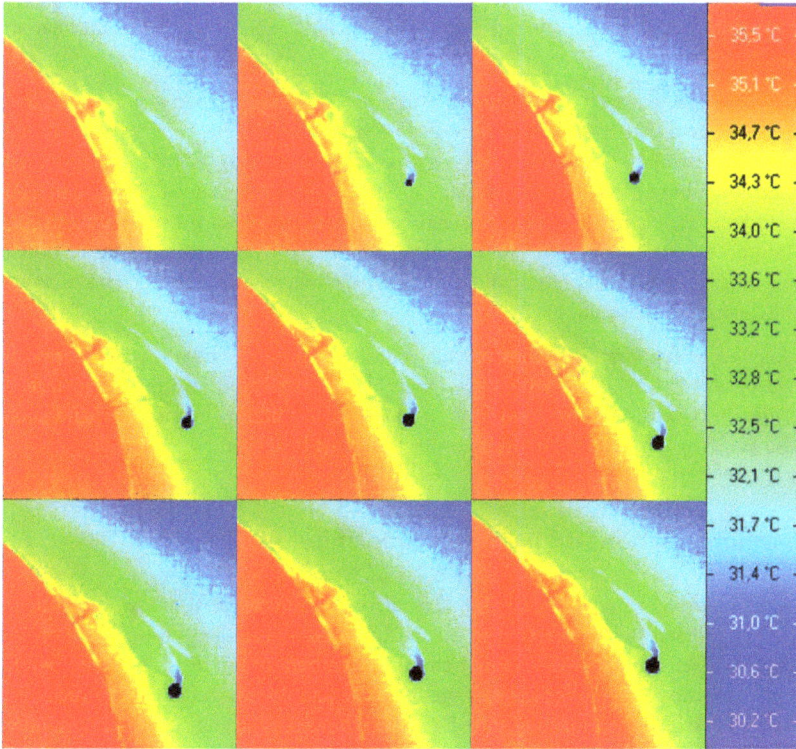

Figure 4. Sequence of thermographic images showing the production of a drop during feeding and the subsequent cooling of the abdomen in an *Anopheles stephensi* female. The insect fed on a human host ($T^\circ_{host} = 36^\circ$ C, $T^\circ_{environment} = 23^\circ$ C). Images were taken every 5 seconds.

6. A novel significance of prediuresis

Even though the occurrence of prediuresis and the elimination of fresh blood have been largely reported, it has been always considered just a way of concentrating erythrocytes and reducing the insect weight for take-off [30]. Nevertheless, two puzzling aspects of prediuresis in mosquitoes remained unsolved. The first one is the elimination during feeding of some of the just ingested blood containing erythrocytes [29]. It is widely accepted that strong selective pressures made blood-sucking insects minimize their contact time with a host in order to reduce the risk of being predated [1]. Thus, throwing away some of the food they ingest appears, at first glance, as a maladaptive strategy. From a point of view of thermoregulation, however, this "waste" makes sense, since it allows a quick increase in the volume (and evaporative surface) of the droplet and perhaps the surface properties of the drop, influencing its retention. Thus, the excretion of fresh blood during feeding in mosquitoes can be explained in terms of an adaptive response of evaporative cooling when exposed to thermal stress associated to feeding.

The second puzzling aspect of prediuresis is that not all mosquito species perform it. In fact, it has been shown that species that perform prediuresis need more time to reach repletion during a blood meal than species that do not produce pre-urine [31, 32]. Thus, the production of pre-urine could be seen, again, as a maladaptive strategy. However, an increase in feeding time could represent a trade-off between feeding quickly and avoiding overheating in species that are particularly sensitive to thermal stress. Others may be less sensitive or, as *Aedes* minimize the consequences of thermal stress by synthetizing more heat-shock proteins as, for example, *Anopheles* mosquitos.

Drop-keeping as evaporative cooling mechanism is in accordance with the particular position adopted by *Anopheles* species, which keep their abdomen away from the host surface. This causes the drop to be more exposed to the ambient air facilitating evaporation and cooling, and also avoiding the drop to be lost by contact with the host skin.

7. Thermoregulation and pathogens transmission

When anopheline mosquitoes ingest a blood meal from an infected host, mature and functional *Plasmodium* gametocytes are present in the erythrocytes and undergo differentiation in the mosquito midgut, a process that is influenced by temperature. Indeed, high temperatures negatively affect early stages of the parasite life cycle and no exflagellation occurs above 30° C, holding parasites in an inactive state [14]. Later processes such as ookinete formation or migration of sporozoites towards the salivary glands are also influenced by temperature [15, 33, 34]. Furthermore, it has been well demonstrated that different species of *Plasmodium* are thermo-sensitive and that temperature has a direct impact on the incubation period of parasites in the mosquito [13]. On the other hand, the proliferation and dispersion of flaviviruses in *Aedes* mosquitoes is also under the influence of temperature but contrary to *Plasmodium*, this latter constitutes one of the most important factor positively influencing the extrinsic incubation period (*EIP*). It has been shown that high temperatures are important for flaviviruses, acting on the rate of viral multiplication and consequently on the vector competence [35, 36, 37].

Moreover, *Plasmodium* parasites have to cope with the formation of the peritrophic matrix that follows each blood meal, which restrain their penetration through the gut wall [38, 39]. During the process of differentiation, *Plasmodium* ookinetes have to cross the peritrophic matrix and the midgut epithelium, before they turn into oocysts [40]. The time needed for the formation of the peritrophic matrix positively correlates with the vectorial capacity of mosquitoes, taking a longer time in *Anopheles* species than in species of *Aedes* or *Culex* [1, 41]. Thus, for *Plasmodium* parasites, insect's heterothermy could represent an important advantage, since when they enter into the mosquito's body, they are exposed to a rapid fall in temperature, which could immediately trigger exflagellation. Parasites could therefore penetrate the gut wall before the peritrophic matrix is fully formed.

From an evolutionary point of view, it makes sense that *Plasmodium* parasites take an advantage to be associated with species that undergo evaporative cooling, protecting them from lethal temperatures. On the other hand, flaviviruses associated with non drop-keeper species would benefit from a necessary warmer environment.

Evaporative cooling could also protect from heat stress the symbiotic microorganisms associated to mosquitoes and that can play an important role in haematophagous insects [10]. *Asaia* bacteria have been found in high density in the gut of *Anopheles stephensi* females as well as in ovaries [11]. Recently many genera have been identified in the midgut of natural populations of *Anopheles gambiae* [42]. In particular, the abundance of *Enterobacteriaceae* in the mosquito midgut has been found to correlate significantly with the *Plasmodium* infection status [42].

8. Thermoregulation and thermotolerance in mosquitoes

Finally, it is possible to speculate on two further implications of our interpretation of the functionality of prediuresis as thermoregulatory mechanisms. The first one concerns how environmental temperature may affect the survival of less thermotolerant mosquitoes. If we consider that the species that perform evaporative cooling could be more sensitive to heat, any change in the environmental temperature, due to local or global warming, would have a higher impact on them than on species that do not perform it, as for example *Culex spp.* that feed quickly and do not perform prediuresis while feeding [43]. It can be predicted that such species have been selected to reduce the contact time with their host and consequently to be more thermotolerant to temperature increases. Indeed, *Aedes aegypti* and its ability to produce Hsps represent an example of this [20].

The second implication of our finding is related to the control of mosquito populations. Prediuresis has deeper physiological consequences than just diuresis. In addition to excretion, it implies blood concentration and thermoregulation. The exploitation of the knowledge about excretion physiology to control disease vector insects by interfering with the function of Malpighian tubules has been already proposed for other haematophagous insects [44], and the same can be expected for mosquitoes. In this case, blocking or delaying the production of urine would have a double impact on disease transmission by affecting microorganisms transmitted by prediuresis [45, 46] and/or affecting the survival of mosquitoes exposed to overheating.

9. Conclusion

Anopheles mosquitoes are capable to perform thermoregulation by evaporative cooling during blood intake. This mechanism protects the insect itself, as well as the associated microorganisms (both symbionts and parasites) from thermal stress. Thus, prediuresis which plays such different roles in the mosquito physiology, appears one more time as an interesting possible target for the control of disease vectors.

Acknowledgements

We are very grateful to Catherine Bourgouin and the CEPIA staff (Institut Pasteur, France) for providing us anopheline mosquitoes and rearing advices as well as Rogerio Amino (Institut Pasteur, France) for his valuable comments on the manuscript and helpful discussions. We also thank Fabrice Chandre and Marie-Noelle Lacroix (IRD Montpellier, France) for providing us *Aedes aegypti* eggs. This work received financial support from ANR (EcoEpi), CNRS and the University of Tours (France).

Author details

Chloé Lahondère and Claudio R. Lazzari*

*Address all correspondence to: claudio.lazzari@univ-tours.fr

Institut de Recherche sur la Biologie de l'Insecte, UMR CNRS - Université François Rabelais, Tours, France

References

[1] Lehane MJ. The biology of blood-sucking in insects Cambridge University Press, New York. 2nd ed.; 2005.

[2] Kirby MJ, Lindsay SW. Responses of adult mosquitoes of two sibling species, *Anopheles arabiensis* and *Anopheles gambiae s.s.* (Diptera: Culicidae), to high temperatures. Bulletin of Entomological Research 2004; 94 441-448.

[3] Muirhead Thomson CR. The reactions of mosquitoes to temperature and humidity. Bulletin of Entomological Research 1938; 125-140.

[4]   Lanciani CA, Le TM. Effect of temperature on the wing length body-weight relation-ship in *Anopheles quadrimaculatus*. Journal of the American Mosquito Control Assoca-tion 1995; 11 241-243.

[5]   Lyimo EO, Takken W, Koella JC. Effect of rearing temperature and larval density on larval survival, age at pupation and adult size of *Anopheles gambiae*. Entomoligia Ex-perimentalis et Applicata 1992; 63 265-271.

[6]   Rueda LM, Patel KJ, Axtell RC, Stinner RE. Temperature-dependent development and survival rates of *Culex quinquefasciatus* and *Aedes aegypti* (Diptera: Culicidae). Journal of Medical Entomology 1980; 27 892-898.

[7]   Clements AN. The biology of mosquitoes. Chapman & Hall, London, UK, Vol. 1; 1992.

[8]   Mellanby K. The influence of athmospheric humidity on the thermal death point of a number of insects. Journal of Experimental Biology 1932; 9 222-231.

[9]   Eldridge BF. Effect of temperature and photoperiod on blood-feeding and ovarian development in mosquitoes of *Culex pipiens* complex. American Journal of Tropical Medicine and Hygiene 1968; 17 133-140.

[10]   Brooks MA. Symbiotes and nutrition of medically important insects. Bulletin of the World Health Organisation 1964; 31 555-559.

[11]   Favia G, Ricci I, Damiani C, Raddadi N, Crotti E, Marzorati M, Rizzi A, Urso R, Bru-setti L, Borin S, et al. Bacteria of the genus *Asaia* stably associate with *Anopheles ste-phensi*, an Asian malarial mosquito vector. Proceeding of the National Academy of Science of the United States of America 2007; 104 9047-9051.

[12]   Gusmão DS, Santos AV, Marini DC, Russo ES, Peixoto AMD, Bacci MJr, Berbert-Mo-lina MA, Lemos, FJA. First isolation of microorganisms from the gut diverticulum of *Aedes aegypti* (Diptera: Culicidae): new perspectives for an insect-bacteria association. Memorias do Instituto Oswaldo Cruz 2007; 102 919-924.

[13]   Boyd MF. Epidemiology: factors related to the definitive host. In Malariology. ed Boyd MF, W.B. Saunders & Co, Philadelphia, Vol 1; 1949.

[14]   Ogwan'g RA, Mwangi JK, Githure J, Were JBO, Roberts CR, Martin SK. Factors af-fecting exflagellation of in-vitro cultivated *Plasmodium falciparum* gametocytes. Amer-ican Journal of Tropical Medicine and Hygiene 1993; 49 25-29.

[15]   Vanderberg JP, Yoeli M. Effects of temperature on sporogonic development of *Plas-modium berghei*. Journal of Parasitology 1966; 52 559-564.

[16]   Jones JC, Pilitt DR. Blood-feeding behavior of adult *Aedes aegypti* mosquitoes. Biologi-cal Bulletin 1973; 145 127-139.

[17]   Weathersby AB, Ah HS, Mccall JW. Mosquitoes feeding on engorged mosquitoes. Mosquito News 1971; 31 110-111.

[18] Heinrich, B. The hot-blooded insects : strategies and mechanisms of thermoregulation Harvard University Press, Cambridge, Massachusetts; 1993.

[19] May ML. Insect thermoregulation. Annual Review of Entomology 1979; 24 313-349.

[20] Benoit JB, Lopez-Martinez G, Patrick KR, Phillips ZP, Krause TB, Denlinger, DL. Drinking a hot blood meal elicits a protective heat shock response in mosquitoes. Proceeding of the National Academy of Science of the United States of America 2011; 108 8026-8029.

[21] Gross TL, Myles KM, Adelman ZN. Identification and characterization of heat shock 70 genes in *Aedes aegypti* (Diptera: Culicidae). Journal of Medical Entomology 2009; 46 496–504.

[22] Benoit JB, Lopez-Martinez G, Phillips ZP, Patrick KR, Denlinger DL. Heat shock proteins contribute to mosquito dehydration tolerance. Journal of Insect Physiology 2010; 56 151–156.

[23] Lahondère C, Lazzari CR. Mosquitoes cool down during blood feeding to avoid overheating. Current Biology 2012; 22, 40–45.

[24] Adams PA, Heath JE. An evaporative cooling mechanism in *Pholus achemon*. Journal of Research on the Lepidoptera 1964; 3 69-72.

[25] Mittler TE. The excretion of honey-dew by *Tuberolachnus salignus* (Gmelin) (Homoptera: Aphididae). Proceeding of the Royal Entomological Society, Series A General Entomology 1958; 33 49-55.

[26] Heinrich B. Heat-exchange in relation to blood-flow between thorax and abdomen in bumblebees. Journal of Experimental Biology 1976; 64 561-585.

[27] Heinrich B. Keeping a cool head - honeybee thermoregulation. Science 1979; 205 1269-1271.

[28] Prange HD. Evaporative cooling in insects. Journal of Insect Physiology 1996; 42 493-499.

[29] Chege GMM, Beier JC Blood acquisition and processing by three *Anopheles* (Diptera: Culicidae) species with different innate susceptibilities to *Plasmodium falciparum*. Journal of Medical Entomology 1998; 35(3) 319-323.

[30] Briegel H, Rezzonico L. Concentration of host blood protein during feeding by Anopheline mosquitoes (Diptera, Culicidae). Journal of Medical Entomology 1985; 22 612-618.

[31] Vaughan JA, Noden BH, Beier JC. Concentration of human erythrocytes by Anopheline mosquitoes (Diptera, Culicidae) during feeding. Journal of Medical Entomology 1991; 28 780-786.

[32] Chadee DD, Beier JC, Mohammed RT. Fast and slow blood-feeding durations of *Aedes aegypti* mosquitoes in Trinidad. Journal of Vector Ecology 2002; 27 172-177.

[33] Ball GH, Chao J. Temperature stresses on mosquito phase of *Plasmodium relictum*. Journal of Parasitology 1964; 50 748-752.

[34] Noden BH, Kent MD, Beier JC. The impact of variations in temperature on early *Plasmodium falciparum* development in *Anopheles stephensi*. Parasitology 1995; 111 539-545.

[35] Davis NC. The effect of various temperatures in modifying the extrinsic incubation period of the yellow fever virus in *Aedes aegypti*. American Journal of Epidemiology 1932; 16 163-176.

[36] Hardy JL, Houk EJ, Kramer LD, Reeves WC. Intrinsic factors affecting vector competence of mosquitoes for arboviruses. Annual Review of Entomology 1983; 28 229-262.

[37] Kramer LD, Ebel GD. Dynamics of flavivirus infection in mosquitoes. Advances in Virus Research 2003; 60 187-232.

[38] Baton LA, Ranford-Cartwright LC. How do malaria ookinetes cross the mosquito midgut wall? Trends in Parasitology 2005; 21 22-28.

[39] Freyvogel TA, Staeubli W. The formation of the peritrophic membrane in Culicidae. Acta Tropica 1965; 22 118-147.

[40] Sinden RE. *Plasmodium* differentiation in the mosquito. Parassitologia 1999; 41 139-148.

[41] Devenport M, Jacobs-Lorena M. The peritrophic matrix of hematophagous insects. In Biology of Disease Vectors, ed. W.C. Marquardt Elsevier Academic Press, Amsterdam; 2005.

[42] Boissière A, Tchioffo MT, Bachar D, Abate L, Marie A, Nsango SE, Shahbazkia HR, Awono-Ambene PH, Levashina EA, Christen R, Morlais I. Midgut microbiota of the malaria mosquito vector *Anopheles gambiae* and interactions with *Plasmodium falciparum* infection. Public Library of Science Pathogens 2012; 8(5): e1002742. doi: 10.1371/journal.ppat.1002742

[43] Vaughan JA, Azad AF Passage of host immunoglobulin-G from blood meal into hemolymph of selected mosquito species (Diptera, Culicidae). Journal of Medical Entomology 1988; 25 472-474.

[44] Santini MS, Ronderos JR. Allatotropin-like peptide released by Malpighian tubules induces hindgut activity associated with diuresis in the Chagas disease vector *Triatoma infestans* (Klug). Journal of Experimental Biology 2007; 210 1986-1991.

[45] Sadlova J, Reishig J, Volf P. Prediuresis in female *Phlebotomus* sandflies (Diptera: Psychodidae). European Journal of Entomology 1998; 95 643-647.

[46] Blow JA, Turell MJ, Walker ED, Silverman AL. Post-bloodmeal diuretic shedding of hepatitis B virus by mosquitoes (Diptera: Culicidae). Journal of Medical Entomology 2002; 39 605-612.

Chapter 4

Bacterial Biodiversity in Midguts of *Anopheles* Mosquitoes, Malaria Vectors in Southeast Asia

Sylvie Manguin, Chung Thuy Ngo,
Krajana Tainchum, Waraporn Juntarajumnong,
Theeraphap Chareonviriyaphap,
Anne-Laure Michon and Estelle Jumas-Bilak

Additional information is available at the end of the chapter

1. Introduction

Factors allowing the development of a pathogen to reach the infecting stage in a mosquito are poorly known. On the 528 species of mosquitoes recorded within the *Anopheles* genus [1], only 70 to 60 are able to transmit parasites responsible for malaria and filariasis [2, 3]. In vector-parasite interactions, the mosquito gut represents the first point of contact between parasites ingested and the vector epithelial surfaces. In the midgut, the parasites will have the opportunity to undergo their life cycle, but of the tens of thousands of *Plasmodium* gametocytes ingested by mosquitoes, less than five oocysts might be produced [4]. The factors responsible for this drastic reduction are still poorly understood. Recent studies showed that one of these factors concerns the primordial role played by the bacteria naturally present in mosquito midgut. Then, there is a growing interest on bacterial biodiversity in *Anopheles* mosquitoes and particularly those based on the identification of bacteria to be used for malaria transmission blocking based on bacterial genetic changes to deliver antiparasite molecules or paratransgenic approach [5-13]. Recent studies reported the presence of symbiotic bacteria, such as *Pantoea agglomerans* or *Asaia* in midgut lumen with anti-*Plasmodium* effector proteins that render host mosquitoes refractory to malaria infection [6, 10, 13]. Engineered *P. agglomerans* strains were able to inhibit *Plasmodium falciparum* development by 98% [13]. Other studies showed that insects with an important microbiota seem more resistant to infections and certain bacteria, such as *Enterobacter* sp. (Esp Z) inhibit partially or totally ookinete, oocyst and sporozoite formation [14-16]. In *Anopheles albimanus*, co-infections with the bacteria, *Serratia marcescens*, and *Plasmodium vivax* resulted in only 1% of mosquitoes being infected with oocysts, compared with 71% infection for control mosquitoes without bacteria [17]. A recent meta-taxogenomic study provides an in-depth description of the microbial communities in the midgut of *Anopheles gambiae* exposed to *P. falciparum* infection and the links between microbiota and parasitic status by comparing midgut microbiota in *P. falciparum*-positive and *P. falciparum*-negative individuals. Authors found significant correlation between the high enterobacterial content and malaria infection. Despite conflicting results on the role of enterobacteria, it has now clearly been established that bacteria present in *Anopheles* populations have a great influence on parasite transmission [18].

In Thailand and Vietnam, malaria is a public health priority with a strong prevalence of this disease in forested regions, in particular along the international borders with Myanmar and Cambodia respectively. In these malaria endemic areas, another parasitic disease occurs, Bancroftian lymphatic filariasis (BLF) for which only limited data are available [2]. Malaria and BLF are mosquito-borne diseases with *Plasmodium* species, especially *P. falciparum*, *P. vivax*, and rural strains of *Wuchereria bancrofti* sharing the same *Anopheles* vector species. In Southeast Asia, *Anopheles* vectors belong to species complexes with different involvement in the transmission of pathogens [19]. Few sibling species of the Dirus and Minimus Complexes and the Maculatus Group are involved in malaria and BLF, but specific role of each sibling species and factors influencing this role have never been studied due to the lack of reliable methods for species identification, now available [20-22]. As mosquito microbiota is one of the factors influencing pathogen transmission, this chapter is presenting the biodiversity of bacteria in the midgut of field-collected adults of 10 *Anopheles* species, topic less studied compared to the large number of studies presenting bacteria in the defense against parasites in laboratory conditions.

1.1. Midgut microbiome of mosquitoes

Many insects contain large communities of diverse microorganisms that probably exceed the number of cells in the insect itself [23]. More specifically, complex microbiotae have been described in mosquito midgut reporting the presence of numerous Gram-negative rods, including *Serratia marcescens*, *Klebsiella ozaenae*, *Pseudomonas aeruginosa*, *Escherichia coli*, *Enterobacter* spp. [14]. Recently, three metagenomic studies provided a more comprehensive picture of the diversity of midgut microbiota in *Anopheles gambiae*, the main malaria vector in Africa [18, 24, 25]. In wild caught adults of *Anopheles* species, the microbiota showed the common presence of *Pseudomonas* and *Aeromonas* species reported from at least five species among which malaria vectors (Table 1). The following five genera, *Asaia*, *Bacillus*, *Chryseobacterium*, *Klebsiella*, and *Pantoea* have been reported from four field collected *Anopheles* species, while *Serratia* and *Stenotrophomonas* were identified in three species (Table 1). At least three mosquito-specific bacterial species, isolated from the midgut of main malaria vectors of the Gambiae Complex, have been described, such as *Thorsellia anophelis* [26], *Janibacter anophelis* [27] and *Elizabethkingia anophelis* [28]. The first of the three species represents a new genus and species found predominant in the midgut of *Anopheles arabiensis* [29], the same *Anopheles* species in which *J. anophelis* was isolated. The third newly described species is closely related to *Elizabethkingia meningoseptica* as they share 98.6% similarity, and both species have been found in the midgut of *Anopheles gambiae* [11, 28]. The latter species, *E. meningoseptica*, was also isolated from diseased birds, frogs, turtles, cats, being most likely an agent of zoonotic infections, as well as a human meningitis especially in newborn infants [30]. Bacteria of the genus *Asaia* have also been associated with *Anopheles* species, in particular field-collected *An. gambiae, An. funestus, An. coustani* and *An. maculipennis* (Table 1), as well as a colony of *An. stephensi* in which *Asaia* bacteria was dominant and stably associated [9]. The presence of *Asaia* species in *Anopheles* could serve as candidate for malaria control based on the production of antiparasite molecules in mosquitoes for use in paratransgenic control of malaria [6, 9, 31]. Other bacterial species have been defined as antimalarial agents, especially those producing prodigiosin, a pigment produced by various bacteria, including *S. marcescens* [14].

The number of bacteria not only varied between individuals but also changed markedly during development, depending on both the stage of development and the blood-feeding status of the mosquitoes [31]. The normal midgut microbiota of *Anopheles* mosquitoes need to be further identified [5] as only few studies have reported the microbiota of wild caught malaria vectors (Table 1) [5-7, 9, 11, 12, 17, 24, 26-29, 31-35]. Further investigations of gut microbiota, especially of wild-caught insect vectors, might contribute to understanding the annual and regional variations recorded for vector transmitted diseases [17] and yield novel vector-control strategies [14].

1.2. Exploring bacterial communities by 16S PCR-TTGE

Bacterial communities are classically assessed through culture-dependent methods based on colony isolation on solid medium, sometimes after enrichment by growth in liquid medium. But, it is now obvious that the microbial diversity is poorly represented by the cultured fraction, and culture have been shown to explore less than 1% of the whole bacterial diversity in environment samples [36]. Thanks to sophisticated biotechnological and computational tools of the metagenomics, molecular ecology offers the potential of determining microbial diversity in an ecosystem by assessing the genetic diversity. The complete metagenomic approach will give the total gene content of a community, thus providing data about biodiversity but also function and interactions [37]. For the purpose of biodiversity studies, metagenomics can focus on one common gene shared by all members of the community. The most commonly used culture-independent method relies on amplification and analysis of the 16S rRNA genes in a microbiota [38].

The 16S rRNA genes are widely used for documentation of the evolutionary history and taxon assignment of individual organisms because they have highly conserved regions for construction of universal primers and highly variable regions for identification of individual species [39]. The notion developed by Woese that rRNA genes could identify living organisms by reconstructing phylogenies resulted in the adoption of 16S rRNA gene in microbiology [39]. Its universality and the huge number of sequences stored in databases have established 16S rRNA gene as the "gold standard" not only in microbial phylogeny, systematics, and identification but also microbial ecology [40].

Bacteria genera (species)	Anopheles									Total Anopheles species
	albimanus	arabiensis	coustani	darlingi	dureni	funestus	gambiae	maculipennis	stephensi	
Achromobacter (A. xylosoxidans)						[31]			[5, 34]	2
Acidovorax (A. temperans)		[12]								1
Acinetobacter sp. (A. hemolyticus, A. radioresistens)						[24]			[34]	2
Aeromonas sp. (A. hydrophila)			[24]*	[35]		[24]	[12, 24]		[5]	5
Anaplasma (A. ovis)		[12]								1
Asaia spp. (A. bogorensis, A. siamensis)		[24]				[24]	[9, 24]	[9]		4
Bacillus spp. (B. cereus, B. coagulans, B. megaterium, B. mucoides, B. silvestris, B. simplex, B. thuringensis)		[12]				[31]	[31]		[34]	4
Bordetella									[5]	1
Brevundiumonas (B. diminuta)						[31]				1
Cedecea (C. davisae)						[31]	[31]			2
Chryseobacterium (C. indologenes)		[24]				[24]	[24]		[34]	4
Citrobacter (C. freundii)									[34]	1
Enterobacter spp. (E. amnigenus, E. cloacae, E. sakazaki)	[17]								[34]	2
Ehrlichia		[12]								1
Erwinia (E. ananas, E. chrysanthenum)						[31]	[31]			2
Escherichia (E. coli, E. senegalensis)		[12]				[31]				2
Elizabethkingia (E. anophelis, E. meningoseptica)							[11, 28]			1
Flavobacterium (F. resinovorum)						[31]				1
Gluconobacter (G. cerinus)						[31]				1
Janibacter (J. anophelis, J. limosus)		[12, 27]								1
Klebsiella spp. (K. pneumoniae)				[33]		[31]	[31]		[32]	4
Kluyvera (K. cryocrescens)						[31]				1
Leuconostoc (L. citreum)									[34]	1
Leminorella (L. grimontii)									[34]	1
Morganella (M. morgani)							[31]			1
Mycoplasma (M. wenyonii)		[12]								1
Myroides									[5]	1
Nocardia (N. corynebacterioides)		[12]								1
Paenibacillus sp.		[12]								1
Pantoea (P. agglomerans, P. stewartii)				[35]		[31]	[11, 31]		[7]	4

Bacteria genera (species)	Anopheles									Total Anopheles species
	albimanus	arabiensis	coustani	darlingi	dureni	funestus	gambiae	maculipennis	stephensi	
Pseudomonas spp. (P. aeruginosa, P. mendosina, P. pseudoflava, P. putida, P. stutzeri, P. synxantha, P. testosteroni)				[35]	[33]	[29, 31]	[12, 31]		[5, 34]	5
Salmonella spp. (S. choleraesuis, S. enteritidis)						[31]	[31]			2
Serratia (S. marcescens, S. nematodiphila, S. odorifera, S. proteamaculans)	[17]	[12]						[32, 34]		3
Sphingobacterium (S. multivorum)							[11]			1
Spiroplasma sp.					[12]					1
Stenotrophomonas (S. maltophilia)		[12]				[31]	[11, 12]			3
Thorsellia (T. anophelis)		[26, 29]								1
Vibrio (V. metschnikovii)		[12]								1
Xenorhabdus (X. nematophila)									[34]	1
Zymobacter							[24]			1

°, An. gambiae s.l. or s.s.; *, For Osei-Poku et al (2012) [24], genera with low frequency were not considered in this table.

Table 1. Bacterial genera isolated from the midgut of wild-caught adults of 9 Anopheles species linked to the associated reference numbers.

The complete 16S rRNA gene (1500 bp) gives the accurate affiliation to a species in most cases. In metagenomics, the amplified fragments are shorter, ranging from 200 to 400 bp, but contain nine hypervariable regions (V1-V9) [41], which compensate the lack of information due to the small sequence size by a high rate of mutation. In most studies, the V3 region located in the 5' part of the gene is chosen [42]. However, the phylogenetic information is sometimes insufficient to achieve species identification. Depending on the bacterium, sequences provide identification to the genus or family level only. Consequently, the diversity of the community is not described by a list of bacterial species but by a list of operational taxonomic units (OTUs) corresponding to the lower taxonomic level being accurately identified. The 16S rRNA gene, in spite of some recognized pitfalls [43], remains today the most popular marker for studying the specific diversity in a bacterial community. Alternative markers can also be proposed such as rpoB [40] but universal rpoB PCR primers allowing the exploration of the whole bacterial diversity cannot be designed (Jumas-Bilak E, personal data) and the databases remain poor in rpo sequences.

Molecular approaches for assessing biodiversity avoid the bias of cultivability but displayed several pitfalls that should be evaluated and considered for a sound interpretation of the data. Particularly, DNA should be recovered and amplified from all the genotypes in the community, i.e. extraction and PCR should be as universal as possible. Special attention should be given to Firmicutes and Actinobacteria because they display thick and resistant cell wall. The extraction efficiency should be tested on a wide panel of bacteria to scan a large range of bacterial types. Extraction is generally improved by the use of large-spectrum lytic enzymes and/or by a mechanical grinding [44, 45]. The PCR itself is another cause of limitations in the molecular approaches. It often praises for its detection sensitivity but this sensitivity can fail when complex samples are analyzed. For example, detection thresholds of 10^3-10^4 CFU (colony forming units)/mL are currently described for universal PCR and migration in denaturing gels [44-46]. The detection limit cannot be easily assessed as it depends on both CFU/g count of each OTU and the relative representation of OTUs in the community. Minor populations of less than 1% of total population are generally undetectable for denaturing-gel-based methods used in microbial ecology [45, 47, 48].

In biodiversity studies, the different 16S rRNA genes representative of the community are amplified by PCR and then separated and identified either by cloning and Sanger sequencing or by direct pyro-sequencing [38]. Tools for sequence-specific separation after bulk PCR amplification, such as T-RFLP (Terminal-Restriction Fragment Length Polymorphism) [49], D-HPLC (Denaturing High Performance Liquid Chromatography) [50], CDCE (Constant Denaturing Capillary Electrophoresis) [51], SSCP (Single Stranded Conformation Polymorphism) [52], DGGE (Denaturing Gradient Gel Electrophoresis) [53], TGGE (Temperature Gradient Gel Electrophoresis), [48] and TTGE (Temporal Temperature Gradient Gel Electrophoresis) [47], can also be used. Methods based upon separation in denaturing electrophoresis allow the comparison of microbiotae with low or medium diversity [54]. They easily provide a "fingerprint" of the community diversity and therefore they are suitable for the follow-up of large collection of samples.

PCR-TTGE is a PCR-denaturing gradient gel electrophoresis that allows separation of DNA fragments in a temporal gradient of temperature [47, 55]. PCR amplicons of the same size but with different sequences are separated in the gel. In a denaturing acrylamide gel, DNA denatures in discrete regions called melting domains, each of them displaying a sequence specific melting temperature. When the melting temperature (Tm) of the whole amplicon is reached, the DNA is denatured creating branched molecules. This branching reduces DNA mobility in the gel. Therefore, amplicons of the same size but with different nucleotide compositions can be separated based on differences in the behavior of their melting domains. When DNA is extracted and amplified from a complex community, TTGE leads to the separation of the different amplicons and produces a banding pattern characteristic of the community. Counting bands on the TTGE profile provides a diversity score that roughly corresponds to the number of molecular species in the sample. The banding profile can be further analyzed by measuring distance migration of bands and comparing with patterns from known species. This comparison allows the affiliation of band to some representative species. Affiliation of all bands can be achieved by cutting bands from the gel, extracting DNA from bands and sequencing. A method associating migration distances measurement and sequencing of selected bands has shown its efficiency in describing bacterial communities of low complexity such as the gut microbiota of neonates [45]. Such an approach is simple enough and cost-effective to survey bacterial communities on a wide range of samples [56].

This chapter presents the bacterial biodiversity in the midguts of malaria vectors from Thailand and Vietnam based on the amplification of the V3 region of the 16S rRNA gene, separation of amplicon by TTGE and sequencing. The bacterial biodiversity among specimens and species in relation to the collection site are discussed.

2. Material and methods

2.1. Mosquito collections and species identification

In Thailand, populations of *Anopheles* mosquitoes were collected from three different sites located in malaria endemic area along the Thai-Myanmar border (Figure 1). One study site is in Pu Teuy, a village located in Sai Yok District, Kanchanaburi Province, western Thailand (14° 17′N, 99° 01′E). The rural site is located in mountainous terrain mostly surrounded by forest. The main water body near the collection site is a narrow, slow running stream, bordered with native vegetation [57]. This stream represents the main larval habitat for *An. minimus* s.l. [58]. A total of 1,330 malaria cases were reported in 2011 in the Sai Yok District with a prevalence of 389 cases of *P. falciparum* (44.7%) and 481 cases of *P. vivax* (55.3%) with a mortality rate per 100,000 inhabitants of 0.71 [59]. The second site located in Mae Sod District, Tak Province, is in the northern part of Thailand (16° 67′N, 98° 68′E). This is a forested area associated to agricultural fields and small streams. In 2011, 1,876 malaria cases were reported in this district with 187 cases of *P. falciparum* (28.3%) and 473 cases of *P. vivax* (71.7%). The mortality rate per 100,000 was of 0.56 [59]. The third site in Sop Moei District is the most southern district of Mae Hong Son Province (17° 86′N, 97° 96′E). This mountainous province is located north of Tak Province with a high malaria transmission occurring from June to August, during the rainy season [60]. In 2011, 1,643 malaria cases were found in this district due to *P. falciparum* with 419 cases (45.0%) and *P. vivax* with 511 cases (55.0%) and a mortality rate per 100,000 of 0.41 [59].

The specimens from Vietnam were collected from six sites located in Dak Ngo Commune, Tuy Duc District, Dak Nong Province (11°59′N, 107°42′E - central Highlands) where 848 malaria cases were reported in 2011, of which, 322 cases (54.9%) were caused by *P. falciparum*, 209 cases (35.6%) by *P. vivax* and 56 cases (9.5%) were mixed infections [61]. This province was named in 2004 after integrating parts from northern area of Binh Phuoc Province and southern area of Dak Lak Province. The average temperature in this province is around 24° C with the rainy season ranging from May to October and the dry season from November to April. The climate is favorable for agriculture, especially coffee, pepper and rubber plantations. Crops of coffee, pepper or cashew nuts were normally cultivated around houses. Villages were surrounded by cassava, corn and rice fields and located in the fringe forest. Every year, during harvest period, workers from neighbourhood come to work in the field, which generate high population movements in this area.

Anopheles mosquitoes were morphologically sorted by taxon before using specific AS-PCR assays for species identification within the complex or the group [20-22]. Each individual was split in two pieces, head-thorax for species identification and abdomen for midgut bacteria analysis.

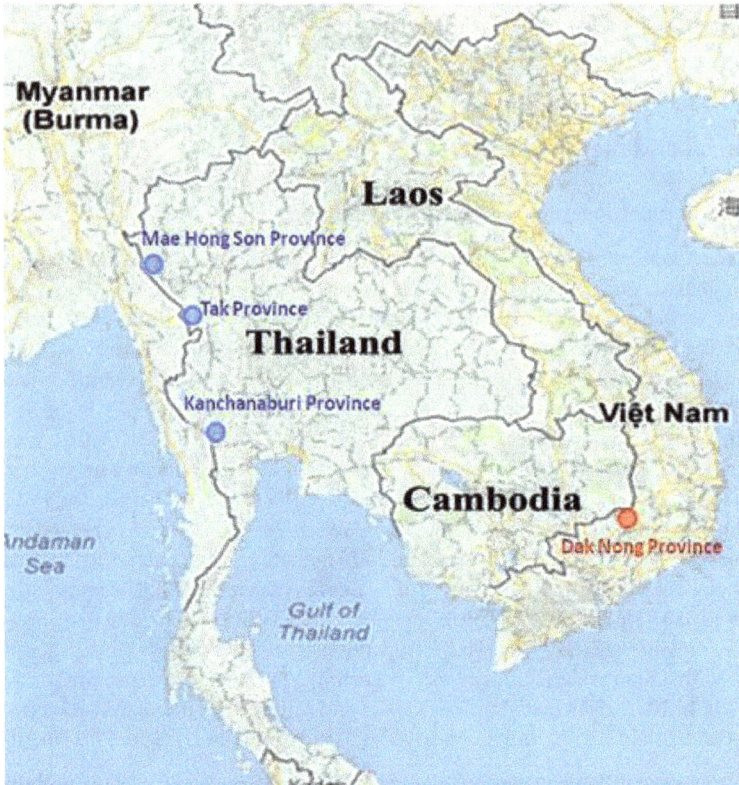

Figure 1. Map of Southeast Asia showing the locations of three provinces in Thailand (blue dots) and the province in Vietnam (red dot) where the mosquito collections were implemented.

2.2. DNA extraction

Mosquitoes stored at -20°C were surface rinsed twice in purified water prepared for injectable solution, and abdomen was thoroughly disrupted using a tissue crusher device in 150 µl of TE buffer. DNA was extracted using the Master Pure Gram Positive DNA purification kit as recommended by the supplier (Epicentre Biotechnologics, Madison, USA).

2.3. PCR

The V2–V3 region of the 16S rRNA gene of bacteria in the samples was amplified using the primers HDA1/HDA2 [45]; HDA1: 5′-ACTC CTA CGG GAG GCA GCA GT-3′, HDA2: 5′-GTA TTA CCG CGG CTG CTG GCA-3′. A 40-bp clamp, named GC (5′-CGC CCG GGG CGC GCC

CCG GGC GGG GCG GGG GCA CGG GGG G-3′) flanked the 5′ extremity of HDA1 [47] in order to form HDA1-GC. PCR was performed using an Eppendorf thermal cycler® (Eppendorf, Le Pecq, France) and 0.5 ml tubes. The reaction mixture (50 µl) contained 2.5 units of Taq DNA Polymerase (FastStart High fidelity PCR system, Roche, Meylan, France), 0.2 mM of each primer and 1 µl of DNA in the appropriate reaction buffer. Amplification was 95°C for 2 min, 35 cycles of 95°C for 1 min, 62°C for 30 s, 72°C for 1 min and 7 min at 72°C for final extension. To avoid contamination, solutions were prepared with sterile DNA-free water and preparation of the mastermix, addition of template DNA and gel electrophoresis of PCR products were carried out in separate rooms. PCR amplification was checked by DNA electrophoresis in 1.5% agarose gels containing ethidium bromide and visualized under ultraviolet light.

2.4. TTGE migration

TTGE was performed using the DCode universal mutation detection system (Bio-Rad Laboratories, Marne-la-Coquette, France) in gels that were 16 cm × 16 cm by 1 mm. The gels (40 ml) were composed of 8% (wt/vol) bisacrylamide (37.5:1), 7 M urea, 40 µl of N,N,N′,N′-tetramethylethylenediamine (TEMED), and 40 mg ammonium persulfate (APS). Gels were run with 1X Tris–acetate–EDTA buffer at pH 8.4. The 5 µl of DNA was loaded on gel with 5 µl of in-house dye marker (saccharose 50%, Bromophenol Blue 0.1%) using capillary tips. Denaturing electrophoresis was performed at 46 V with a temperature ramp from 63°C to 70°C during 16 h (0.4°C/h) after a pre-migration of 15 min at 20 V and 63°C. Gels were stained with ethidium bromide solution (5 µg/ml) for 20 minutes, washed with de-ionized water, viewed using a UV transillumination system (Vilbert-Lourmat, France) and photographed.

2.5. TTGE band sequencing and OTU affiliation

TTGE bands were excised and the DNA was eluted with 50 µl of elution buffer (EB) of the Qiaquick PCR purification kit (Qiagen, Courtabeuf, France) overnight at 37°C before PCR amplification with HDA1/HDA2 used without GC clamp. The reaction conditions were identical to those described above. PCR products were sequenced on an ABI 3730xl sequencer (Cogenics, Meylan, France). Each sequencing chromatograph was visually inspected and corrected. The sequences were analyzed by comparison with Genbank (http://www.ncbi.nlm.nih.gov/) and RDPII databases (http://rdp.cme.msu.edu/) using Basic Local Alignment Search Tool (BLAST) and Seqmatch programs, respectively. The reference sequence with the highest percentage was used for OTU affiliation. A sequence was affiliated to a species-level OTU when the percent of sequence similarity was above 99.0%, as previously proposed [62]. This value is over the recognized cut-off value for the delineation of species [63], but warrants high stringency for species-level OTU affiliation. Below 99.0%, the sequence is affiliated to the genus of the reference sequence with the highest percentage. When several species reference sequences match equally, affiliation was done to the genus level. For example, sequence with 99.5% in similarity to the species *Aeromonas caviae* and *Aeromonas hydrophila* was only assigned to the genus *Aeromonas*. Low cut-off is not defined for the genus delineation since affiliation to a higher taxonomic rank such as family or order will be done considering the taxonomic frame of the clade using Greengenes database [64]. On each TTGE gel, about

50% of the bands were sequenced, the others being affiliated to an OTU by comparison of their migration distance with that of sequenced bands.

2.6. Phylogeny

The sequences for phylogenetic analysis were selected in the GenBank database using BLAST program and taxonomy browser (http://www.ncbi.nlm.nih.gov). The sequences were then quality checked using SEQMATCH program in the 16S rDNA-specialized database, RDPII (http://rdp.cme.msu.edu). Sequences were aligned using the ClustalX program [65], and the alignment was manually corrected to exclude gaps and ambiguously aligned regions. Maximum-likelihood (ML) phylogenetic analysis was performed using PhyML v2.4.6 [66], the model being General Time Reversible plus gamma distribution plus invariable site. ML bootstrap support was computed on 100 reiterations using PhyML.

3. Results

3.1. *Anopheles* species

Among the 175 specimens of *Anopheles* collected in Thailand and Vietnam, a total of 10 species were identified including six species per country of which two, *An. maculatus* and *An. dirus*, were common to both countries (Table 2). Eight species out of 10 belong to a group or a complex of which the sibling species were identified using the appropriate PCR assay (see Material and Methods). The Maculatus Group was represented by two species, *An. maculatus* and *An. sawadwongporni*, the latter collected in Thailand only. Within the Dirus Complex, three species were identified, *An. dirus*, *An. baimaii* and *An. scanloni*, the latter two were also collected in Thailand, as well as two species of the Minimus Complex, *An. minimus* and *An. harrisoni*. Three additional species were collected in Vietnam, *An. gigas* belonging to the Gigas Complex, *An. barbumbrosus*, and *An. crawfordi*. Among the 10 collected species, the former seven species of the Maculatus Group, Dirus and Minimus Complexes are defined as important malaria vectors and the latter three species have not been reported as being involved in malaria transmission [19, 67].

3.2. PCR-TTGE profiles and diversity index in midgut bacterial communities of *Anopheles*

The midgut microbiota of 175 specimens of *Anopheles* mosquitoes was investigated by 16S rRNA gene PCR-TTGE anchored in the V3 hypervariable region. A representative gel is given in Figure 2. TTGE profiles were obtained for 144 samples, 31 samples (17.7%) giving no amplification in PCR or a faint PCR signals leading to non-detectable TTGE profiles. Negative results suggested a low bacterial inoculum rather than a total absence of bacteria in the corresponding samples. Most negative samples came from Vietnam mosquitoes (n=26), compared to Thailand (n=5), and seemed to be unrelated to the *Anopheles* species. Finally, V3 16S PCR-TTGE approach led to the description of a microbial community for about 80% of the specimens analyzed and therefore appeared as an efficient tool to investigate midgut bacterial diversity in a large population of mosquitoes.

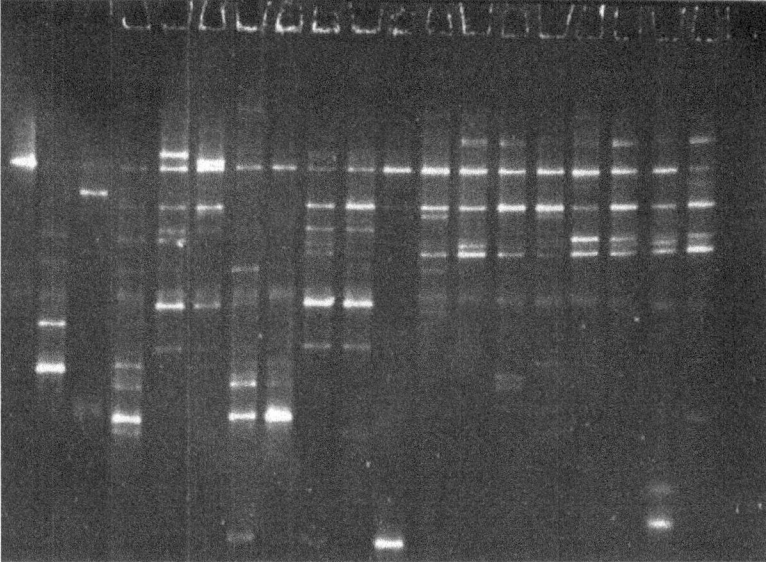

Figure 2. Representative TTGE analysis of V3 16S rRNA gene PCR products amplified from midgut samples of *Anopheles* mosquitoes from Thailand. Each lane corresponded to a specimen microbiota.

A raw diversity index that globally reflects the bacterial diversity in a sample is classically evaluated by counting the bands in TTGE profiles. At a first glance, the number of bands on TTGE profiles (Figure 2) ranged from 1 to 10 suggesting that the bacterial diversity per specimen ranged from 1 to 10 OTUs. However, sequencing showed that bands with different distance of migration could belong to the same OTU. This atypical phenomenon was observed for bacteria displaying sequence heterogeneity among their 16S rRNA gene copies. For instance, members of the genus *Acinetobacter* as well as most members of the genera affiliated to the family *Enterobacteriaceae* displayed a high level of 16S rRNA gene heterogeneity leading to complex banding patterns in V3 16S PCR-TTGE. Considering that *Acinetobacter* and *Enterobacteriaceae* were prevalent in our samples, the raw diversity index drastically overestimated the bacterial diversity. Therefore, a refined diversity index was calculated after affiliation of each band to an OTU by sequencing or by comparative approach (see Material and Methods).

The refined diversity index showed a low bacterial diversity per specimen with an average of 1.5 OTU per specimen. Most positive samples displayed a diversity index of 1 or 2 (Figure 3). Five OTUs is the maximal biodiversity per specimen observed in our population of *Anopheles* mosquitoes. Figure 3 showed that the number of OTUs per specimen differed slightly between populations from different origin, with an average of 1.7 and 1.3 OTU per specimen in Thailand and Vietnam, respectively. Considering mosquito species, the average diversity varied between 0 for *An. sawadwongporni* and 3 for *An. harrisoni* (Table 2).

	COUNTRY		VECTORS									NON VECTORS		
			Maculatus			Minimus		Dirus						
	Thailand (n=75)	Vietnam (n=100)	An. maculatus (n=28)	An. maculatus (n=11)	An. sawadwongporni (n=1)	An. minimus (n=37)	An. harrisoni (n=13)	An. baimaii (n=4)	An. scanloni (n=3)	An. dirus (n=6)	An. dirus (n=23)	An. gigas (n=24)	An. barbumbrosus (n=13)	An. crawfordi (n=12)
Acinetobacter			14			10	10	1	1		11	18	3	5
Aeromonas						8								
Asaia			2				4							
Bacillus			1					1						1
Cellvibrio*											1			
Chromobacterium*						1								
Chryseobacterium							1	1					1	
Citrobacter						1								
Corynebacterium*														1
Cronobacter*						5								
Diaphorobacter*						1								
Diplorickettsia*											1	1		
Elizabethkingia						4				1				
Enhydrobacter*													1	
Enterobacter				1		11		1		1	2			
Escherichia						1								
Gluconacetobacter*							2							
Kluyvera							3							
Microbacterium*													1	
Moraxella*			1								1			2
Nitrincola*												3		
Pantoea						1								
Pseudomonas				8		1	8		1	1				2
Psychrobacter*												1		
Raoultella*						2	9				2			
Riemerella*													1	
Serratia				8		6			1	2				3
Shewanella*							1							
Sphingomonas*			20								16	8	1	1
Staphylococcus*												1	1	
Stenotrophomonas											2			
Diversity Index	1.7	1.3	1.3	1.8	0	1.5	3	0.6	1.3	1.2	1.7	1.4	0.6	0.3

Table 2. Bacterial genera detected in midgut of *Anopheles* species caught in Thailand (blue) and Vietnam (red) with the number of specimens carrying each genus. Diversity index links to *Anopheles* species and origin is given at the bottom of the table. Genera described for the first time in *Anopheles* are marked with asterisk. Vertical lines delineated, from left to right, both countries with their respective number of *Anopheles* specimens, and groupings of *Anopheles* species, such as the Maculatus Group, the Minimus and Dirus Complexes, and the non-vector species including the Gigas Complex and 2 additional species.

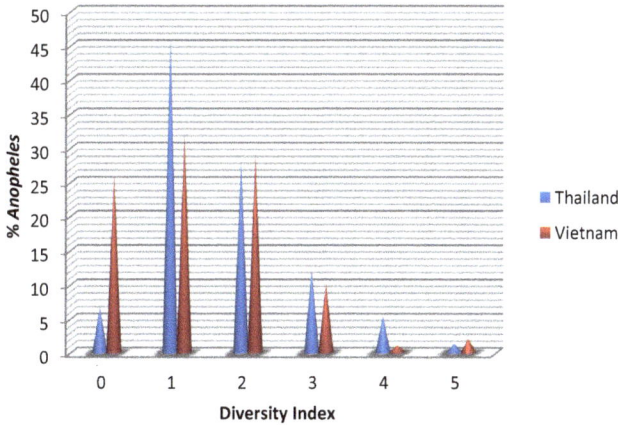

Figure 3. Distribution of the *Anopheles* mosquito populations from Thailand and Vietnam according to their refined diversity index

3.3. Bacterial diversity in the whole population of *Anopheles* mosquitoes

16S rRNA gene PCR-TTGE is focused on hypervariable region V3 produced sequences of about 200 bp, which are generally not informative enough for species affiliation. Consequently, we presented here the bacterial diversity to the genus level. However, probable species affiliation will be proposed for several genera when the phylogenetic signal of the V3 region was significant.

Contrasting with the low diversity per specimen, OTU diversity in the whole population was high with the detection of 31 different bacterial genera (Table 2) distributed in four phyla, *Proteobacteria, Bacteroidetes/Chlorobi, Firmicutes* and *Actinobacteria. Proteobacteria* largely dominated the midgut microbiota of *Anopheles* mosquitoes with 232 OTUs in the population studied. Their diversity encompassed *Alpha, Beta-* and *Gamma* superclasses of *Proteobacteria*.

The gamma-proteobacterial genera *Acinetobacter, Pseudomonas, Enterobacter, Serratia* and *Raoultella* were widely detected in our populations. A total of 40% of specimens and 70% of *Anopheles* species were colonized by members of the genus *Acinetobacter*, which therefore could be considered as a 'core genus' of the midgut microbiota of *Anopheles*. The sequences affiliated to the genus *Acinetobacter* were identified to the species level by a phylogenetic approach (Figure 4). The *Anopheles* midgut microbiota included 6 main species, *Acinetobacter baumannii, Acinetobacter calcoaceticus, Acinetobacter johnsonii, Acinetobacter soli, Acinetobacter guillouiae* and *Acinetobacter junii*, the two latter being more represented. The genus *Acinetobacter* belongs to the order *Pseudomonadales* in gamma-proteobacteria together with *Pseudomonas* (*Pseudomonas fluorescens* and *Pseudomonas alcaligenes*), *Moraxella, Enhydrobacter, Psychrobacter* and *Cellvibrio. Enterobacteriales* was the second main order of gamma-proteobacteria represented in the midgut microbiota of *Anopheles*. In enterobacteria, the species affiliation could not be achieved since genera are very close together in 16S rRNA gene phylogeny, particularly for *Enterobacter* and its relatives *Cronobacter* and *Pantoea*. Members of gamma-proteobacteria of the orders *Legionellales* (*Diplorickettsia*), *Oceanospirillales* (*Nitrincola*), *Alteromonadales* (*Shewanella*), *Xanthomonadales* (*Stenotrophomonas*) and *Aeromonadales* (*Aeromonas*) were also detected showing the very wide diversity of gamma-proteobacteria in the midgut microbiota of *Anopheles*.

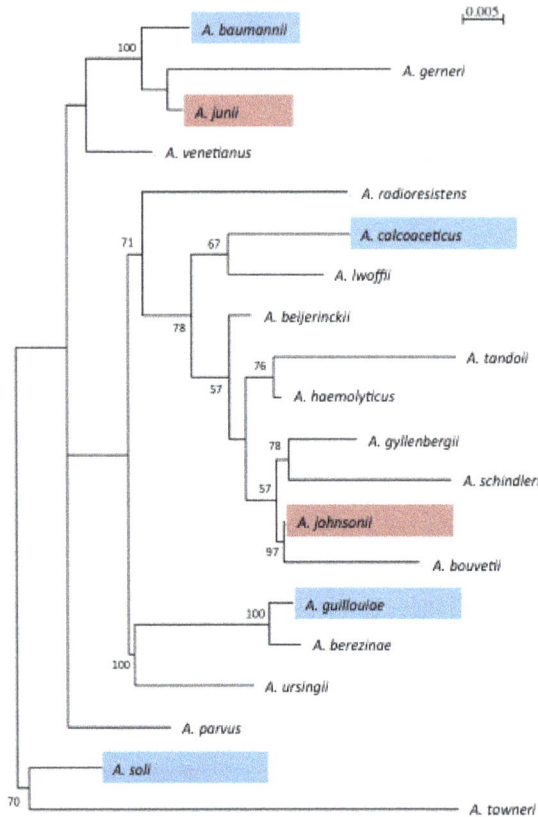

Figure 4. Maximum Likelihood phylogenetic tree of the genus *Acinetobacter*. Lineages of strains detected in the microbiota of *Anopheles* mosquitoes are in color, blue for Thailand, red for Vietnam. Bootstrap percentages (>50 %) after 100 resamplings are shown. Bar: 0.5 % sequence divergence.

The diversity was lower in alpha- and beta-proteobacteria. However, the genus *Sphingomonas* that belonged to *Alphaproteobacteria*, was the second main genus detected in this study (26% of the *Anopheles* species colonized) mostly represented by sequences affiliated or related to the species *Sphingomonas aromaticivorans* and *Sphingomonas glacialis*. Acetic-acid bacteria (*Asaia* and *Gluconacetobacter*) belonged to *Alphaproteobacteria* and were sporadically represented as well as *Chromobacterium* and *Diaphorobacter*, the two members of *Betaproteobacteria*.

Beside *Proteobacteria*, the phyla *Bacteroidetes/Chlorobi*, *Actinobacteria* and *Firmicutes* were represented by only few genera: 15, 9 and 5 respectively. *Chryseobacterium, Elizabethkingia* and *Riemerella*, which colonized only 8 mosquitoes, belonged to *Bacteroidetes/Chlorobi* and class *Flavobacteriia*. Sequences affiliated to the genus *Elizabethkingia* could not be related with certainty to *Elizabethkingia anophelis*, because the V3 region did not discriminate between this *Anopheles*-specific species and the human pathogen *Elizabethkingia meningoseptica*. *Bacillus* and *Staphylococcus* (*Firmicutes*), *Corynebacterium* and *Microbacterium* (*Actinobacteria*) were the sole Gram-positive genera found in the population of *Anopheles* mosquitoes. The most related species were *Bacillus cereus, Corynebacterium freiburgense* and *Microbacterium trichothecenolyticum*. The *Staphylococcus* sequences found in two mosquitoes were identical to those of a strain isolated in the midgut of the ladybug *Harmonia axyridis* and were linked to the species *Staphylococcus sciuri*.

3.4. Bacterial associations and relationship

Acinetobacter spp. was present in all mosquito specimens except in *An. maculatus* and *An. dirus* from Thailand. Specimens of these two *Anopheles* species were mainly colonized by *Pseudomonas* and *Serratia* (Table 2). When the microbiota of each specimen is considered (data not shown), the pair *Pseudomonas / Serratia* never co-habited with *Acinetobacter* in the same midgut. *Pseudomonas* strains associated with *Serratia* were related to the species *P. fluorescens* whereas *P. alcaligenes* was never associated with *Serratia* and inhabited midguts colonized with *Acinetobacter*. These results suggested that the association *P. fluorescens / Serratia* might specifically inhibit the colonization of *Anopheles* midgut by *Acinetobacter*.

Negative relationships between *Sphingomonas* and enterobacteria were also suggested in Table 2 for mosquitoes from Vietnam. Considering each specimen, we always observed the absence of enterobacteria when *Sphingomonas* colonized the midgut (data not shown).

3.5. Comparison of bacterial diversity in the midgut of *Anopheles* from Thailand and Vietnam

Table 2 and Figure 5 showed the differential distribution of bacterial genera according to the geographic origin of mosquitoes. Eight genera were shared between specimens from Thailand and Vietnam and corresponded to genera with high prevalence such as *Enterobacter, Serratia, Pseudomonas* and *Acinetobacter*. In Thailand, each of these four genera colonized more than 10% of specimens, each of the genera *Raoultella, Cronobacter, Aeromonas, Elizabethkingia* and *Asaia* colonized 3 to 10% of the specimens, and 10 other genera colonized 2% or less of the specimens (Figure 5A).

Except for the core genus *Acinetobacter*, main genera found in Thailand were not prevalent in specimens from Vietnam, *Enterobacter, Serratia, Pseudomonas, Raoultella*, and *Asaia* colonizing each 2% or less of the Vietnam specimens (Figure 5B). *Cronobacter, Aeromonas* and *Elizabethkingia* were not detected in *Anopheles* mosquitoes from Vietnam. Except for the genus *Acinetobacter* again (40%), the more prevalent genera in specimens from Vietnam appeared origin-specific. Indeed, *Sphingomonas* and *Moraxella* present in *Anopheles* from Vietnam at 36% and 3% respectively, were not detected in mosquitoes from Thailand (Figure 5B). When the species forming the genus *Acinetobacter* were considered, we observed again an origin-specific distribution with *A. junii* and *A. johnsonii* dominating the microbiota of mosquitoes from Vietnam but absent from the Thailand samples. Gut microbiota of mosquitoes from Thailand displayed a wider *Acinetobacter* diversity with four species represented, *A. baumannii*, *A. calcoaceticus*, *A. soli* and *A. guillouiae* (Figure 4). In the same phylogenetic clade of *Acinetobacter*, bacterial lineages from Thailand mosquitoes differed from bacterial lineages of Vietnam mosquitoes. For instance, the lineages *A. baumannii* and *A. junii* belonged to the same clade in the 16S rRNA gene tree but inside this clade, each lineage was origin-specific (Figure 4).

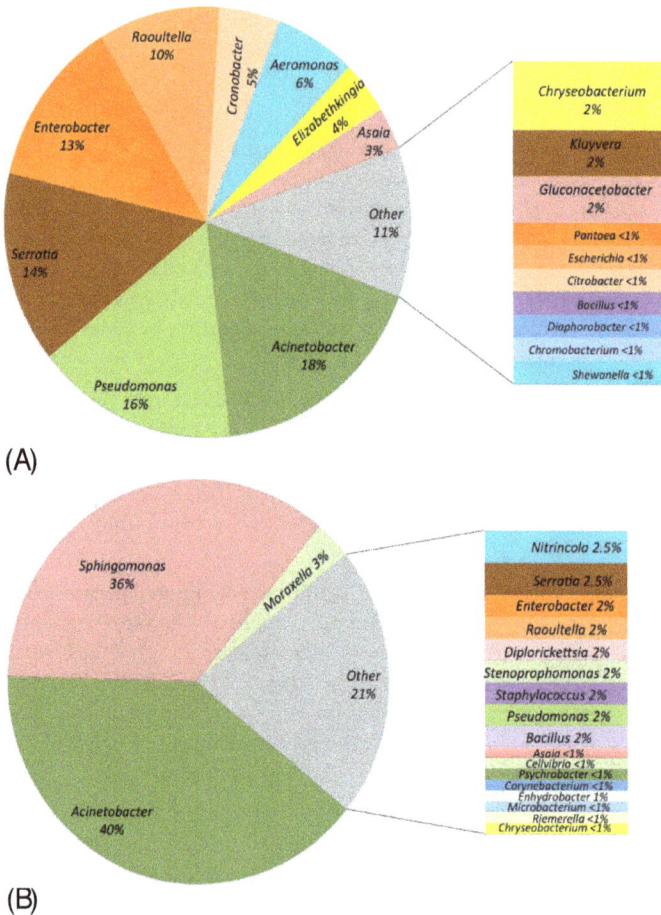

Figure 5. Repartition in genera of OTU assigned bands obtained by PCR-TTGE from 175 specimens of *Anopheles* mosquitoes from Thailand (A) and from Vietnam (B).

Considering bacterial taxa higher than the genus, the microbiotae of *Anopheles* from Thailand and Vietnam were both dominated by *Pseudomonadales* (Figure 6) due to the general high prevalence of *Acinetobacter*. *Enterobacteriaceae* largely dominated the microbiota of *Anopheles* from Thailand but contributed little to bacterial diversity in *Anopheles* from Vietnam.

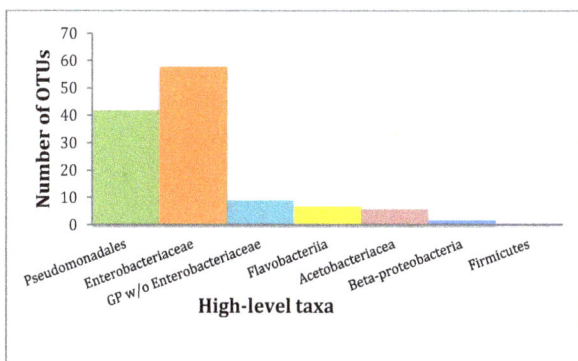

(A)

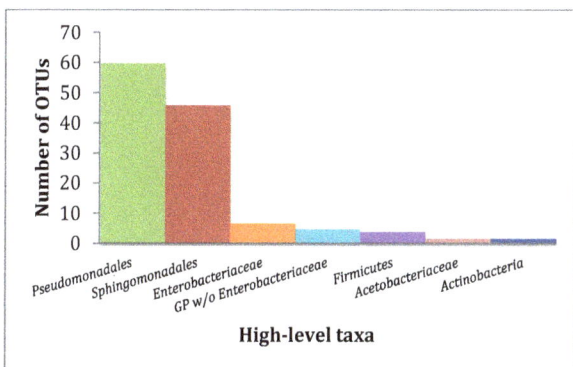

(B)

Figure 6. Repartition in significative high-level bacterial taxa of OTU from 175 specimens of *Anopheles* mosquitoes from Thailand (A) and from Vietnam (B). GP for *Gammaproteobacteria*.

This low prevalence of enterobacteria in the midgut of *Anopheles* from Vietnam was particularly noteworthy (Fig. 6B). In opposite, *Sphingomonadales* was the major high-level taxon in Vietnam specimens but absent from Thailand specimens. Therefore, the ratio *Enterobacteriaceae / Sphingomonadales* appeared as a signature differentiating Thailand and Vietnam *Anopheles* specimens. Other signatures, which should be confirmed with more specimens, were *Betaproteobacteria* and *Actinobacteria* in specimens from Thailand and Vietnam, respectively.

3.6. Links between microbiota composition and *Anopheles* species or species complexes

Table 2 showed the distribution of bacterial genera according to the species of *Anopheles*. To evaluate the link between bacteria and host species, we first compared the microbiotae of the same mosquito species but from different origins. Specimens of *An. maculatus* gave a good model for this comparison because it was enough represented in both geographic sites (Figure 7). The two groups of microbiotae differed clearly, in particular considering the origin-specific signature, i.e. the ratio *Enterobacteriaceae / Sphingomonadales* (Figure 7). Therefore, the case of *An. maculatus* indicated that the microbiota composition was influenced by sampling geographic sites rather than *Anopheles* species. Comparison of the microbiotae between *An. dirus* from Thailand and Vietnam resulted in the same conclusion (Table 2).

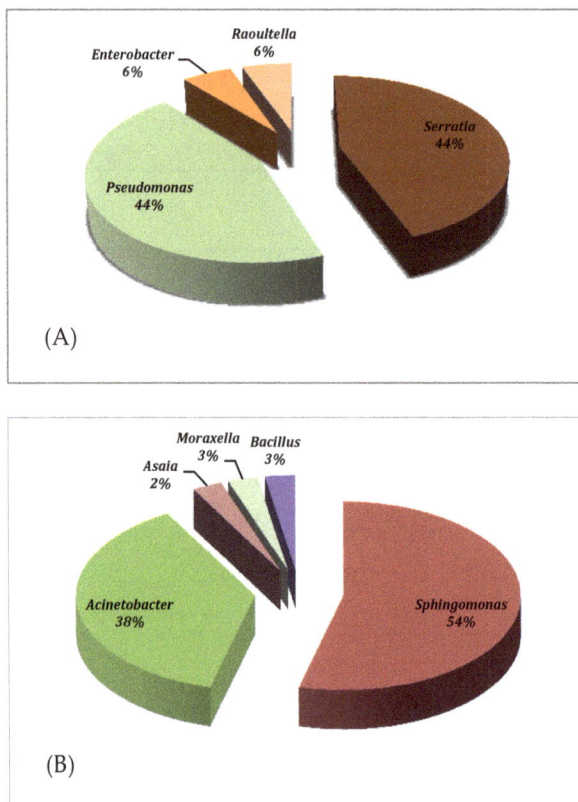

Figure 7. Comparison of the microbiota of *An. maculatus* caught in Thailand (n=11) (A) and in Vietnam (n=28) (B).

Sibling species within a group or a complex have been linked to the microbial content of the midgut. As previously observed for the species *An. maculatus*, the corresponding complex displayed a non-specific microbiota but its bacterial colonization is influenced by the geographic origin. Similar situation was observed in the Dirus Complex for which the shared bacterial genera were *Acinetobacter* and *Enterobacter*, as well as for *An. gigas* of the Gigas Complex with shared bacteria belonging to the dominating genera *Acinetobacter* and *Enterobacter*.

In the Minimus Complex, *An. minimus* and *An. harrisoni* were colonized by 18 different bacterial genera but only three were shared by both species. Two shared genera corresponded to bacteria widely represented in the whole population, *Acinetobacter* and *Pseudomonas*, while the third one, *Raoultella*, seemed to be more specific, represented in two and nine specimens of *An. minimus* and *An. harrisoni* respectively, showing its higher association to the latter species.

4. Discussion

To our knowledge, this study describes the midgut microbiotae of the largest population of field-collected *Anopheles* species with 10 species (Table 2) when the literature shows 9 analyzed species, *An. gambiae* being the most studied species of all (Table 1). Thereby, 16S rRNA gene PCR-TTGE focused on hypervariable region V3 proves its efficiency to study microbiota of *Anopheles* mosquitoes. This method, that presents a relative low resolution, is efficient to follow bacterial communities with low to moderate diversities. This limit is due to the number of bands that can be separated within the length of the gel. Optimization of TTGE conditions allows separation of bands by a minimum of 0.1 mm over all the gel length. Therefore, TTGE would be difficult to interpret if the diversity exceeds 25 to 30 OTUs [45]. Microbiotae of *Anopheles* displays TTGE profiles that do not exceed 10 bands but the profiles have been interpreted with difficulties due to heterogeneities in rRNA genes for most bacteria in the mosquito midgut ecosystem. At the genomic level, rRNA genes are generally organized in multigene families [68] in which sequences show low variability within species, subspecies or genome [69]. However, intra-genomic heterogeneity in the form of nucleotide differences between 16S rRNA gene copies are described in relation to fine-tuning of the ribosome function to optimize bacterial niche fitness [70]. In PCR-TTGE, heterogeneities lead to multiple bands for a single OTU and then to an overestimation of OTU diversity. This pitfall has been avoided here by band sequencing that led to the definition of a refined diversity index drastically lowered in comparison with the raw diversity index. The level of ribosomal heterogeneity in bacteria genome from midgut of mosquitoes suggested adaptation processes in a rather instable niche.

With the development of high-output sequencing, twenty-one century metagenomics consider fingerprint approaches as obsolete. However, these methods remain of great interest to give a snapshot of microbiota in large populations of hosts. Thereby, we described herein the midgut microbiotae of 175 specimens of 10 *Anopheles* species with a sequencing effort of less than 150 reads compared to 5 millions of reads estimated for the same study by pyrosequencing. A pyrosequencing study of the midgut microbiota of *An. gambiae* (30 laboratory breed and two field-collected mosquitoes) has been recently published [18]. Authors described bacteria belonging to 26 phyla, among which, five represented more than 99% of the total microbiota: *Proteobacteria, Bacteroidetes, Actinobacteria, Firmicutes,* and *Fusobacteria.* Except the latter, four phyla corresponded to those described in this study, suggesting that PCR-TTGE explored the majority of bacterial populations in the microbiota. Among 147 OTUs detected by pyrosequencing, only 28 genera had an abundance of >1% in at least one mosquito midgut [18]. This is in accordance with our results describing 31 bacterial genera in the microbiota of field-collected *Anopheles.* Fourteen of the 31 genera have been previously detected in diverse studies on field-collected *Anopheles* (Table 1). Then, we would like to highlight the fact that 17 bacterial genera were described herein for the first time (Table 2), 6 (32%) and 12 (60%) from the populations of Thailand and Vietnam respectively, suggesting that the bacterial diversity associated to midgut of *Anopheles* remains underestimated. It is noteworthy that twice as many new genera were found in specimens from Vietnam compared to Thailand. Newly described genera were scarcely represented in few specimens except for *Sphingomonas* found in 46 specimens belonging to five species from Vietnam and *Raoultella* found in 13 specimens belonging to 3 species from Thailand and Vietnam. Of note the genus *Sphingomonas* has been detected by pyrosequencing in the midgut of a population of *An. gambiae* maintained in standard insectary conditions [18].

The gut microbiota of mosquitoes presented a large inter-specimen variability but was dominated by few genera, *Acinetobacter, Pseudomonas, Enterobacter, Serratia, Raoultella* and *Sphingomonas.* Among them, *Acinetobacter* was considered as a mosquito midgut core genus because it was detected in most specimens. *Acinetobacter, Pseudomonas* and *Sphingomonas* also belong to the *An. gambiae* midgut core microbiota defined by Boissière et al. [18]. *Asaia* was found in all samples by pyrosequencing but its relative abundance showed great variations ranging from 0.04 to 98.95% according the *An. gambiae* specimen [18]. We detected *Asaia* in only 6 specimens of *An. maculatus* and *An. harrisoni.* Again, our result compared to pyrosequencing data suggested that PCR-TTGE failed to detect minority and/or low loaded populations. This low resolution is certainly a limit but we also see it as a benefit because the majority taxa detected by TTGE probably corresponds to true colonizers of the midgut and not to transient or contaminant bacteria.

Anopheles-associated bacterial species recently described were not detected or identified with confidence in this study. Members of the genus *Elizabethkingia* detected in *Anopheles* from Thailand could not be identified as *E. anophelis* owing to its relatedness in 16S rRNA gene sequence with *E. meningosepticum.* Of note, *Thorsellia anophelis* has been detected in mosquitoes used in the optimization step of this study but not in mosquitoes included in the study population.

In spite of the large inter-specimen variability, sub-populations from different geographic origins exhibit drastically different midgut microbiotae. High prevalence of *Enterobacteriacea* and absence of *Sphingomonas* spp. characterize microbiotae of *Anopheles* caught in Thailand whereas *Anopheles* in Vietnam displayed high prevalence of *Sphingomonas* and low rate of enterobacteria. Similar differences in enterobacteria prevalence have been described in *An. gambiae* originating from two sampling sites in Cameroon [18]. Composition of the midgut microbiota seems unrelated to *Anopheles* species, except for *Raoultella* and *An. harrisoni* but their relationship needs to be confirmed on additional specimens. Some positive and negative associations of bacteria suggested complex interactions in the microbiota. The most striking result was the pair *P. fluorescens* / *Serratia* which never co-habited with *Acinetobacter*. *Pseudomonas fluorescens* is well known as a great anti-microbial and bacteriocin-like substances producer [71] exhibiting negative effect on diverse Gram-negative bacteria and biofilm formation [72]. The bacteriocins are narrow-spectrum toxins that typically kill bacteria related to the producing strain as is the case for *P. fluorescens* and *Acinetobacter*, which both belong to the order *Pseudomonadales*. Moreover, bacteriocins can play an important role in the fitness of a strain by killing or inhibiting bacterial co-inhabitants that compete for the limited resources probably found in the midgut environment [71]. Similar antagonism was observed between *Sphingomonas* and enterobacteria in mosquitoes from Vietnam. *Sphingomonas* is a sparsely known genus but antimicrobial activities against *Candida* have been described recently [73]. Culture of the natural isolates of *P. fluorescens*, *Serratia*, *Acinetobacter* and *Sphingomonas* should confirm these potential antagonisms and give insights about their mechanism.

Antagonism against enterobacteria is of particular interest because it has been suggested that mosquitoes harboring *Enterobacteriacae* are more likely to be infected by *P. falciparum* [18]. In our collection, *An. minimus* specimen KAN-27 from Pu Teuy, Kanchanaburi was infected by *P. falciparum* and displayed a microbiota containing exclusively enterobacteria that belonged to four genera, *Pantoea, Enterobacter, Cronobacter* and *Escherichia*. This specimen displayed the highest enterobacterial diversity of the *Anopheles* collection and the core genus *Acinetobacter* was not detected. Identification of the *Enterobacter* species in our samples will be the next step with the search for *Enterobacter* (Esp_Z), which was reported to inhibit *P. falciparum* development in *An. gambiae* [15]. As the microbiota might have an impact on pathogen development in *Anopheles* mosquitoes and disease transmission, more studies need to be done for better understanding the role of some specific bacteria in wild mosquito populations before developing potential method of control.

5. Conclusion

Based on the analysis of the midgut microbiota of 10 field-caught *Anopheles* species from Thailand and Vietnam, we described 17 bacterial genera for the first time in *Anopheles* mosquitoes, suggesting that the bacterial diversity associated to midgut of *Anopheles* remains underestimated. Low bacterial diversity ranging from one to three per specimen was found which contrasted with a high OTU diversity in the whole *Anopheles* population that presented 31 different bacterial genera distributed in four phyla, *Proteobacteria, Bacteroidetes/Chlorobi, Firmicutes,* and *Acinetobacteria*. More specifically, the association of *Pseudomonas* and *Serratia* never co-habited with *Acinetobacter* in the same mosquito midgut. The same presence/absence was observed between *Sphingomonas* and enterobacteria. Midgut microbiota was drastically different for the *Anopheles* from Thailand compared to those from Vietnam showing the importance of the geographic origin. The ratio *Enterobacteriaceae* / *Sphingomonadales* appeared as a signature differentiating the *Anopheles* specimens from Thailand and Vietnam.

Acknowledgements

We are thankful to Naritsara Malaithong and Wanapa Ritthison, students of the Department of Entomology (Kasetsart University, Bangkok, Thailand) for their involvement in the optimization step of this study. This study was funded by the French Ministry of Foreign Affairs in the framework of the "Partenariat Hubert Curien" - PHC Thai project 20627SD.

Author details

Sylvie Manguin[1*], Chung Thuy Ngo[1,2], Krajana Tainchum[3], Waraporn Juntarajumnong[3], Theeraphap Chareonviriyaphap[3], Anne-Laure Michon[4] and Estelle Jumas-Bilak[4]

*Address all correspondence to: sylvie.manguin@ird.fr

1 Institut de Recherche pour le Développement (IRD), Faculté de Pharmacie, Montpellier, France

2 National Institute of Veterinary Research, Ha Noi, Viet Nam

3 Department of Entomology, Faculty of Agriculture, Kasetsart University, Bangkok, Thailand

4 University Montpellier, Equipe Pathogènes et Environnements, Faculté de Pharmacie, Montpellier, France

References

[1] Harbach RE. *Anopheles* classification. Mosquito Taxonomic Inventory, http://mosqui-to-taxonomic-inventory.info/, accessed on 8 November 2012.

[2] Manguin S, Bangs MJ, Pothikasikorn J, Chareonviriyaphap T. Review on global co-transmission of human *Plasmodium* species and *Wuchereria bancrofti* by *Anopheles* mosquitoes. Infection, Genetics and Evolution : journal of molecular epidemiology and evolutionary genetics in infectious diseases 2010;10:159-177.

[3] Manguin S, Carnevale P, Mouchet J, Coosemans M, Julvez J, Richard-Lenoble D, et al. Biodiversity of malaria in the world. Paris, France: John Libbey Eurotext; 2008.

[4] Al-Olayan EM, Williams GT, Hurd H. Apoptosis in the malaria protozoan, *Plasmodium berghei*: a possible mechanism for limiting intensity of infection in the mosquito. International Journal for Parasitology 2002;32:1133-1143.

[5]   Chavshin AR, Oshaghi MA, Vatandoost H, Pourmand MR, Raeisi A, Enayati AA, et al. Identification of bacterial microflora in the midgut of the larvae and adult of wild caught *Anopheles stephensi*: a step toward finding suitable paratransgenesis candidates. Acta Tropica 2012;121:129-134.

[6]   Damiani C, Ricci I, Crotti E, Rossi P, Rizzi A, Scuppa P, et al. Mosquito-bacteria symbiosis: the case of *Anopheles gambiae* and *Asaia*. Microbial Ecology 2010;60:644-654.

[7]   Dinparast Djadid N, Jazayeri H, Raz A, Favia G, Ricci I, Zakeri S. Identification of the midgut microbiota of *An. stephensi* and *An. maculipennis* for their application as a paratransgenic tool against malaria. PloS One 2011;6:e28484.

[8]   Dong Y, Das S, Cirimotich C, Souza-Neto JA, McLean KJ, Dimopoulos G. Engineered *Anopheles* immunity to *Plasmodium* infection. PLoS Pathogens 2011;7:e1002458.

[9]   Favia G, Ricci I, Damiani C, Raddadi N, Crotti E, Marzorati M, et al. Bacteria of the genus *Asaia* stably associate with *Anopheles stephensi*, an Asian malarial mosquito vector. Proceedings of the National Academy of Sciences of the United States of America 2007;104:9047-9051.

[10] Favia G, Ricci I, Marzorati M, Negri I, Alma A, Sacchi L, et al. Bacteria of the genus *Asaia*: a potential paratransgenic weapon against malaria. Advances in Experimental Medicine and Biology 2008;627:49-59.

[11] Lindh JM, Borg-Karlson AK, Faye I. Transstadial and horizontal transfer of bacteria within a colony of *Anopheles gambiae* (Diptera: Culicidae) and oviposition response to bacteria-containing water. Acta Tropica 2008;107:242-250.

[12] Lindh JM, Terenius O, Faye I. 16S rRNA gene-based identification of midgut bacteria from field-caught *Anopheles gambiae* sensu lato and *A. funestus* mosquitoes reveals new species related to known insect symbionts. Applied and Environmental Microbiology 2005;71:7217-7223.

[13] Wang S, Ghosh AK, Bongio N, Stebbings KA, Lampe DJ, Jacobs-Lorena M. Fighting malaria with engineered symbiotic bacteria from vector mosquitoes. Proceedings of the National Academy of Sciences of the United States of America 2012;109:12734-12739.

[14] Azambuja P, Garcia ES, Ratcliffe NA. Gut microbiota and parasite transmission by insect vectors. Trends in Parasitology 2005;21:568-572.

[15] Cirimotich CM, Dong Y, Clayton AM, Sandiford SL, Souza-Neto JA, Mulenga M, et al. Natural microbe-mediated refractoriness to *Plasmodium* infection in *Anopheles gambiae*. Science 2011;332:855-858.

[16] Dong Y, Manfredini F, Dimopoulos G. Implication of the mosquito midgut microbiota in the defense against malaria parasites. PLoS Pathogens 2009;5:e1000423.

[17] Gonzalez-Ceron L, Santillan F, Rodriguez MH, Mendez D, Hernandez-Avila JE. Bacteria in midguts of field-collected *Anopheles albimanus* block *Plasmodium vivax* sporogonic development. Journal of Medical Entomology 2003;40:371-374.

[18] Boissiere A, Tchioffo MT, Bachar D, Abate L, Marie A, Nsango SE, et al. Midgut microbiota of the malaria mosquito vector *Anopheles gambiae* and interactions with *Plasmodium falciparum* infection. PLoS Pathogens 2012;8:e1002742.

[19] Manguin S, Garros C, Dusfour I, Harbach RE, Coosemans M. Bionomics, taxonomy, and distribution of the major malaria vector taxa of *Anopheles* subgenus *Cellia* in Southeast Asia: An updated review. Infection, Genetics and Evolution : journal of molecular epidemiology and evolutionary genetics in infectious diseases 2008;8:489-503.

[20] Garros C, Koekemoer LL, Coetzee M, Coosemans M, Manguin S. A single multiplex assay to identify major malaria vectors within the African *Anopheles funestus* and the Oriental *An. minimus* groups. American Journal of Tropical Medicine & Hygiene 2004;70:583-590.

[21] Walton C, Handley JM, Kuvangkadilok C, Collins FH, Harbach RE, Baimai V, et al. Identification of five species of the *Anopheles dirus* complex from Thailand, using allele-specific polymerase chain reaction. Medical and Veterinary Entomology 1999;13:24-32.

[22] Walton, C, Somboon, P, O'Loughlin, S. M, Zhang, S, Harbach, R. E, Linton, Y. M, et al. Genetic diversity and molecular identification of mosquito species in the *Anopheles maculatus* group using the ITS2 region of rDNA. Infection, Genetics and Evolution: journal of molecular epidemiology and evolutionary genetics in infectious diseases (2007); 7, 93-102.

[23] Dillon RJ, Dillon VM. The gut bacteria of insects: nonpathogenic interactions. Annual Review of Entomology 2004;49:71-92.

[24] Osei-Poku J, Mbogo CM, Palmer WJ, Jiggins FM. Deep sequencing reveals extensive variation in the gut microbiota of wild mosquitoes from Kenya. Molecular Ecology 2012;21:5138-5150.

[25] Wang Y, Gilbreath TM, 3rd, Kukutla P, Yan G, Xu J. Dynamic gut microbiome across life history of the malaria mosquito *Anopheles gambiae* in Kenya. PLoS One 2011;6:e24767.

[26] Kampfer P, Lindh JM, Terenius O, Haghdoost S, Falsen E, Busse HJ, et al. *Thorsellia anophelis* gen. nov., sp. nov., a new member of the Gammaproteobacteria. International Journal of Systematic and Evolutionary Microbiology 2006;56:335-338.

[27] Kampfer P, Terenius O, Lindh JM, Faye I. *Janibacter anophelis* sp. nov., isolated from the midgut of *Anopheles arabiensis*. International Journal of Systematic and Evolutionary Microbiology 2006;56:389-392.

[28] Kampfer P, Matthews H, Glaeser SP, Martin K, Lodders N, Faye I. *Elizabethkingia anophelis* sp. nov., isolated from the midgut of the mosquito *Anopheles gambiae*. International Journal of Systematic and Evolutionary Microbiology 2011;61:2670-2675.

[29] Briones AM, Shililu J, Githure J, Novak R, Raskin L. *Thorsellia anophelis* is the dominant bacterium in a Kenyan population of adult *Anopheles gambiae* mosquitoes. The ISME Journal 2008;2:74-82.

[30] Bernardet JF, Vancanneyt M, Matte-Tailliez O, Grisez L, Tailliez P, Bizet C, et al. Polyphasic study of *Chryseobacterium* strains isolated from diseased aquatic animals. Systematic and Applied Microbiology 2005;28:640-660.

[31] Straif SC, Mbogo CN, Toure AM, Walker ED, Kaufman M, Toure YT, et al. Midgut bacteria in *Anopheles gambiae* and *An. funestus* (Diptera: Culicidae) from Kenya and Mali. Journal of Medical Entomology 1998;35:222-226.

[32] Jadin J. [Role of bacteria in the digestive tube of insects, vectors of plasmodidae and trypanosomidae]. Annales des Sociétés Belges de Médecine Tropicale, de Parasitologie, et de Mycologie 1967;47:331-342.

[33] Jadin J, Vincke IH, Dunjic A, Delville JP, Wery M, Bafort J, et al. [Role of *Pseudomonas* in the sporogenesis of the hematozoon of malaria in the mosquito]. Bulletin de la Société de Pathologie Exotique et de ses filiales 1966;59:514-525.

[34] Rani A, Sharma A, Rajagopal R, Adak T, Bhatnagar RK. Bacterial diversity analysis of larvae and adult midgut microflora using culture-dependent and culture-independent methods in lab-reared and field-collected *Anopheles stephensi*-an Asian malarial vector. BMC Microbiology 2009;9:96.

[35] Terenius O, de Oliveira CD, Pinheiro WD, Tadei WP, James AA, Marinotti O. 16S rRNA gene sequences from bacteria associated with adult *Anopheles darlingi* (Diptera: Culicidae) mosquitoes. Journal of Medical Entomology 2008;45:172-175.

[36] Riesenfeld CS, Schloss PD, Handelsman J. Metagenomics: genomic analysis of microbial communities. Annual Review of Genetics 2004;38:525-552.

[37] Tyson GW, Chapman J, Hugenholtz P, Allen EE, Ram RJ, Richardson PM, et al. Community structure and metabolism through reconstruction of microbial genomes from the environment. Nature 2004;428:37-43.

[38] Nossa CW, Oberdorf WE, Yang L, Aas JA, Paster BJ, Desantis TZ, et al. Design of 16S rRNA gene primers for 454 pyrosequencing of the human foregut microbiome. World Journal of Gastroenterology : WJG 2010;16:4135-4144.

[39] Woese CR. Bacterial evolution. Microbiological Reviews 1987;51:221-271.

[40] Case RJ, Boucher Y, Dahllof I, Holmstrom C, Doolittle WF, Kjelleberg S. Use of 16S rRNA and rpoB genes as molecular markers for microbial ecology studies. Applied and Environmental Microbiology 2007;73:278-288.

[41] Van de Peer Y, Chapelle S, De Wachter R. A quantitative map of nucleotide substitu-
      tion rates in bacterial rRNA. Nucleic Acids Research 1996;24:3381-3391.

[42] Jany JL, Barbier G. Culture-independent methods for identifying microbial commun-
      ities in cheese. Food Microbiology 2008;25:839-848.

[43] von Wintzingerode F, Gobel UB, Stackebrandt E. Determination of microbial diversi-
      ty in environmental samples: pitfalls of PCR-based rRNA analysis. FEMS Microbiolo-
      gy Reviews 1997;21:213-229.

[44] Le Bourhis AG, Dore J, Carlier JP, Chamba JF, Popoff MR, Tholozan JL. Contribution
      of *C. beijerinckii* and *C. sporogenes* in association with *C. tyrobutyricum* to the butyric
      fermentation in Emmental type cheese. International Journal of Food Microbiology
      2007;113:154-163.

[45] Roudiere L, Jacquot A, Marchandin H, Aujoulat F, Devine R, Zorgniotti I, et al. Opti-
      mized PCR-Temporal Temperature Gel Electrophoresis compared to cultivation to
      assess diversity of gut microbiota in neonates. Journal of Microbiological Methods
      2009;79:156-165.

[46] Temmerman R, Masco L, Vanhoutte T, Huys G, Swings J. Development and valida-
      tion of a nested-PCR-denaturing gradient gel electrophoresis method for taxonomic
      characterization of bifidobacterial communities. Applied and Environmental Micro-
      biology 2003;69:6380-6385.

[47] Ogier JC, Son O, Gruss A, Tailliez P, Delacroix-Buchet A. Identification of the bacteri-
      al microflora in dairy products by temporal temperature gradient gel electrophoresis.
      Applied and Environmental Microbiology 2002;68:3691-3701.

[48] Zoetendal EG, Akkermans AD, De Vos WM. Temperature gradient gel electrophore-
      sis analysis of 16S rRNA from human fecal samples reveals stable and host-specific
      communities of active bacteria. Applied and Environmental Microbiology
      1998;64:3854-3859.

[49] Kitts CL. Terminal restriction fragment patterns: a tool for comparing microbial com-
      munities and assessing community dynamics. Current Issues in Intestinal Microbiol-
      ogy 2001;2:17-25.

[50] Penny C, Nadalig T, Alioua M, Gruffaz C, Vuilleumier S, Bringel F. Coupling of de-
      naturing high-performance liquid chromatography and terminal restriction fragment
      length polymorphism with precise fragment sizing for microbial community profil-
      ing and characterization. Applied and Environmental Microbiology 2010;76:648-651.

[51] Thompson JR, Randa MA, Marcelino LA, Tomita-Mitchell A, Lim E, Polz MF. Diver-
      sity and dynamics of a north atlantic coastal Vibrio community. Applied and Envi-
      ronmental Microbiology 2004;70:4103-4110.

[52] Ege MJ, Mayer M, Normand AC, Genuneit J, Cookson WO, Braun-Fahrlander C, et al. Exposure to environmental microorganisms and childhood asthma. The New England Journal of Medicine 2011;364:701-709.

[53] Muyzer G, de Waal EC, Uitterlinden AG. Profiling of complex microbial populations by denaturing gradient gel electrophoresis analysis of polymerase chain reaction-amplified genes coding for 16S rRNA. Applied and Environmental Microbiology 1993;59:695-700.

[54] Roudiere L, Lorto S, Tallagrand E, Marchandin H, Jeannot JL, Jumas-Bilak E. [Molecular fingerprint of bacterial communities and 16S rDNA intra-species heterogeneity: a pitfall that should be considered]. Pathologie-Biologie 2007;55:434-440.

[55] Yoshino K, Nishigaki K, Husimi Y. Temperature sweep gel electrophoresis: a simple method to detect point mutations. Nucleic Acids Research 1991;19:3153.

[56] Jacquot A, Neveu D, Aujoulat F, Mercier G, Marchandin H, Jumas-Bilak E, et al. Dynamics and clinical evolution of bacterial gut microflora in extremely premature patients. The Journal of Pediatrics 2011;158:390-396.

[57] Chareonviriyaphap T, Prabaripai A, Bangs MJ, Aum-Aung B. Seasonal abundance and blood feeding activity of *Anopheles minimus* Theobald (Diptera: Culicidae) in Thailand. Journal of Medical Entomology 2003;40:876-881.

[58] Kengluecha A, Singhasivanon P, Tiensuwan M, Jones JW, Sithiprasasna R. Water quality and breeding habitats of anopheline mosquito in northwestern Thailand. Southeast Asian Journal of Tropical Medicine & Public Health 2005;36:46-53.

[59] MoPH. Report of Vector Borne Disease. In: Department DC, editor: Ministry of Public Health, Bangkok, Thailand; 2011.

[60] Thimasarn K, Jatapadma S, Vijaykadga S, Sirichaisinthop J, Wongsrichanalai C. Epidemiology of Malaria in Thailand. Journal of Travel Medicine 1995;2:59-65.

[61] IMPEQN. Malaria cases reported in 2011 - The Central and Highland provinces. Institute of Malaria, Parasite and Entomology sub., Quy Nhon; 2012.

[62] Drancourt M, Bollet C, Carlioz A, Martelin R, Gayral JP, Raoult D. 16S ribosomal DNA sequence analysis of a large collection of environmental and clinical unidentifiable bacterial isolates. Journal of Clinical Microbiology 2000;38:3623-3630.

[63] Stackebrandt E, Goebel BM. Taxonomic note: a place for DNA-DNA reassociation and 16S rRNA sequence analysis in the present species definition in bacteriology. International Journal of Systematic Bacteriolgy 1994;44:846-849.

[64] McDonald D, Price MN, Goodrich J, Nawrocki EP, DeSantis TZ, Probst A, et al. An improved Greengenes taxonomy with explicit ranks for ecological and evolutionary analyses of bacteria and archaea. The ISME Journal 2012;6:610-618.

[65] Thompson JD, Gibson TJ, Higgins DG. Multiple sequence alignment using ClustalW and ClustalX. Current protocols in bioinformatics / editoral board, Andreas D Baxevanis [et al] 2002;Chapter 2:Unit 2 3.

[66] Guindon S, Delsuc F, Dufayard JF, Gascuel O. Estimating maximum likelihood phylogenies with PhyML. Methods of Molecular Biology 2009;537:113-137.

[67] Sinka ME, Bangs MJ, Manguin S, Chareonviriyaphap T, Patil AP, Temperley WH, et al. The dominant *Anopheles* vectors of human malaria in the Asia-Pacific region: occurrence data, distribution maps and bionomic précis. Parasites & Vectors 2011;4:89.

[68] Acinas SG, Marcelino LA, Klepac-Ceraj V, Polz MF. Divergence and redundancy of 16S rRNA sequences in genomes with multiple rrn operons. Journal of Bacteriology 2004;186:2629-2635.

[69] Liao D. Gene conversion drives within genic sequences: concerted evolution of ribosomal RNA genes in bacteria and archaea. Journal of Molecular Evolution 2000;51:305-317.

[70] Roger F, Lamy B, Jumas-Bilak E, Kodjo A, Marchandin H. Ribosomal Multi-Operon Diversity: An Original Perspective on the Genus *Aeromonas*. PloS One 2012;7:e46268.

[71] Loper JE, Hassan KA, Mavrodi DV, Davis EW, 2nd, Lim CK, Shaffer BT, et al. Comparative genomics of plant-associated *Pseudomonas* spp.: insights into diversity and inheritance of traits involved in multitrophic interactions. PLoS Genetics 2012;8:e1002784.

[72] Guerrieri E, Bondi M, Sabia C, de Niederhausern S, Borella P, Messi P. Effect of bacterial interference on biofilm development by *Legionella pneumophila*. Current Microbiology 2008;57:532-536.

[73] Lee LH, Cheah YK, Nurul Syakima AM, Shiran MS, Tang YL, Lin HP, et al. Analysis of Antarctic proteobacteria by PCR fingerprinting and screening for antimicrobial secondary metabolites. Genetics and Molecular Research, 2012;11:1627-1641.

Vector Control: Current Situation, New Approaches and Perspectives

Distribution, Mechanisms, Impact and Management of Insecticide Resistance in Malaria Vectors: A Pragmatic Review

Vincent Corbel and Raphael N'Guessan

Additional information is available at the end of the chapter

1. Introduction

Malaria is still a major burden causing the death of nearly 655,000 people each year, mostly in children under the age of five, and affecting those living in the poorest countries [1]. Currently, the major obstacles to malaria control and elimination are the absence of a protective vaccine, the spread of parasite resistance to anti-malarial drugs and the mosquito resistance to insecticides [2]. Controlling mosquito vectors is fundamental to reduce mosquito-borne diseases by targeting vectorial capacity and hence the transmission. Vector control through the use of chemicals for mosquito bed nets and indoor residual spraying is still the cornerstone of malaria prevention [1]. Unfortunately, the extensive use of insecticides since the 1950s has led to the development of strong resistance worldwide hence representing a major public health problem where insecticidal vector control is implemented. Here, we propose to review the current level, distribution and mechanisms of insecticide résistance in malaria vectors and address their impact on the efficacy of vector control interventions. Strategies to prevent and/or delay the spread of insecticide resistance in natural mosquito populations are also discussed.

2. Definition of resistance

According to the *World Health Organization* (WHO), resistance is defined as the ability of an insect to withstand the effects of an insecticide by becoming resistant to its toxic effects by means of natural selection and mutations [3]. This definition differs from that provided by the *Insecticide Resistance Action committee* (IRAC) (www.irac-online.org) that gathers independent scientists and experts belonging to Agrochemical Companies who define operational (field) resistance as a heritable change in the sensitivity of a pest population that is reflected in the repeated failure of a product to achieve the expected level of control when used according to the label recommendation for that pest species. The IRAC definition, although pragmatic, is less "sensitive" with the scope to implement early *Insecticide Resistance Management* (IRM) strategies in the field. In both cases however, appropriate tools (biological, biochemical and/or molecular) are needed to identify the mechanisms involved and to conduct surveillance at individual and/or population levels [4].

Resistance has been observed in more than 500 insect species worldwide among which more than 50 *Anopheles* species (Diptera: Culicidae) are responsible for the transmission of malaria parasites to humans [5]. Resistance is a heritable character that relies on a genetic basis. Resistance results from the selection of a genetic modification in one or several genes occurring by migration and/or mutation. For example, when a mosquito population is exposed to an insecticide A, the individuals having resistant genes to this insecticide A survive and reproduce until the resistant allele becomes almost fixed. The use of insecticides for agricultural purposes and more recently for public health has played pivotal step in the selection of resistance in malaria vectors [6]. Resistance can involve several physiological and/or behavioural changes. Changes in the insecticide target site that reduce its binding to insecticides (known as target-site resistance) is the best understood type of resistance mechanism and molecular diagnostics to detect this resistance mechanism are now integrated into insecticide resistance monitoring strategies in malaria control programmes [7, 8]. Enhanced insecticide metabolism that lowers the amount of insecticide reaching the target site (known as metabolic resistance) is more complex but recent advances have identified key enzymes responsible for insecticide detoxi-fication, paving the way for the development of molecular markers for this type of resistance mechanism [9, 10]. Other physiological changes (e.g. reduce penetration through cuticular resistance) and/or behavioural changes in the mosquito population were identified but their impact on the efficacy of insecticides is still poorly understood.

It is commonly accepted that the enhanced metabolism and target site modifications are responsible for high level of insecticide resistance in malaria vectors. To date, malaria vectors have developed resistance to the main chemical classes used in public health (i.e. pyrethroids, DDT, carbamates and organophosphates) (table 1) and the occurrence of cross-resistance[1] and multiple resistance[2] represent a serious threat to achieving the Millennium Development Goals for malaria control (i.e 75% reduction of global malaria cases by 2015). Surveillance and routine monitoring campaigns to assess the level and type of resistance are essential to help Malaria Control Programme (MCPs) to design more effective and sustainable malaria vector control strategies at an operational scale [4].

3. History of resistance to public health insecticides

Since the humans used chemicals for crop protection and/or the prevention of vector borne diseases, cases of resistances have been reported [11, 12]. Insecticides used for malaria control

---

1**Cross resistance:** occurs when a resistance mechanism, which allows insects to resist one insecticide, also confers resistance to another insecticide. Cross resistance can occur between insecticides from different chemical classes.

2**Multiple resistance:** occurs when insects develop resistance to several compounds by expressing multiple resistance mechanisms. The different resistance mechanisms can combine to provide resistance to multiple classes of products.

have included organochlorine, organophosphorus, carbamate, and pyrethroid insecticides, with the latter now taking increasing market share for both indoor residual spraying and Long Lasting Insecticidal mosquito Nets (LLINs) programmes [13]. Resistance has naturally tended to follow the use and switches of these insecticides [5].

Insecticides	Molecular target	Resistance mechanisms		References
		target site	enzymatic mechanisms	
Pyrethroids, type I	sodium channel	Kdr and super Kdr mutations	monooxygenases + esterases	[10,61,62]
Pyrethroids, Type II	sodium channel	Kdr mutations	monooxygenases + esterases	[10,61,62]
Organochlorates	sodium channel	Kdr mutations	GS-tranferases + monooxygenases	[10,61,62]
N-alkyl-amides	sodium channel	no resistance reported against insect of public health importance		
Organophosphates	acetylcholinesterase	Ace1 R mutation	esterases + GS-tranferases + monooxygenases	[10,59,63-67]
Carbamates	acetylcholinesterase	Ace1 R mutation		[10,59,63-67]
Neonicotinoids	nicotinic acetylcholine receptor	not reported	monooxygenases	[68,69]
Spinosad	nicotinic acetylcholine receptor	not reported		
Cyclodienes, Lindane, Bicyclic phosphates	GABA receptor	Rdl mutation	GS-transferases	[62,70]
Phenylpyrazoles	GABA receptor	Rdl mutation	GS-transferases	[62,70]
Avermectines	GABA receptor	undiscribed	monooxygenases + esterases	[62,70]
Insect Growth Regulators	Ecdysone agonist/disruptor or inhibitor of ATP synthase, chitin biosynthesis or lipid synthesis	no resistance reported against insect of public health importance		
Bacillus thuringiensis var. israelensis	microbial disruptors of insect midgut membranes	reported against Culex pipiens s.l. but non discribed		[71]

Table 1. Mechanisms of insect resistance to the main insecticide families of public health interest

Historically, DDT was first introduced for mosquito control and malaria eradication programme in 1946. The first case of DDT resistance was reported in *An. sacharovi* in Greece in 1953 and was followed by dieldrin resistance in 1954 [15]. Onset of resistance was marked by deterioration in malaria control that has continued for more than 30 years with sporadic epidemics of disease [16]. Resistance in *An. sacharovi* has been later reported in Bulgaria, Lebanon, Iran, Iraq, and Syria [12]. Pronounced DDT resistance appeared in *An. stephensi* in Iran and Iraq when full scale house spraying operations began in 1957 and dieldrin resistance appeared three years later. In India, house-spraying of DDT and Lindane (HCH) under the public health programme was introduced in the 1950s. Resistance of the main malaria vector *An. culicifacies* to dieldrin developed in 1958 [17] and resistance to DDT in 1959 [18], but the malaria control programme continued until 1965-1966 when both DDT and HCH failed to control outbreaks of malaria [19]. As a result, malathion was introduced in some areas in 1969 with some success but *An. culicifacies* rapidly developed resistance by 1973 [20]. Malathion resistance resulted in colossal epidemics of malaria in 1975 with 4 million cases reported as compared with 125,000 in 1965. The experience in Pakistan was similar with DDT resistance appearing in 1963. The importance of the resistance was not recognized until outbreaks of malaria began in 1969 and neither DDT nor HCH was effective. By 1975, malaria cases were reported in Pakistan to number 100 million as compared to 9,500 in 1961 [12]. DDT resistance in *An. culicifacies* was reported in Sri Lanka in 1968 resulting in a severe epidemic of malaria

[21]. This vector is now resistant to DDT, dieldrin, organophosphates, carbamates and pyrethroids [11].

Similar trend was noted in Central America and the Caribbean. Dieldrin spraying against *An. albimanus* begun in 1956 and widespread resistance appeared in 1958 [12]. A return to DDT spraying produced generalized resistance by 1960 [18]. The carbamate propoxur was employed in El Salvador, Guatemala, Honduras and Nicaragua in 1970 and resistance developed by 1974. *An albimanus* now exhibits multiple resistances to DDT, dieldrin, lindane and other chemical recently used in public health [22].

Much less information is however available for South East Asian malaria vectors, most probably because resistance monitoring was not carried out in routine before the 80s. In Vietnam, DDT resistance was found in 1989 in *An. epiroticus* of the Sundaicus Complex and is still occurring [23]. From 1990 till 2000, pyrethroid resistance was almost absent in all tested species except in some populations of *An. vagus* and *An. minimus s.l.* [24]. In Thailand, no evidence of insecticide resistance in malaria vectors was present before 1985 [25]. In 1986, development of physiological resistance to DDT was detected in *An. aconitus* from the north where DDT was commonly used for malaria control. One year later, DDT resistance was found in field collected mosquitoes of *An. philippinenis*, *An. nivipes* and *An. aconitus* from the same northern region. Between 1990 and 1997, DDT resistance has been detected in the three primary malaria vectors *An. dirus s.l.*, *An. minimus s.l.* and *An. maculatus s.l.* and permethrin resistance was suggested in a population of *An. minimus s.l.* from northern Thailand, based however on a lower discriminative dosage (0.25%) of permethrin than that used today [25].

In Africa, resistance was initially found in *An. gambiae* in Bobo Dioulasso by 1967 (Burkina Faso), hence less than 7 years after the end of DDT use for malaria control [12]. DDT resistance was found in neighbouring countries including Cote d'Ivoire, Nigeria and Mali [26] and was then reported in most of Central and East African countries [27]. Strong association was observed between the level of DDT resistance in malaria vectors and the amount of DDT use for cotton protection [28]. Regarding BHC/dieldrin, the first cases of resistance were reported in Nigeria in 1954 hence only few months after the introduction of this molecule for malaria control. Initially found in very limited geographical areas, dieldrin resistance has spread in areas free of any insecticide treatments [29]. Few years later, resistance was reported in Bobo-Dioulasso and Cote d'Ivoire [30]. Today, resistance to BHC/dieldrin is still widespread in wild field anopheline populations despite its abandon in public health for many decades [31]. As for DDT, dieldrin resistance in malaria vectors arose and persisted from intensive use of pesticide for agricultural practices and in some specific settings due to public health programmes [32, 33].

After the 80s, DDT has been more or less abandoned worldwide and replaced by organophosphate (OP), pyrethroids and, to lesser extent, carbamates. However, insecticide resistance continued to be a problem, and vector control operations were affected, particularly in India, Africa and Latin America, by extensive use of agricultural pesticides. OP resistance, either in the form of broad-spectrum OP resistance or malathion-specific resistance was found in the major malaria vector species worldwide [12]. Pyrethroids were introduced in late 70s in public health and increasingly used in the 90s; however, cases of resistance were rapidly reported in the main malaria vectors worldwide including *An. albimanus* [34], *An. darlingi* [35], *An. culicifacies* [36], *An. stephensi* [37], *An. gambiae* [38], *An. funestus* [39] and *An minimus* [40]. Despite a sporadic use (compared to DDT and pyrethroids), resistance to carbamates was earlier reported in several mosquito species including *An. albimanus* [41], *An. atroparvus* [42], *An. sacharovi* [5] and *An. gambiae* [43]. Carbamate resistance is now spreading in malaria vectors especially in West Africa where it has been reported in Cote d'Ivoire [44], Burkina Faso [45, 46], Benin [47] and Nigeria [48]. Increased level of carbamate resistance in African mosquito populations is worrying for malaria control because these chemicals are increasingly used in replacement to pyrethroids for Indoor Residual Spraying (IRS) [49].

It is obvious that insecticide resistance in malaria vectors is increasing worldwide due to the increasing selection pressure on mosquito populations caused by the presence of urban, domestic and/or agricultural pollutants in the environment [50]. Transversal and longitudinal monitoring surveys are essential to address the spatio-temporal changes in resistance (dynamic) and to design appropriate strategies for a better control of resistant malaria vector populations worldwide.

4. Resistance mechanisms

The various mechanisms that enable insects to resist the action of insecticides can be grouped into four distinct categories including metabolic resistance, target-site resistance, reduce penetration and behavioral avoidance. These mechanisms that are shown in the figure 1 are briefly described in the following sections.

4.1. Metabolic resistance

Metabolic resistance is the most common resistance mechanism that occurs in insects. This mechanism is based on the enzyme systems which all insects possess to help them to detoxify naturally occurring xenobiotics/insecticides. It is commonly accepted that insect detoxification systems derived from the plant-insect evolutionary arm race and several insect detoxification enzymes have been associated to the detoxification of plant toxins and all types of chemicals, including insecticides [51]. Over-expression of enzymes capable of detoxifying insecticides or amino acid substitutions within these enzymes, which alter the affinity of the enzyme for the insecticide, can result in high levels of insecticide resistance (see [52] for review). Increased expression of the genes encoding the major xenobiotic metabolizing enzymes is the most common cause of insecticide resistance in mosquitoes. Over expression of detoxyfing enzymes can occur as the result of gene amplification (e.g. duplication) or due to changes in either trans-acting regulator elements or in the promoter region of the gene [5, 53, 54]. The consequence is a significant increase of enzyme production in resistant insects that enables them to metabolize or degrade insecticides before they are able to exert a toxic effect. Three categories of enzymes, namely esterases, P450s and glutathione-S-transferases are known to confer resistance to insecticides in insect pest such as malaria vectors. These large enzyme families contain multiple enzymes with broad overlapping substrate specificities, and one member of the family might

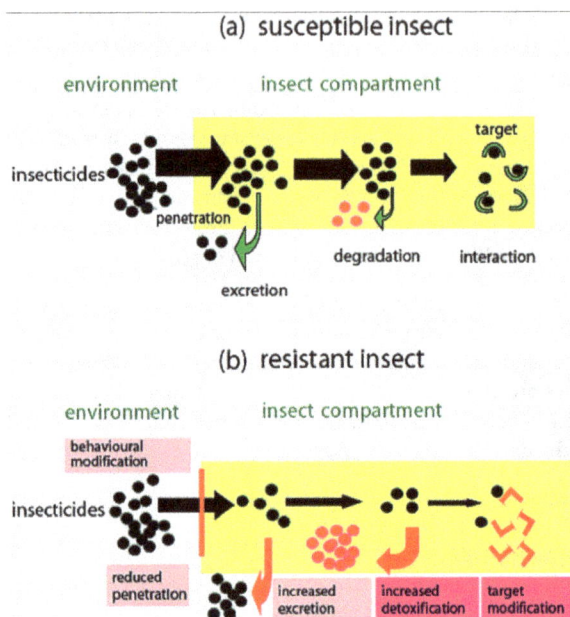

Figure 1. Scheme of potential behavioral and physiological changes associated with insecticide resistance in malaria vectors; (a) susceptible insect; (b) resistant insect (source ; see [14])

be capable of metabolizing limited number of insecticides. Similarly, the level of resistance conferred can vary from low to very high and may differ from compound to compound. Metabolic resistance mechanisms have been identified in mosquito populations for all major classes of insecticides currently used for vector control, including organochlorine, organo-phosphates, carbamates, and pyrethroids.

Esterases. One of the most common metabolic resistance mechanisms is that of elevated levels, or activity, of esterase enzymes which hydrolyze ester bonds or sequester insecticides. A striking example comes from studies on *Culex quinquefasciatus* that resist to a broad range of OP insecticides. In this species, multiple copies of EST-genes was already found hence enabling it to overproduce this type of enzyme [55]. In contrast to the situation in *Culex*, a number of *Anopheles* species (ie *An. culicifacies, An. stephensi* and *An. arabiensis*) have a non-elevated esterase mechanism that confers resistance specifically to malathion through increased rates of metabolism. Malathion resistance in *Anopheles* spp was associated with an altered form of esterase that specifically metabolizes the molecule at a much faster rate than that in susceptible counterparts [56, 57]. Although Carboxylesterase (CCEs) have been mostly associated to organophosphate resistance in mosquitoes, their role in pyrethroid resistance is probable. Indeed, the ability of esterases to metabolize pyrethroids has been suggested in mosquitoes [58, 59] even if no specific mosquito CCE has yet been validated as a pyrethroid metabolizer

[50]. Clearly much more information is needed on the esterase-mediated resistance in malaria vectors.

P450s. Cytochrome P450-dependent monooxygenases are an important and diverse family of enzymes involved in the metabolism of numerous endogenous and exogenous compounds. P450 belong to six families and increased transcription of genes belonging to the CYP4, CYP6, and CYP9 has been observed in various insecticide-resistant species from different taxa [60]. There is increasing number of reports demonstrating elevated P450 monooxygenase activities in insecticide-resistant mosquitoes, frequently in conjunction with altered activities of other enzymes. In most cases where a link between insecticide resistance and elevated P450 activity has been shown, the CYP gene belongs to the CYP6 family. Since the publication of the *An. gambiae* genome [61], P450s were extensively studied in the primary malaria vector in Africa. A total of 111 P450 enzymes were identified [62] and, as in other insects, only a small number of these enzymes are capable of detoxifying insecticides. However, higher activity of enzymes and/or expression of detoxification genes in insecticide resistant colonies do not necessarily correlate with insecticide resistance. For example, some authors have shown elevated transcript levels of an adult-specific CYP6 P450 gene, CYP6Z1, in pyrethroid-resistant strain *of An. gambiae* [63, 64] and *An. funestus* [65]. Further validation studies conducted in *An. gambiae* showed that cyp6z1 was however not capable to metabolize pyrethroids but was capable to metabolize DDT [66]. Another study showed that CYP6z2 displays broad substrate specificity, which may be associated with xenobiotics metabolism and detoxification [67]. Despite, CYP6Z2 being able to bind to permethrin and cypermethrin, this gene does not metabolise any of these insecticides. Microarray-based approaches have lately identified three new "candidate" P450 genes that were found to be repeatedly over-produced in pyrethroid resistant populations of *An. gambiae*: CYP6M2, CYP6P3 and CYP6Z2 [68-70]. All of these genes encode for enzymes that are able to bind to type I and type II pyrethroids but only CYP6P3 and CYP6M2 showed to metabolize the insecticides [10, 71]. More recently, some authors demonstrated that CYP6M2 is also capable of metabolizing the organochlorine insecticide DDT in *An. gambiae*, hence demonstrating the first evidence for a metabolic cross-resistance in malaria vectors [9]. Interestingly the putative ortholog of *An. gambiae* CYP6P3, CYP6P9, as being the prime candidate for conferring pyrethroid resistance, have been identified in *An. funestus* [72, 73] but only the CYP6P9 showed to metabolize types I and II pyrethroids [74]. Recent works showed that over-production of CYP6P9 in *An. funestus* result from gene duplication [72]. In *An. minimus* mosquito, CYP6AA3 and CYP6P7 were up-regulated in pyrethroid-resistance population of Thailand [75] and seem to possess activities toward pyrethroid degradation [76, 77].

Glutathione S-transferases (GSTs). Glutathione transferases (GSTs) are multifunctional enzymes involved in the detoxification of many endogenous and xenobiotic compounds. Conjugation of Glutathione (GSH) to such organic molecules enhances solubility, thus facilitating their eventual elimination [78]. Elevated GST activity has been implicated in resistance to at least four classes of insecticides in insects. Higher enzyme activity is usually due to an increase in the amount of one or more GST enzymes, either as a result of gene amplification or more commonly through increases in transcriptional rate, rather than qualitative changes in individual enzymes [52]. At least six classes of insect GSTs have been identified in *An. gambiae* [79], found in several large clusters on all three chromosomes. The Delta and Epsilon classes found exclusively in insects are the largest classes of insect GSTs. Members of both classes have been implicated in resistance to all the major classes of insecticide. The primary role of GSTs in mosquito insecticide resistance is in the metabolism of DDT to DDE (non toxic products), although they also have a secondary role in organophosphate resistance [80]. GST-based DDT resistance is common in a number of anopheline species including *An. gambiae* [81-83], reflecting the heavy use of this insecticide for malaria control over several decades. Molecular biology and *in vitro* expression studies showed that *aggst3-2* was over expressed in resistant strain of *An. gambiae* and that recombinant *aggst3-2* was very efficient at metabolizing DDT [84]. Most studies of GSTs suggested that regulation occurs at the transcriptional level. Several regulatory elements have been identified in the promoter regions of GSTs that may mediate their induction but the significance of these findings is unclear. Genetic mapping of the major genes controlling GST-based DDT resistance in *An. gambiae* provided however evidence for a trans-acting regulator [84], although in this species, mutations in promoter elements of the Epsilon GST cluster are also associated with resistance [81]. It has been suggested that GSTs may play a role in pyrethroid resistance by detoxifying lipid peroxidation products induced by pyrethroids and/or by protecting from insecticide exposure induced oxidative stress [85]. Furthermore, GST might confer secondary role in pyrethroid resistance by sequestering the insecticide hence reducing the total *in vivo* concentration of insecticide [86].

Despite the great advance obtained recently in the identification of the role of detoxifying enzymes in insecticide resistance, force is to note that the function of >90% of metabolic genes is still unknown. Although only a limited number of resistance mechanisms have been implicated to date, the diversity within enzyme families involved in metabolic resistance is likely to contribute substantially to resistance to many insecticide classes. Further functional genomics and post-genomic technology are needed to reveal the contributions of hitherto unsuspected enzymes in insecticide metabolism and/or sequestration and to identify the causal mutations associated with metabolic resistance in mosquitoes. The contribution that these enzymes make towards various insecticide resistance phenotypes in malaria vectors is yet to be elucidated.

4.2. Target-site resistance

The second most common resistance mechanism encountered in insects is target-site resistance. Insecticides generally act at a specific site within the insect, typically within the nervous system (e.g. OP, carbamate, DDT and pyrethroid insecticides). The site of action can be modified in resistant strains of insects such that the insecticide no longer binds effectively. Reduce sensitivity of the target receptors to insecticide results from non-silent point mutations in the gene encoding the protein. For example, the target site for OP and carbamate insecticides is acetylcholinesterase (AChE) in the nerve cell synapses. Several mutations in the gene encoding for an acetylcholinesterase have been found in insects" [87] which result in reduced sensitivity to inhibition of the enzyme by these insecticides [88, 89]. In malaria vectors, the

G119S mutation (i.e. glycine to serine substitution at position 119) responsible for carbamate and OP resistance has been reported in *An. gambiae* and *An. albimanus,* essentially at the heterozygous state [90]. Recent sequence analysis of some resistant mosquitoes collected in Benin revealed the presence of a duplication of the *ace-1* gene in both A*n*. *A. gambiae* M and S forms [91]. In addition, mutations at a single codon (position 302) in the Rdl (resistance to dieldrin) gene encoding one receptor subunit, from an alanine residue to a serine (or more rarely to a glycine), have been documented in dieldrin-resistant insect species [92] including the malaria vectors *An. stephensi* [93], *An. gambiae s.l.* [94] and *An. funestus* [31]. Similarly, mutations in the amino acid sequence in the voltage-gated sodium channels of nerve cell membranes leads to a reduction in the sensitivity of the channels to the binding of DDT and pyrethroid insecticides [95]. Alterations in the target site that cause resistance to insecticides are often referred to as knockdown resistance (*kdr*) in reference to the ability of insects with these alleles to withstand prolonged exposure to insecticides without being 'knocked-down" [96]. One of the most common amino acid replacements associated with pyrethroid resistance in malaria vectors is a substitution of the leucine residue found at codon 1014 with either phenylalanine (1014F) [97] or serine (1014S) [98] in the Voltage-Gated Sodium Channel (VGSC). Interestingly, residue 1014 does not appear to interact directly with the insecticide but is predicted to alter channel activation kinetics [99]. Note that a *de novo* mutation (N1575Y) recently emerged within domains III-IV of voltage gate sodium channel in pyrethroid resistant populations of *An. gambiae* and seems to occurs only in a single long-range haplotype, also bearing 1014F allele [100]. It has been suggested that the N1575Y mutation may compensates for deleterious fitness effects of 1014F and/or confers additional resistance to pyrethroid insecticides.

4.3. Reduced penetration

Modifications in the insect cuticle or digestive tract linings that prevent or slow the absorption or penetration of insecticides can be found is some resistant insects. This resistance mechanism is not specific and can affect a broad range of insecticides. Reduced uptake of insecticide, often referred to as cuticular resistance, is frequently described as a minor resistance mechanism. Certainly for pests where the major route of insecticide delivery is via ingestion, this is likely to be the case. However, for malaria control, where insecticides are typically delivered on bed nets or on wall surfaces, uptake of insecticides is primarily through the appendages. An increase in the thickness of the tarsal cuticle, or a reduction in its permeability to lipophilic insecticides, could have a major impact on the bioavailability of an insecticide *in vivo*. Examples of reduced-penetration mechanisms are however limited; cuticular resistance was reported for the domestic Fly *Musca domestica* [101] and the lymphatic filariasis vector *Culex quinque-fasciatus* [102]. In *Anopheles*, microarrays studies have recently identified two genes, cplcg3 and cplcg4, encoding cuticular proteins that were upregulated in pyrethroid resistant strains from four populations and two different species (i.e. *An. gambiae* and *An. stephensi*) ([69, 103, 104]. Recently, measures of mean cuticle thickness in a laboratory strain of *An. funestus* using scanning electron microscopy (SEM) showed that the mean cuticle thickness was significantly greater in pyrethroid tolerant mosquitoes than their susceptible counterparts [105]. Clearly much more work is required in order to identify the significance of cuticular resistance in phenotypic resistance.

4.4. Behavioural resistance

Insecticide resistance in mosquitoes is not always based on biochemical mechanisms such as metabolic detoxification or target site mutations, but may also be conferred by behavioural changes in response to prolonged exposure to an insecticide. Behavioural resistance does not have the same "importance" as physiological resistance but may be considered to be a contributing factor, leading to the avoidance of lethal doses of an insecticide [106, 107]. For example, the first study on the irritant effect of DDT residual deposits was conducted using *Anopheles quadrimaculatus* where females were found to be irritated shortly after making contact with the treated surfaces resulting in a rapid escape response from a treated house prior to taking a blood meal [108]. This type of response can be further divided into direct contact excitation (sometimes referred to as 'irritancy') and non-contact spatial repellency that is used when insects move away from the insecticide-treated area before making direct contact [106, 109]. Examples of behavioral resistance or avoidance are few. Change in vector composition (i.e. switch from *An. minimus* to *An. harrisoni*) has been observed following implementation of ITNs in a village form central Vietnam [110]. With regard to *An. funestus*, recent findings showed a shift from indoor to outdoor biting preferences in Tanzania in relation to increasing coverage of pyrethroid-impregnated net [111]. Significant changes in the host-seeking behavior of the *An. funestus* population was confirmed in Benin (West Africa) where scaling up of LLINs at community level induced a change from night biting to early-morning biting behaviour [112]. It is unclear however whether adaptation of malaria vectors species to insecticidal based vector control interventions such as LLIN may result from a phenotypic plasticity or from selected behavioral traits (see Durnez & Coosemans for details).

5. Method to detect insecticide resistance

Currently most resistance monitoring is dependent on bioassays, using fixed insecticide concentrations and exposure times, and the data is reported as percentage mortality and/or Knock Down (KD) effect. The World Health Organisation (WHO) has defined diagnostic doses (i.e. twice the dosage that killed 100% susceptible mosquitoes of a given species) for most insecticides used in malaria control and produces susceptibility test kits consisting of exposure chambers and insecticide treated filter papers [113-115]. Although simple to perform, these diagnostic dose assays provide limited information and several alternative methods for detecting resistance are available (Table 2). These alternative assays generally detect specific resistance mechanisms, and should always be performed as an addition, not a substitute, to bioassays, to avoid the risk that unknown resistance mechanisms go undetected. It should be noted that none of the current methods listed in Table 2 are suitable for detecting cuticular and/or behavioural resistance. Regular monitoring for insecticide resistance is essential in order to react proactively to prevent insecticide resistance from compromising control. If the frequency of resistance alleles is going to build up unchecked, resistance may eventually become 'fixed' in the populations. Once resistance reaches very high levels, strategies to restore susceptibility are unlikely to be effective.

Method	Advantages	Disadvantages
Bioassays using WHO defined diagnostic doses of insecticide	Standardized, simple to perform, detect resistance regardless of mechanism	Lack sensitivity and provide no information about level and type of resistance (except when using with synergists), to be done on live mosquitoes
Dose response bioassays	Provides data on level of resistance in population, regardless of mechanism	Require large numbers of alive mosquitoes, and data from different groups not readily comparable
Biochemical assays to detect activity of enzymes associated with insecticide resistance	Provides information on specific mechanisms responsible for resistance	Requires cold chain. Not available for all resistance mechanisms, sensitivity and specificity issues for some assays (e.g. GST)
Molecular assays to detect resistant alleles	Very sensitive. Can detect recessive alleles and therefore provide an 'early warning' of future resistance.	Requires specialized and costly equipment. Only available for a limited number of resistance mechanisms.

Table 2. Methods for detecting insecticide resistance (source: see [6])

5.1. Bioassays

Guidelines for test procedures and interpretation of results are available from the WHOPES[3] (see http://www.who.int/whopes/resistance/en/). It is important that the mosquitoes used for the bioassays are standardized for age, sex and physiological status as all of these can affect the outcome of the tests. Typically either adults raised from isofemale lines or F1 progeny from field collected blood fed females are used. The limitations and advantages of these two alternatives have recently been discussed [116].

These diagnostic dose assays are simple to perform and provide standardized data sets that, assuming the guidelines are followed, can be readily compared to identify temporal and/or geographical variations in the resistant status of malaria vector populations. However, it is important to recognize some of the limitations of these susceptibility tests. As only a single concentration of insecticide is used, the results do not provide any information about the level of resistance in a population. For example if 50 % of population A and 20 % of population B were killed after exposure to the diagnostic dose of permethrin, it cannot be concluded that population B is more resistant than population A. The results only indicate that both populations are resistant (according to WHO definitions if there is < 80 % mortality, the population is defined as resistant) and that, subject to tests of significance, there is a higher frequency of

---

3 World Health Organization Pesticide Evaluation Scheme

resistant individuals in population B than in A. Dose response assays would be needed to compare the levels of resistance in two populations (e.g. by measuring the Resistant Ratios and their 95% confidence intervals). For pyrethroids, median knock down time (MKDT) is also a useful quantifiable variable [117]. Similarly, the results of these tests cannot be used to compare the levels of resistance to two different insecticides. If 50 % mortality was observed after exposure to the diagnostic dose of permethrin (0.75 %) whereas mortality was 70% after exposure to the diagnostic dose of deltamethrin (0.05%), it is not correct to state that the population is more resistant to permethrin than deltamethrin. Again, all that can be stated is that the population is resistant to both insecticides.

Partly due to the limitations of the diagnostic dose assays described above and partly due to the difficulties that are sometimes incurred in obtaining a regular supply of the insecticide impregnated papers from WHO, an alternative bioassay methodology has been developed [118] and is being adopted by some monitoring programmes. This method, known as the CDC bottle bioassay, uses glass bottles coated with a known concentration of insecticide. As these test kits are assembled in the users own laboratory, the concentration of insecticide can be readily adjusted enabling dose response curves to be developed to compare two or more strains. A caveat to this is that the flexibility, and the potential variation in the insecticide grade used in the tests, impairs comparison of results between two separate studies.

Both WHO diagnostic doses and CDC bottle bioassays can be modified to incorporate synergists. Synergists such as piperonyl butoxide, that block the activity of two major detoxification enzyme families, can be used to explore the role of different resistance mechanisms. If resistance is due to increased metabolism, exposure to an appropriate synergist prior to insecticide bioassays should increase the level of mortality observed.

5.2. Biochemical tests

Biochemical tests to detect alterations in activities of enzyme families associated with insecticide resistance have been available for over two decades and are sometimes used in combination with insecticide bioassays [119]. These assays employ model substrates to record the overall activity of glutathione transferases, carboxylesterases or cytochrome P450s in individual insects. Biochemical assays are also available to detect target site resistance to organophosphate and carbamate insecticides caused by insensitive acetylcholinesterase (AChE). The enzymatic reaction produces a colour change that is generally visible to the naked eye and hence these assays do not require access to expensive equipment (spectrophotometer is appropriate). However, it is important that the mosquitoes are kept on ice from the point of collection to the performance of the assay and this can often pose logistical challenges. Furthermore, there are sensitivity and specificity issues that limit the utility of some of these assays. For example, with over 100 different cytochrome P450 enzymes in malaria vectors, an assay that measures the total level or activity of this enzyme family may not have the sensitivity to detect over production of the single or small number of P450 enzymes that are thought to be involved in pyrethroid metabolism. This may explain the lack of significant correlation observed in many studies between cytochrome P450 activity and bioassay mortality results [120, 121]. In addition not all members of the enzyme family will have the same affinity for the model substrates used in these assays (e.g. CDNB (1-chloro 2-4, dinitrobenzene) is the substrate typically used to assess glutathione transferase activity but the Epsilon class of GSTs which are responsible for DDT resistance have relatively low activity with this substrate). In order to incorporate data from resistance monitoring into evidence based decisions on appropriate insecticide based interventions for malaria control, it is clearly essential that the data is both reliable and accessible. Although guidelines for conducting the various assays exist, there is little consensus on the number of sites and frequency with which resistance monitoring should occur [122]. It is clear that resistance is a dynamic trait, and wide fluctuations in resistance levels throughout the malaria transmission season have been reported [116, 123, 124]. Resistance can also be very focal, particularly when vector composition differs between sites [125], hence a minimum number of sampling sites should be established, taking into account patterns of vector distribution and insecticide usage. The WHO/AFRO African Network for Vector Resistance was established in 2000 and amongst its objectives was the important goal of improving the dissemination of resistance data. Accordingly a database was established to store the results of resistance monitoring activities by the African Network for Vector Resistance (ANVR) members but until recently, this database was not readily accessible by outside users. The recent establishment of new data base (see section 6), as an online centralized resource for collating data on insecticide resistance in disease vectors and the integration of this with the ANVR database, will hopefully ensure that both published and unpublished data on resistance in malaria vectors are more readily available to all interested parties.

5.3. Molecular tests

A multitude of molecular assays have been developed to detect *kdr* alleles in malaria mosquitoes, several of which were recently compared in a study by Bass et al (see [126]). These are routinely used by research laboratories monitoring for insecticide resistance and are gradually being incorporated into some national malaria control resistance monitoring programmes. Unfortunately, despite the recent identification of the key enzymes responsible for metabolic resistance to pyrethroids in *An gambiae* and *An funestus*, there are currently no simple DNA based assays to detect these resistance mechanisms. Detection of these genes is presently dependent on RNA based approaches using relatively sophisticated equipment (e.g. RT-qPCR). Assays to detect the genetic mutation(s) responsible for the resistance phenotype in individual insects can provide an early warning of the emergence of resistance which may not have been detectable by bioassays that can only record the population response. The presence of a single individual with an allele known to confer resistance should be cause for concern as experience dictates that resistance can spread very rapidly in a population unless the selection pressure is eased and/or the genetic cost associated with the resistant allele is high. Conversely, a negative result from a molecular assay should not lead to complacency. As discussed above, molecular assays are presently only available for target site resistance and the failure to detect *kdr* clearly cannot be interpreted as an absence of resistance in a population. Hence molecular assays should be seen as a complement rather than a substitute for bioassays.

6. Current distribution of insecticide resistance

Insecticide resistance has been reported in the main malaria vectors worldwide. Resistance is however not uniformly distributed among vector species and can greatly differ from one village, province, country, region and continent to another. Unfortunately, the highest levels of insecticide resistance were reported in Africa where malaria burden is still the highest in the world [1]. Resistance to pyrethroids, the gold standard insecticides used for LLIN and IRS will be extensively discussed in the present chapter as it remains a real and ever-present danger to future success of malaria vector control. Note that more information on the distribution of insecticide resistance in malaria vectors can be found in *Anobase,* http://anobase.vector-base.org/ir/; *MARA* http://www.mara.org.za; *Arthropod Pesticide Resistance Database,* http://www.pesticideresistance.org.; and IR mapper, http://www.irmapper.com.

6.1. Africa

Although the occurrence of insecticide resistance in malaria vectors in Africa is not a "new" event (see section 2.), the speed at which pyrethroid-resistance recently evolved in field populations is worrying as it may jeopardize the current malaria vector control initiatives carried out in the continent. As shown in figure 2, pyrethroid resistance in *Anopheles* sp. is widespread but not uniformly distributed among the different countries. In the 49 African countries that have been investigated (see [6] for details), 15 did not report any data on resistance in the last 10 years i.e. Algeria, Botswana, Democratic Republic of Congo, Djibouti, Sierra Leone, Lesotho, Liberia, Libya, Maurice, Mauritania, Namibia, Rwanda, Somalia, Swaziland, Tunisia. If a lot of data has been generated in West Africa (as far as *An. gambiae s.l.* is concerned), a lack of information is globally observed in Central, Eastern and Austral Africa. It is obvious that the frequent conflicts that has occurred in the last decades in some African countries has rendered difficult the conduct of routine monitoring surveys by NMCP, International Organisation (WHO/ANVR) and/or research institutions.

Globally, pyrethroid resistance is high in *An. gambiae s.l.* in West Africa including Benin [127], Burkina Faso [128], Guinea Konakry ([129], Ghana [130], Mali [131], Niger [132], Nigeria [133] and Cote d'Ivoire [134]). In this region, pyrethroid resistance is predominant in *An. gambiae s.s.,* compared to *An. arabiensis.* Surprisingly, susceptibility to pyrethroids (permethrin and/or deltamethrin) was reported in *An. gambiae* s.l. in Guinea Bissau [135] despite the presence of the L1014F mutation. In Central Africa, pyrethroid resistance/tolerance is widespread in *An. gambiae s.l* in Cameroon [136-138], Chad [116, 139], Gabon [140, 141], Equatorial Guinea [8] and Sudan [142, 143]. In Chad, North Cameroon and Sudan, pyrethroid resistance is present essentially in *An. arabiensis,* which is consistent with the higher prevalence of this mosquito species in more arid areas with higher mean annual temperatures [144]. In East and Austral Africa, *An. gambiae* and *An. arabiensis* populations are mostly susceptible to pyrethroids in Tanzania [145, 146], Mozambique [147] and Madagascar [148], but highly resistant in eastern Uganda [149, 150], Ethiopia [151], Kenya [152, 153], Zambia [154], South Africa [155] and the Gwave Region of Zimbabwe [120]. Regarding *An. funestus,* most of the literature reporting pyrethroid resistance comes from South Africa [39, 156] and Mozambique [157-159], most probably because *An. funestus* is the main malaria vector in these countries. The data available

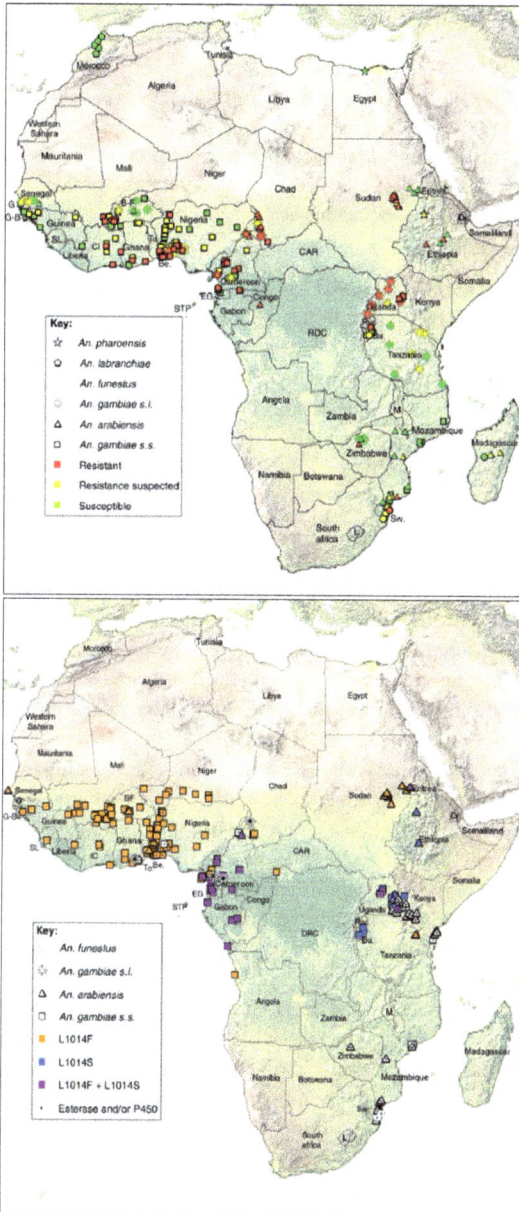

Figure 2. Maps showing the distribution of pyrethroid-resistance in African malaria vectors; A) status of pyrethroid resistance according to WHO criteria ; B) Target site (*kdr*) and metabolic resistance reported for a given mosquito species (Source; see [6]).

in other African countries is very limited in partly due to the difficulty to colonize *An. funestus* species in laboratory. Pyrethroid resistance/tolerance was detected in Malawi [160, 161] and suspected in Obusi and Kassena-Nankana Regions from Ghana [121, 162] and Benin [163] whereas full susceptibility to permethrin and deltamethrin was found in Burkina Faso [164] and Tanzania [145]. There is a lack of information on secondary vectors e.g. *An. moucheti* and *An. nili* which can play important role in malaria transmission in specific settings (e.g. Cameroon, Congo, Côte d'Ivoire). Regarding other vectors species, full susceptibility to pyrethroids has been reported in *An. labranchiae* in Morocco [165] and in *An. pharoensis* in Egypt [166] and Ethiopia [167].

In Africa, the L1014F mutation is widespread (figure 2) and predominant in the molecular S form compared to the M form, except in Benin [168], Guinea Equatorial [8] and Niger [132]. Some authors suggested that the *kdr* alleles may have arisen from at least four independent mutation events in the *An. gambiae* S-form [169]. Regarding the M form, it is not clear whether the *kdr* mutation resulted from an introgression from the S form only [170, 171] and/or from independent mutation events, has recently suggested for Bioko Island [172]. The second mutation, a leucine–serine substitution at the same codon (L1014S), was identified first in a colony of *An. gambiae s.l.* from Kenya [98]. This substitution has been lately reported in Burundi [173], Cameroon [136, 138], Gabon [174], Equatorial Guinea [175], Uganda [176], Republic of Congo [177] and Angola [140], mainly in co-occurrence with the 1014F *kdr* allele. Although some authors have reported that the 1014S allele may confer lower level of pyrethroid resistance than the 1014F allele [178], its spread from eastern to central Africa and more recently to West Africa [124, 179] suggest a survival advantage of mosquitoes sharing this mutation in presence of pyrethroids. So far, the L1014S substitution has always been detected in the S molecular form [180] but recent findings showed the occurrence of the 1014S allele in the M form in Equatorial Guinea [181] and Cameroon [182]. In these two countries, the 1014S allele was present at very low frequencies, alone or associated with the L1014F allele. It is currently impossible to know whether the *kdr* alleles have arisen first in Cameroon or Equatorial Guinea. The higher frequency of the 1014S allele in the S form compared with the M form could either be attributed to an introgression from the S taxon or to a *de novo* mutation. Regarding the sister taxa *An. arabiensis*, both of these mutations were reported in Western [124], Central [183] and Eastern Africa [184]. Interestingly, a new *kdr* mutation (N1575Y) occurring within domains III-IV of voltage gate sodium channel was found in both S and M molecular forms of *An. gambiae* and occurs upon a 1014F haplotypic background only [100]. Additive resistance of *1575Y* was demonstrated for permethrin and DDT in both molecular forms of *An. gambiae*. The prevalence of the 1575Y mutation has increased in West Africa in the last years hence indicating that the 1014F-1575Y haplotype is under strong selection pressure (Djégbé pers. com). It is possible that besides the 1014F/1014S *kdr* mutation, other mutations in the para-type sodium channel gene might be needed for mosquitoes to survive after exposure to a discriminating concentration of an insecticide. Further investigation is needed to better address the distribution and the role of the N1575Y mutation in pyrethroid resistance as well as to assess the fitness benefits conferred by this allele on the L1014F mutation in malaria vectors.

Beyond the spread of *kdr* alleles, metabolic-based resistance due to detoxifying enzymes namely oxidase, the GST (epsilon) and CCE families have expanded in African malaria vectors.

In *An. gambiae s.l.* metabolic resistance involving increased levels of P450 has been reported at least in Kenya [185], Cameroon [186], Benin [69], Nigeria [69], Ghana [70], Mozambique [147], South Africa [187] and Zimbabwe [120]. Up to now, only genes encoding CYP6P3 and CYP6M2 P450 enzymes have been clearly involved in cellular mechanisms known to metabolize deltamethrin and permethrin [10, 71].These genes were found over-expressed in pyrethroid-resistant *An. gambiae* populations from Benin, Nigeria and Ghana [69, 70], mainly in co-association with the *kdr* L1014F allele. In *An. funestus*, pyrethroid resistance involving increased activity of P450 monooxygenase and/or GST was demonstrated in South Africa [157], Mozambique [188] and Malawi [161].

To conclude, the immense challenge in Africa will be not to manage and control *kdr*-resistant mosquitoes only but to deal with the development of "multiple resistant" populations that could resist to different class of insecticides used in public health. One other issue is the occurrence and development of carbamate resistance in some countries (eg Benin, Nigeria) where this chemical class is in use for IRS through the PMI programme [47, 48]. The spread of carbamate resistance in malaria vectors in Africa is worrying for insecticide resistance management and alternative insecticides, and innovative strategies are urgently needed to better reduce the vectorial capacity of mosquitoes and hence effectively reduce the burden of malaria in the region. Resistance management strategy for malaria control is discussed in section 8.

6.2. South-East Asia and India

The South East Asia Region (SEAR) that account for 13% of the total malaria cases worldwide (2nd position after Africa) [1] is not spare of insecticide resistance in the main malaria vector species.

In the Mekong region, cross-country monitoring of insecticide resistance has been conducted through the MALVECASIA network (http://www.itg.be/malvecasia/) to help MCPs in the choice of insecticide to use at regional level. Large differences in insecticide resistance status were observed among species and countries. *Anopheles dirus s.s.*, the main vector in forested malaria foci, was mainly susceptible to permethrin except in central Vietnam where it showed possible resistance to type II pyrethroids [23]. *Anopheles minimus* s.l. populations were found resistant / tolerant in Vietnam and northern Thailand [189] but almost susceptible in Cambodia and Laos. No *kdr* mutation has been observed so far in these species [190] and pyrethroid resistance seems to result from increased detoxification by esterases and/or P450 monooxygenases [191]. Indeed, increased mRNA expression of two P450 genes, *CYP6P7* and *CYP6AA3*, suspected to metabolize some pyrethroids [76] have been reported in a deltamethrin-resistant population of *An. minimus* in Thailand [75, 192].

Anopheles epiroticus of the Sundaicus Complex showed to be highly resistant to all pyrethroids in the Mekong Delta [23] but susceptible to DDT, except near Ho Chi Minh City. DDT and pyrethroid-resistant populations of *An. subpictus* were reported in Vietnam and Cambodia. Biochemical assays suggest an esterase-mediated pyrethroid detoxification in both *An. epiroticus* and *An. subpictus* whereas DDT resistance in *An. subpictus* might be conferred to a higher GST activity. In Vietnam and Cambodia, *An. vagus* and *An sinensis* showed various levels of pyrethroid resistance and sequence-analysis of the DIIS6 region of the VGSC revealed the presence of the 1014S *kdr* allele [193]. Pyrethroid resistant populations of *An. sinensis* were also reported in the Republic of Korea (ROK) [194] and in China [195]. In China, cypermethrin resistance in *An. sinensis* was associated with the presence of both 1014F and L1014C substitutions, whereas only 1014F and 1014S mutations were found in the ROK and Vietnam, respectively. In Indonesia, molecular analysis carried out in field mosquito samples revealed the presence of the 1014F allele in the four main malaria vectors i.e. *An. sundaicus, An. aconitus, An. subpictus* and *An. vagus* [196]. At the present time, it is difficult to speculate on the relative contribution of the *kdr* mutations *versus* metabolic detoxification on pyrethroid and DDT resistance in malaria vectors from the SEA region and more work are needed to establish a clear trend.

Insecticide resistance is known to be widespread in other part of Asia such as India. In this country, resistance has a long history (see section 2) and it represents a big challenge for malaria vector control. Among the *Anopheles* species, *An. culicifacies s.l.*, the major vector of malaria in most parts of the country, has developed strong resistance to pyrethroids [36], DDT [197, 198], dieldrin/HCH [199], and malathion [198]. The 1014F mutation, which generates the *kdr* phenotype was detected in pyrethroid and DDT resistant *An. culicifacies s.l.* populations sometimes in co-occurrence with the 1014S mutation [197]. Note that a novel mutation V1010L (resulting from G-to-T or -C transversions) in the VGSC was recently identified in Indian *An. culicifacies* and was tightly linked to 1014S substitution [197]. Elevated activities of GST seem to play also an important role in DDT-resistance in this mosquito species [82]. Similarly, strong level of pyrethroid resistance due to the presence of both 1014F and 1014S mutations was found in the urban malaria vector *An. stephensi* particularly in the Rajasthan District [200]. Other vectors that are reported to be resistant to pyrethroid, DDT and/or dieldrin/HCH in India are *An. annularis, An. subpictus* and *An. philippinensis* [201]. In contrast, *An. minimus* has still not showed pyrethroid and DDT resistance [202].

The same trend was noted in Sri Lanka where the main malaria vectors species, i.e. *An. culificifacies s.l.* and *An. subpictus* have developed DDT, pyrethroid and malathion resistance in several districts [203, 204]. However, the main mechanisms associated with DDT and malathion resistance in *An. culicifacies s.l.* and *An. subpictus* are primarily metabolic and involve carboxylesterases (malathion) or monooxygenases and GSTs (for DDT) [205, 206]. An altered acetylcholinesterase conferring organophosphate resistance has been suspected in both vector species [205].

In the delta region of Bangladesh, the *An. sundaicus* malaria vector is fully susceptible to DDT but other malaria vectors such as *An. philippinensis, An. maculatus s.l.*, and *An. aconitus* have all developed resistance to DDT [207]. *Anopheles aconitus*, additionally, has been reported to be resistant to dieldrin/HCH. Bhutan records *An. maculatus s.l.* as resistant to DDT, but there is no record of its resistance to any other insecticides [207]. Two vectors of malaria in Nepal, *An. maculatus s.l.* and *An. aconitus*, also have developed resistance to DDT whereas only malathion resistance was reported in *An. stephensi* in Pakistan [208]. Finally, in Iran and Turkey, *An. stephensi* and *An. sacharovi* showed resistance to DDT and dieldrin but both species are mostly susceptible to pyrethroids [209-211].

6.3. Latin America

The countries of the Amazon Basin (Bolivia, Brazil, Colombia, Ecuador, Guyana, Peru, Surinam and Venezuela) carry the greatest burden of malaria in the Americas. The primary vectors of this disease in the Amazon basin are *An. darlingi* and *An. albimanus*. Surprisingly, much less data on insecticide resistance is available for these two mosquito species comparatively to African and/or Asian malaria vector species [212].

In Colombia, DDT resistance was reported in the late 80's in some populations of *An. darlingi* in the districts of Quibdó and close to the Atrato River [213, 214]. Successive insecticide susceptibility evaluations revealed resistance to pyrethroids in both *An. darlingi* and *An. albimanus* mainly in the Chocó State [215]. In *An. darlingi*, increased levels of both Multi function Oxidase (MFO) and Non specific Esterase (NSE) were reported in a deltamethrin and DDT-resistant population, hence suggesting a possible involvement of these detoxifying enzymes in cross resistance to DDT and deltamethrin [35]. Note that various levels of resistance to organophosphate and pyrethroids were also reported in the secondary malaria vector *An. nuneztovari* [216].

In neighboring countries, DDT, permethrin and deltamethrin resistance was found in laboratory colonized populations of *An. albimanus* from Guatemala, whereas full susceptibility was noted in field populations from El Salvador and Belize [217, 218]. The colonies from Guatemala showed significant increase in the specific activity of esterase and/or oxidase as measured by spectrophotometer suggesting their potential involvement in pyrethroid-resistance [34, 217]. In Peru, monitoring campaigns carried out since 2000 showed that *An. albimanus* was the only Anopheline species to exhibit pyrethroid-resistance [219].

In Mexico, high level of DDT resistance and low levels of resistance to organophosphate, carbamate and pyrethroid insecticides were detected in field populations of *An. albimanus* in Chiapas, prior to a large-scale resistance management project [220]. Biochemical assays revealed that the DDT resistance was caused by elevated levels of GST activity leading to increased rates of metabolism of DDT to DDE [22], whereas carbamate resistance was attributed to an altered acetylcholinesterase (AChE). More recent studies conducted in the southern Yucatan Peninsula showed high levels of DDT, deltamethrin and pirimiphos-methyl resistance in the *An. albimanus* populations tested [221]. Biochemical tests revealed elevated levels of GST, P450 and esterases activities that could be involved in DDT and pyrethroid-resistance. As for carbamate, pirimiphos-methyl resistance was strongly correlated with the presence of an insensitive acetylcholinesterase.

To our knowledge, it is the main "published" information available on the distribution, levels and mechanisms of resistance (i.e. accessible through Medline and pub med) in malaria vectors in Latin America. It is then essential to strengthen the capacity of all Latin America countries that suffering from malaria to make insecticide monitoring in routine to obtain much accurate information on the insecticide resistance situation in the malaria vectors. This will provide stake holders with useful information for the implementation of more effective and sustainable malaria control programmes in the region.

7. Impact of pyrethroid-resistance on programmatic malaria control

Few operational reports exist that measure the impact of pyrethroid resistance on epidemiological outcomes of malaria, owing to body of factors that mislead the attributable component
of resistance. Where tentative evidence is provided in most cases, the design of the study has
been observational and the effect of confounding factors can never be excluded with confidence, making difficult the interpretation of data.

Most probably, the only clearest evidence of control failure being directly linked to pyrethroid
resistance was reported from the borders of Mozambique and South Africa. In 1996, the malaria
control programme in KwaZulu Natal switched from using DDT to deltamethrin for indoor
spraying. Within four years, notified malaria cases had increased about four fold, *An. funestus* had re-appeared and was observable emerging alive from pyrethroid sprayed houses.
Bioassays showed that this species was resistant to pyrethroids but susceptible to DDT [39]. A
decision was taken to switch back to DDT spraying and, within the two years after this switch
was made, *An. funestus* was no longer observed emerging alive from insecticide sprayed
houses. The combination of DDT and antimalarial drugs in KwaZulu-Natal has resulted in a
91% decline in the malaria incidence rate [222, 223]. There is no doubt that that the emergence
of pyrethroid resistance and the avoidance of its effects by switching to DDT, has been of major
operational importance [224].

Additional evidence was brought on the island of Bioko on the West African Coast. A malaria
control strategy based on IRS with lambdacyhalothrin was launched by the Bioko Island
Malaria Control Project (BIMCP) funded by the Government of Equatorial Guinea and a
consortium of private donors led by Marathon Oil Corporation. One round of IRS using the
pyrethroid deltamethrin (K-Orthrine WP50, Bayer Crop Sciences, Isando, South Africa) failed
to curtail an increase in the population density of *An. gambiae* M form because of evidence in
the rise of the knock-down resistance (*kdr*) gene in this species [8]. The programme switched
to carbamate insecticide before a substantial decline in the mosquito population, transmission
index and malaria prevalence in children was seen. Nevertheless, in an observational study
such as this, the possible contribution of other confounding factors to the failure of pyrethroid
IRS cannot be overlooked so the direct consequence of the *kdr* frequency is unclear.

Another programmatic study was conducted in the highland provinces of Burundi. Between
2002 and 2005, a well targeted vector control programme (conducted in foot of valleys only)
combining IRS with pyrethroids and/or PermaNet 1.0 LLINs was initiated in one of the most
affected island provinces, Karuzi [225]. Initially, one round per year of pyrethroid-IRS was
carried out in all human dwellings and cattle sheds before the seasonal increase in transmission. LLIN distribution preceded the first IRS round in the same year. The S-form of *An.
gambiae* was the predominant vector species in Karuzi District and showed resistance to
pyrethroids due to the *kdr* mutation. The entomological data showed that the intervention,
overall, effectively reduced *Anopheles* density by 82% and malaria transmission was decreased
by 90% despite high frequencies of the L1014S allele in the local *An. gambiae* population [173].

In a more recent observational study conducted in Malawi, the impact of pyrethroid resistance on operational malaria control has been assessed with more controversial evidence of

resistance impacting pyrethroid-based vector control [161]. In this trial, pyrethroid-LLINs were distributed to communities in 2007 followed by a pilot campaign of IRS with lambda-cyhalothrin supported by the President's Malaria Initiatives between 2008-2010 within districts. A series of sentinel sites were established during these periods to track the effect of the increase in pyrethroid resistance in the local malaria vectors (*An. gambiae* and *An. funestus*) and assess any impact on malaria transmission and prevalence of infection. Pyrethroid resistance had been selected over the 3 years of the programme in these two major malaria vectors with the resistance in the later vector (i.e; *An. funestus*) being metabolically-mediated and involving the up-regulation of two duplicated P450s. The selection of resistance over 3 years had however not triggered a major increase in parasite prevalence in Malawian children, but it may have reduced the benefit of introducing IRS alone in several districts [161]. The impact of this pyrethroid resistance on the ability of LLIN and IRS to reduce malaria infection in Malawi needs to be further elucidated.

Similarly, in the Dielmo Village of Senegal, a longitudinal study of inhabitants was carried out between January, 2007, and December, 2010 [226]. In July, 2008, deltamethrin-LLINs were provided to all villagers and asymptomatic carriage of malaria parasites was assessed from cross-sectional surveys. Overall, the incidence density of malaria attacks decreased from 5.45 per 100 person-months before LLINs distribution in 2007 to 0.41 by August 2010, but increased sharply back to 4.57 between September and December, 2010, i.e, in less than 3 years after the distribution of LLINs. Within the same time frame, the malaria vector became gradually resistant to pyrethroids and the prevalence of the 1014F *kdr* resistance allele increased from scratch, i.e. 8% in 2007 to 48% in 2010. Once again, these results should be considered with caution as the study was conducted in an unique village and the conclusions drawn could not be extrapolated or extended to Senegal or other areas of Western Africa. Moreover, the link between the slight rise of pyrethroid resistance and the rebound in malaria cases cannot be established with accuracy and such rebound could be due to other sources of factors totally independent of resistance.

Another recent study reports the presence of pyrethroid-resistance in malaria vectors *versus* the gain in current efforts to control malaria in the Zambia [154]. In line with the Global trend to improve malaria control efforts, a country wide campaign of Olyset Nets and PermaNets (LLIN) distribution was initiated in 1999 and indoor residual spraying with DDT or pyrethroids was reintroduced in 2000 in the country by the NMCP. In 2006, these efforts were strengthened by the PMI. Both major malaria vectors, *An. gambiae* and *An. funestus* were controlled effectively with the ITN and IRS programme in Zambia, maintaining a reduced disease transmission and burden, despite the discovery of DDT and pyrethroid resistance in the country.

There have been extensive randomized controlled trials (RCTs) (phase III) in part of Africa aiming at investigating the efficacy of ITNs for malaria prevention [227], but very few have assessed how pyrethroid resistance might affect the effectiveness of such intervention. RCTs entail a set of communities randomly divided into groups, one that receives the novel form of vector control intervention, and comparison arms that often receive the old form of vector control tools or nothing. The key difficulty is that it is impossible to address the question to whether vector control would produce a smaller reduction in malaria if the vector mosquitoes are resistant than it would have done if they were susceptible, using RCT methods. This is simply because resistance is not an easy factor that can be allocated randomly to some communities and not to others. The distribution of resistance is patchy and its severity seems to differ from one location (village) to another. Moreover there may be more resistance or survival trend of mosquitoes in some villages than others because of variations in the quality of vector control operations, or in mosquito behavior [228, 229]. This is important to mention, because many health scientists regard evidence from randomized-controlled studies as the only reliable basis for decision-making in public health.

The first RCT that investigated the impact of pyrethroid-resistance on LLIN efficacy was conducted in the Korhogo area in the north of Côte d'Ivoire. The trial encompassed multiple villages where the 1014F *kdr* allele frequency was >90% [28] and malaria was endemic. The regular use of conventionally lambdacyhalothrin-treated nets had a significant impact on the entomological inoculation rate (55% reduction) and on malaria incidence in children < 5 (56% reduction of clinical attacks) compared to a control group having no nets [230]. This was the first clear-cut evidence of ITNs continuing to provide effective personal protection against malaria in an area with a very high frequency of *kdr* in the vector population. However, as reported in Ranson et al. [6], the absence of a physical barrier in the control group may have overestimated the impact of pyrethroid treated nets against *kdr* mosquitoes in this study.

More recently, another RCT of LLINs and/or IRS was conducted in 28 villages in southern Benin, from 2007 to 2010 [231]. The objective of the study was to examine whether carbamate-IRS applied every 8 months, as practiced by the PMI programme in Benin provided additional benefit over LLINs (ie Permanet 2.0) in term of malaria prevention and management of pyrethroid resistance in malaria vectors. Results showed that combination of LLINs and IRS did not reduce malaria transmission and morbidity compared to LLIN alone in an area of pyrethroid resistance [124]. Significant increase of 1014F *kdr* frequency was observed in the reference and treated arms only 18 months post intervention hence indicating that LLIN and IRS failed to reduce the spread of the 1014F allele in malaria vectors. The authors suggested that the increase in pyrethroid resistance might have accounted for the reduction of LLIN efficacy at a community level. Clearly, further investigation is needed to assess whether pyrethroid-resistance can reduce efficiency of LLINs and IRS for malaria prevention in Africa.

Given the many obstacles for evaluating the epidemiological impact of resistance, other alternative methods to measure operational impact has been to measure proxy entomological outcomes, such as the relative mortality and feeding success of resistant and susceptible vectors in experimental huts [232, 233]. Although such results can be remarkably clear, and definitively linked to resistance, experimental hut methods have their own limitations owing to the controlled hut structures that differ in many ways to normal houses in rural African context.

An early experimental hut trial of ITNs was conducted in the western African country of Benin. In southern Benin (Ladji), pyrethroid resistance has evolved in the M form of *An. gambiae* mosquitoes that appear to combine the knockdown resistance (*kdr*) gene with oxidase mechanisms [127, 234]. In Ladji, carrier mosquitoes of this resistance were not controlled by pyrethroid treatments in experimental hut trials of ITNs or the leading brands of LLINs, PermaNet 2.0 (Vestergaard Frandsen SA, Aarhus, Denmark) and Olyset (Sumitomo Chemicals, Osaka, Japan) [235]), compared to Malanville in the north where the vector was largely susceptible to pyrethroids [127]. Further household randomized trial conducted in northern susceptible and southern resistance areas demonstrated that lambdacyalothrin-ITNs (regardless the physical condition) lose their capacity to confer personal protection against pyrethroid-resistant An. gambiae [236].

One of the problems associated with many of these studies is that, due to the lack of molecular markers for alternative resistance mechanisms (i.e. metabolic or even cuticular and behavioral), the frequency of kdr alleles is frequently used as a proxy for resistance. It has been recently demonstrated in Southern Benin that kdr by itself in An. gambiae does not seem to bear more malaria parasites than in a susceptible [237] but this conception can be misleading when metabolic or other resistance mechanisms are predominant or combine with kdr to confer resistance. There is an urgent need for properly controlled large-scale trials to assess the impact of pyrethroid resistance on IRS and ITNs in Africa but also in different regions affected by malaria (e.g. Asia and Latin America). Such studies should use both entomological and epidemiological indices and should be conducted in areas where alternative resistance mechanisms are known to be responsible for pyrethroid resistance. Furthermore, these studies must consider the possibility of behavioural resistance as recently suggested in Benin [238] and Tanzania [111] and monitor for changes in key traits such as location of resting and feeding which may impact on the efficacy of current insecticide based interventions.

8. Resistance management strategies

As a general statement, the use of insecticides does not create resistance by itself but select small proportion of individuals having a genetic mutation that allow them to resist and survive the effects of the insecticide. If this advantage is maintained by constant use of the same insecticide, the resistant insects will reproduce and the genetic changes that confer resistance will be transferred to offspring so that they become more prevalent within the population (figure 3). This selection process will take longer time to occur if the gene conferring resistance is rare or present at a low prevalence. Resistance should not be confused with "induction" that can occur after sub-lethal (or low dose) exposure to any insecticide and/or xenobiotic and is not passed on to offspring [239].

8.1. Main factors influencing resistance development

The evolution of insecticide resistance is complex and depends on several genetic, biological and operational factors [240-242]. The biological factors relate by the life cycle of the insect (e.g. rate of reproduction, number of generation/offspring, rate of migration and isolation, etc), while the genetic factors include the intrinsic characteristics of the resistant genes (e.g. mono versus polygenic resistance, dominance, fitness cost and gene interaction). Operational factors concern the treatment itself including the method and frequency of application, dosage and residual activity of the insecticides as well as insecticide coverage.

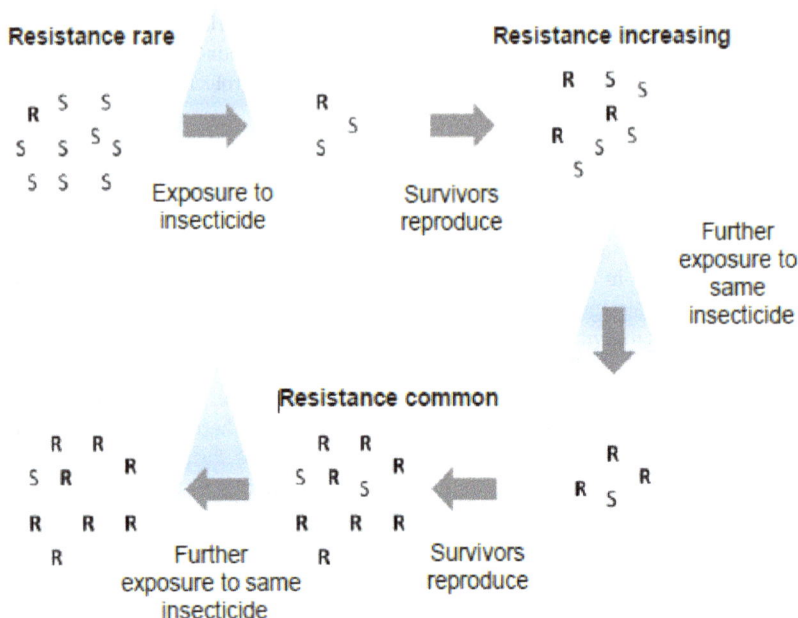

Figure 3. Possible scenario for resistance development in a mosquito population (source; [240])

8.1.1. Biological factors

Rate of reproduction

Insect species that have a short life cycle and high rates of reproduction are likely to develop resistance more rapidly than species that have a lower rate of reproduction, as any resistance genes can rapidly spread throughout the population. Because mosquitoes can produce high number of offspring (i.e. females can lay several hundred eggs during their reproductive life) they are much likely to develop resistance to insecticides than other species.

Population migration / isolation

With mosquitoes, the goal is to eliminate all or the majority of the population, however the greater the selection pressure that is put on a population, the faster susceptibility may be lost. Immigration of individuals possessing susceptible genes from untreated areas can beneficially dilute and compete with the resistance genes in the overall population. An early step in a malaria vector control programme should therefore be to estimate the susceptibility status of vector populations (see section 5 for details) and estimate potential immigration of untreated insects. This can be achieved by using genetic markers to estimate the gene flow (migrants) and genetic structure between populations. For example, an isolated area (e.g. island) where the entire area is treated would have a higher risk of developing resistance as few "susceptible" genotypes would join the treated population. The risk of insecticide resistance developing should be considered when planning a resistance management strategy. Awareness of and coordination with neighboring vector control programmes and agricultural activities should be encouraged, so that the regional and potential "side effect" on the target population is considered.

8.1.2. Genetics factor

Dominance

Resistance genes can range from dominant through semi-dominant to recessive. If dominant or semi-dominant, only one parent needs to possess the characteristic to be fully or partially expressed in the offspring. If recessive, both parents must possess the trait. Fortunately, most resistance mechanisms (e.g. *kdr*) are controlled by recessive or semi-recessive genes, which slows their spread within the population at early stage of resistance development when most individuals are present at heterozygous state. In contrast, when the resistance is genetically dominant, e.g. the $Ace.1^R$ gene conferring cross-resistance to carbamates and OPs [243], it can rapidly become established within the population and will be difficult to manage. Fortunately, strong genetic cost is often associated with dominant resistant gene that can compensate the effect of the dominance and slow down the increase of resistance gene frequency in natural populations [244].

Gene interactions

Epistasis is the non-additive interaction (synergistic *versus* antagonistic) between different loci which contribute to a phenotype [245]. Epistasis between independent loci conferring insecticide resistance is important to investigate as this phenomenon can shape the rate at which resistance evolves and can dictate the level of resistance in the field. Epistasis can be measured in laboratory studies on susceptible and resistant colonies, but without these data, it is generally impossible to predict whether or not it will occur when two genes are being evaluated. Studies of the interactions between resistance loci have been most commonly conducted in house flies [246-248]. Generally, a greater than additive interaction was observed between two loci that were both homozygous resistant, whereas additively (i.e. lack of epistasis) occurs between two loci that were both heterozygous. In mosquitoes, Harstone and colleagues [249] showed multiplicative interactions between *kdr* and P450 detoxification in *Culex pipiens quinquefasciatus* whether the resistance alleles were homozygous or heterozyges. For example, resistance ratio 50 (i.e. LC50 resistant strain/LC50 susceptible strain) to permethrin in the double homozygote mosquitoes (RR50 of 30,000) was much higher than that expected (RR50 of 1,400) by simple additive effect of the two loci. Overall, interactions between independent resistant genes are complex. It is therefore important to better understand the interactions between resistant loci as well as to address how the fitness costs/benefits of the mechanisms can manipulate the observed interactions.

Fitness cost

Populations of insects that have never been exposed to insecticides are usually fully susceptible, and resistance genes within those populations are very rare. This usually occurs through a "fitness cost", which means that insects sharing the resistance allele lack some other attribute or "quality" such that it gives an advantage to the susceptible insects in an insecticide free environment [250]. For example, resistant insects may have lower mating success, be more susceptible to natural enemies [251], or more prone to mortality during over-wintering [252]. Increased production of metabolic enzymes generally shows lower associated fitness cost than those associated with alterations in the structural genes most probably because the primary function of the enzyme is not disrupted [253]. There is good laboratory and field evidence to suggest that the deficit of insecticide selection pressure, in most cases, selects for susceptible genotypes. For example, the absence of homozygote's resistant genotypes in *An. gambiae* populations in West Africa is most probably due to the strong genetic cost associated with the carbamate-resistance allele a*ce.1*^{R} (G119S) [254]. In addition, once resistance in the field has been selected it often rapidly reverts once the insecticide treatment regime is changed. A good example of this occurred in *An. arabiensis* in Sudan, where malathion specific insecticide resistance was selected in the early 1980s through antimalarial house spraying. The development of resistance prompted a switch of insecticide treatment to fenitrothion and the malathion resistance rapidly reverted in the following years. However, reversion rates are variable and may be very slow, particularly when an insecticide has been used for many years. For example, DDT was used extensively for malaria control over a 20 year period up to the 1960s in Sri Lanka to control *An. culicifacies s.l.* and *An. subpictus*. DDT was replaced by malathion in Sri Lanka in the early 1970s when a total and effective ban on DDT use was implemented. Subsequent regular monitoring has shown that DDT resistance has reverted very slowly towards suscept-ibility; around 80% of the adult mosquito population was resistant in the 1970s compared to about 50% in the 1990s. The same is true with the R*dl* gene that was maintained in field mosquito populations despite the abandon of cyclodiene for mosquito control for more than 30 years [33]. Rate of reversion is an important parameter to consider before implementing any resistance management strategy in the field.

8.1.3. Operational factors

In practice, only operational factors such as the insecticide(s) used, the area of coverage (for example for IRS or LLIN), and the timing, rate, and method of application can be manipulated directly to reduce the selection pressure for resistance. Operational factors influence selection by determining the overall fraction of a population exposed (larvae/adults) to a selecting agent and the degree of contact and pick-up of toxicant by exposed pests at what has been termed the "interface between insects and insecticides" [242]. At both stages, operational and intrinsic factors interact in complex ways to establish the net effect of a control treatment on both genetic composition and total population size. Management of resistance therefore entails resolving these interactions to anticipate with some confidence both the suppressive and selective effects of potential control strategies.

Frequency of application, dosage and persistence of effect

How often an insecticide is used is one of the most important factors that influence resistance development [240]. With each use, an advantage is given to the resistant insects within a population. The rate of increase of resistance on any population will generally be faster in the presence of a lower fitness cost and high reproductive and short life cycles producing several generations per season. The length of time that an insecticide remains effective, also called its persistence, is dependent upon the physical chemistry of the insecticide, the type of formulation, the application rate and the substrate. Products which provide a persistent effect provide continual selection pressure in a similar manner to multiple treatments. For example, a space spray will persist for a very short time and will select only against a single generation of mosquitoes. In contrast, a residual wall application (IRS) or Insecticide Treated nets treatment (especially Long Lasting Nets) will persist for months or years providing a selection pressure against many generations of the same insect. For example, repeated application of DDT for indoor residual spraying has contributed to increase the number of DDT-resistant malaria vector species in various geographical settings [255]. Several studies showed however that the use of insecticides in agriculture play a key role in the selection of resistance in mosquitoes [256, 257]. Indeed, most insecticides used in agriculture are of the same chemical classes and have the same targets and modes of action as those used in public health programme. In practice, VC programmes cannot influence the choice of the pesticide used for crop protection and the only thing that can be done is to appropriately select the most judicious insecticide for mosquito control. However, there is more published evidence that public health insecticides can contribute to select for pyrethroid resistance alleles (see section 7 for details). It is obvious that we can expect enhanced selection pressure on resistance genes through the scaling up of LLIN and/or IRS for malaria elimination.

Choice of the insecticide

The speed at which an insecticide effectively kills an insect can also influence the evolution of resistance. All current insecticides approved for ITNs or IRS kill extremely rapidly after contact. While fast-acting conventional insecticides can produce even more effective initial control, they impose enormous selection for resistance by killing young female adults. The consequence is that spectacular initial mosquito control can last as little as a few years, thus providing very poor medium- to long-term disease control [258]. Some authors recently suggest that Late Acting insecticides (e.g. entomofungus) may be a more tactical strategy to manage resistance if female mosquitoes are killed after 2 or more gonotrophic cycles [259]. Indeed, the less the insecticide impact on mosquito fitness, the less the strength of selection, especially if the resistance allele is associated with a strong genetic cost. In theory, it would be possible to create an insecticide that would provide effective malaria control yet never be undermined by the evolution of resistant mosquitoes. However, further studies are required as "proof of principle" i.e. to demonstrate that this strategy can be effective for vector management and malaria prevention in a real setting.

8.2. Resistance management — Strategies and tactics

Historically, the practice of using an insecticide until resistance becomes a limiting factor has rapidly eroded the number of suitable/available insecticides for vector control. Rotations, mosaics, and mixtures have all been proposed as resistance management tools [260, 261] but there are very few "success stories" in public health. Numerous mathematical models have been produced to estimate how these tools could be optimally used [262-264] but these models have rarely been tested under field conditions due to the practical difficulties in estimating changes in resistance gene frequencies (especially for metabolic resistance) in large samples of insects [220]. With the advent of different molecular techniques for resistance-gene frequency estimation, field trials of resistance management strategies have now become more feasible.

8.2.1. Approaches to resistance management

Ideally insecticide resistance management should be undertaken using insecticide based approaches in conjunction with other non-insecticidal vector control methods, i.e. as part of Integrated Vector Management (IVM[4]) [265]. The insecticides used have to be safe to humans and comply with WHO specifications. In practice, most of IVM programmes work well in experimental trials but become challenging when programmes are scaling up into long-term (operational) control. Operationally, the simplest form of resistance management is likely to be "insecticide" based, and this could take several forms.

Rotations

Rotational strategies are based on the rotation over time of two or preferably more insecticide classes with different modes of action. This approach assumes that if resistance to each insecticide is rare, then multiple resistances will be extremely rare [266]. Rotation allows any resistance developed to the first insecticide to decline over time when the second insecticide class is introduced. As for other strategy, rotations are particularly effective if the resistance gene has an associated fitness cost. The timeframe for rotation needs to be sufficiently short to prevent significant levels of resistance to develop to any one rotation partner. Rotations have been successful in many applications in agriculture and are considered to be effective in slowing the evolution of resistance (see [240] for details). The most striking example of "success story" using this strategy was within the framework of the Onchocerciasis Control Programme (OCP) carried in West Africa 40 years ago. Indeed, weekly application of unrelated larvicides in rivers was successful to kill the larvae of the blackfly vector and mitigate the spread of temephos resistance over the 17 years of its implementation [267]. However, the rotation was introduced at early stage of the OCP, as soon as the operators faced temephos resistance problems in pilot localities. As for all IRM strategies, the status of resistance of the insecticide used in the rotation must be known when implementing rotations and the chemicals used should not present any (known) cross-resistance. For LLIN, it is difficult to implement this method knowing that only pyrethroids are recommended so far by WHO for the impregnation [268]. For IRS, the pragmatic approach would be to rotate insecticides annually. Indeed, changing insecticides more than once a year (which could be the case in areas where two spray rounds are conducted each year) is not recommended, because of procurement and other financial and logistical challenges (see [4]). Despite higher cost of implementing rotation than single spray (as available alternatives to pyrethroids —the carbamates organophosphates, insect growth regulators, pyroles —are currently more expensive), this is probably the price to pay to preserve the arsenal of cost-effective insecticides for malaria vector control.

4*Integrated Vector Management* can be defined as "a rational decision making process for the optimal use of resources for vector control". IRM is therefore an integral part of IVM, as only through the active management of insecticide resistance can the available resources be optimally and sustainably used.

Mosaics

Spatially separated applications of different compounds against the same insect constitute a "mosaic" approach to resistance management [240]. Fine scale mosaics can be achieved in malaria vector control programmes, for example, by using two insecticides in different dwellings within the same village. The aim of this strategy is to preserve susceptibility by spatial restriction of insecticides [4]. If such a fine scale mosaic is to be used, careful records of which insecticide was used in each house are essential. Larger scale mosaics have been shown to be effective for the management of pyrethroid resistance in *An. albimanus* in Mexico [22]. Indeed, pyrethroid resistance rose more rapidly in the areas under pyrethroid treatment alone than in the mosaic areas using OP, Pyrethroid and carbamate [240]. Whilst there are some practical difficulties implementing a mosaic in a vector control programme (eg spray with different insecticides, dosages, apparatus, etc), it may offer the advantages of a mixture strategy with lower insecticide inputs and hence cost. The scale at which a mosaic needs to be applied has not been clearly established. In South Africa for example, different insecticides have been used in different types of houses within the same community and this is considered by some to be a mosaic-like strategy [240]. Similarly, mosquito bed nets from panels treated with different insecticides achieve a similar mosaic effect to treating houses with different compounds but on a much finer scale. Industry has recently developed mosaic LLINs containing a pyrethroid insecticide and a synergist (Piperonyl butoxide or PBO an oxidase inhibitor) on the roof to increase efficacy against pyrethroid-resistant malaria vectors. Small scale field trial [235, 269] and mathematical exercises [270] suggested that mosaic LLIN may provide better insecticidal effect against resistant mosquitoes and enhanced community-level protection against malaria compared to "classical" LLIN in area of pyrethroid resistance. Clearly further operational research is required to establish the applicability and effectiveness of mosaics approaches for malaria control.

Mixtures

A mixture is defined by the simultaneous use of two or more insecticides of unrelated mode of action. If two insecticides A and B, with independent resistance mechanisms, are applied together in a mixture, and if resistance to A and resistance to B are both rare, then we expect doubly resistant insects to be extremely rare, and almost all insects resistant to A will be killed by B, and vice versa [266]. This system of "redundant killing" means that resistance to the two insecticides will evolve much more slowly than if either had been used on its own [271]. This approach may be not successful if resistance to one of the components used is already present at a detectable level and/or if linkage disequilibrium is present in the targeted population [4]. Unlike rotations, the effectiveness of mixtures is not directly related to the degree of fitness cost. Rather the mixture aims to overpower resistance instead of preserving susceptibility. However, for mixtures to work well in practice both insecticides need to be used at their full application rate in order that the efficacy and persistence of the two insecticides would be broadly similar (same decay rate). Further, theoretical models suggest that mixtures might delay resistance longer than rotations or broad mosaics [271, 272]. However, mixtures of products were rarely adopted in malaria vector control programmes on grounds of cost, logistics, and safety issue and because of the limited number of recommended compounds available for both

IRS and LLIN. It is not yet clear however how much the addition of a second active ingredient will add to the total cost of manufacturing since the cost of additional insecticide can greatly vary according to the strategy, ie. cost for LLINs would be much lower than that for IRS. For LLIN, previous laboratory and field trials showed interesting prospects for reducing mosquito survival and biting rates with the use of insecticide mixtures applied on mosquito nets against *kdr*-resistant *An. gambiae* in Africa [273, 274]. Other chemicals, such as insect growth regulators (IGR), represent also promising alternative to be included in mixture formulations as they may impact on mosquito longevity, fertility and fecundity [275, 276]. With the development of next-generation of LLIN, combined use of non-pyrethroids and pyrethroids on bed nets is technically achievable and has the potential to provide better control of malaria and prevent further development of pyrethroid-resistance in malaria vectors. Risk assessment and acceptability of such new tools should be however carefully investigated before any trial being implemented at operational level.

Combinations

In this context, combinations expose the vector population to two vector control tools, such that a mosquito that survives contact with one (e.g. LLIN) is exposed to the other one (e.g. IRS), or vice versa. In practice, exposure to two insecticides is not guaranteed but there is some evidence to indicate that this is likely [277]. The effectiveness of combinations in IRM does not depend on the ability to reduce the level of resistance, but on the ability to kill the vector despite the existence of resistance, through the use of another insecticide or intervention, which compensates for resistance [231]. As for other strategy, the combination should not contain insecticides with same mode of action (e.g. avoid pyrethroids for both IRS and LLINs), as this would increase selection pressure rather than reducing it. As combinations require doubling of interventions, cost would be significantly higher than rotations and mosaics. This might nevertheless be warranted in some circumstances, for example where malaria transmission is very high and/or where targeted IRS can help overcome identified resistance to pyrethroids in areas with high LLIN coverage. In practice, combinations would be more easily implemented in countries having sufficient human and financial resources allocated to public health programmes. So far, a small number of observational studies [278-280] and mathematical modeling exercises [263, 264] suggest that VC combination has an added benefit for reduction of the risk of infection because the people not protected by one of the interventions are protected by the other. A recent cluster randomized controlled trial carried out in Benin showed however that neither clinical malaria in children younger than 6 years nor transmission intensity differ between LLIN and carbamate-IRS or Carbamate Treated Plastic Sheeting and the reference group (LLIN alone) and the insecticide combinations did not slow down the evolution of the *kdr* allele in *An gambiae s.s.* compared with LLIN [231]. It was concluded from this study that IRS should be timely implemented (i.e. using appropriate insecticide, dosage and time interval) to ensure optimum efficacy of the IRS intervention over LLIN. Clearly, cost-effectiveness of combined vector control interventions need to be carefully considered to ensure that increased efforts and cost dedicated to combinations effectively contribute to better control and management of pyrethroid-resistant malaria vectors.

9. Conclusions

Insecticide resistance develops in an insect population when individuals carrying genes that allow them to survive exposure to the insecticide pass these genes on. Thus, any activities that control the individuals with the resistance trait will delay the spread of the resistance genes in the population. IRM should then be seen in the context of IVM and should therefore also include activities such as habitat management, community education, and/or larval source management (e.g. biological control). In order to successfully develop and implement any resistance management strategies based on rotations, mosaics, mixtures or combinations, knowledge of the mode of action, chemical properties, and residual life of the available insecticide products is essential. Although insecticides with novel modes of action have recently been introduced in public health (neonicotinoids, pyroles, oxadiazin, etc) few of them appear to have the optimum biological and/or physical properties required for residual wall spray and/or mosquito net. Unfortunately, the exorbitant costs associated with developing and registering new insecticides (see [281] for details) mean that products appear in the more profitable agricultural markets before consideration is given to their public health potential. We have then no other option than to make an appropriate and judicious use of the current insecticides if we want to avoid any disillusion with pyrethroids as we faced before with DDT or dieldrin. The philosopher George Santayana said *"those who cannot remember the past are condemned to repeat it."* Hope it's not too late for malaria vector control.

Author details

Vincent Corbel[1,2*] and Raphael N'Guessan[3,4]

*Address all correspondence to: vincent.corbel@ird.fr

1 Institut de Recherche pour le Développement, Maladies Infectieuses et Vecteurs, Ecologie, Génétique, Evolution et Contrôle (IRD 224-CNRS 5290 UM1-UM2), Benin

2 Department of Entomology, Kasetsart University, Bangkok, Thailand

3 London School of Hygiene & Tropical Medicine, London, UK

4 Centre de Recherches Entomologiques de Cotonou, Cotonou, Benin

References

[1] World Health Organization: WHO malaria report : 2011. In: *WHO Global Malaria Programme.* Edited by Data WLC-i-P. Geneva: WHO; 2011: 259.

[2] Yassine H, Osta MA: *Anopheles gambiae* innate immunity. *Cell Microbiol,* 12(1):1-9.

[3] Davidson G: Insecticide resistance in *Anopheles sundaicus. Nature* 1957, 180(4598): 1333-1335.

[4] World Health Organization: Global Plan for Insecticide Resistance Management in Malaria Vectors (GPIRM). In: *WHO/HTM/GMP/20125.* Edited by Organization WH. Geneva, Switzerland: World Health Organization; 2012: 130.

[5] Hemingway J, Ranson H: Insecticide resistance in insect vectors of human disease. *Annu Rev Entomol* 2000, 45:371-391.

[6] Ranson H, N'Guessan R, Lines J, Moiroux N, Nkuni Z, Corbel V: Pyrethroid resistance in African anopheline mosquitoes: what are the implications for malaria control? *Trends Parasitol* 2011, 27(2):91-98.

[7] Ridl FC, Bass C, Torrez M, Govender D, Ramdeen V, Yellot L, Edu AE, Schwabe C, Mohloai P, Maharaj R *et al*: A pre-intervention study of malaria vector abundance in Rio Muni, Equatorial Guinea: their role in malaria transmission and the incidence of insecticide resistance alleles. *Malar J* 2008, 7:194.

[8] Sharp BL, Ridl FC, Govender D, Kuklinski J, Kleinschmidt I: Malaria vector control by indoor residual insecticide spraying on the tropical island of Bioko, Equatorial Guinea. *Malar J* 2007, 6:52.

[9] Mitchell SN, Stevenson BJ, Muller P, Wilding CS, Egyir-Yawson A, Field SG, Hemingway J, Paine MJ, Ranson H, Donnelly MJ: Identification and validation of a gene causing cross-resistance between insecticide classes in *Anopheles gambiae* from Ghana. *Proc Natl Acad Sci U S A* 2012, 109(16):6147-6152.

[10] Stevenson BJ, Bibby J, Pignatelli P, Muangnoicharoen S, O'Neill PM, Lian LY, Muller P, Nikou D, Steven A, Hemingway J *et al*: Cytochrome P450 6M2 from the malaria vector *Anopheles gambiae* metabolizes pyrethroids: Sequential metabolism of deltamethrin revealed. *Insect Biochem Mol Biol* 2011, 41(7):492-502.

[11] Brown AWA: Insecticide Resistance Mosquitoes: A Pragmatic Rewiew. *J Am Mosq Control Assoc* 1986, 2(2):123-140.

[12] Metcalf RL: Insect resistance to insecticides. *Pesticide Science* 1989, 26(4):333-358.

[13] WHO: Global Insecticide Use for Vector-Borne Disease Control- 4th edition. *In Edited by World Health Organization Geneva: World Health Organization* 2009, WHO/HTM/NTD/WHOPES/GCDPP/2009.6.

[14] Lapied B, Pennetier C, Apaire-Marchais V, Licznar P, Corbel V: Innovative applications for insect viruses: towards insecticide sensitization. *Trends Biotechnol* 2009, 27(4):190-198.

[15] Livadas GA, Georgopoulos G: Development of resistance to DDT by *Anopheles sacharovi* in Greece. *Bull World Health Organ* 1953, 8(4):497-511.

[16] Brown AWA, Haworth J, Zahar AR: Malaria eradication and control from a global standpoint. *Journal of Medical Entomology* 1976, 13(1):1-25.

[17] Patel TB, Ramachandra Rao T, Halgeri AV, Deobhankar RB: A preliminary note on a probable case of dieldrin kesistance in *Anopheles culicifacies* in Thana District, Bombay State. *Indian J Malariol* 1958, 12:367-370.

[18] Brown AW, Pal R: Insecticide resistance in arthropods. *Public Health Pap* 1971, 38(0): 1-491.

[19] Brown AW, Haworth J, Zahar AR: Malaria eradication and control from a global standpoint. *J Med Entomol* 1976, 13(1):1-25.

[20] Rajagopal R: Malathion resistance in *Anopheles culicifacies* in Gujarat. *Indian J Med Res* 1977, 66(1):27-28.

[21] Rawlings P, Herath PR, Kelly S: *Anopheles culicifacies* (Diptera: Culicidae): DDT resistance in Sri Lanka prior to and after cessation of DDT spraying. *J Med Entomol* 1985, 22(4):361-365.

[22] Penilla RP, Rodriguez AD, Hemingway J, Torres JL, Arredondo Jimenez JI, Rodriguez MH: Resistance management strategies in malaria vector mosquito control. Baseline data for a large-scale field trial against *Anopheles albimanus* in Mexico. *Medical and Veterinary Entomology* 1998, 12(3):217-233.

[23] Van Bortel W, Trung HD, Thuan le K, Sochantha T, Socheat D, Sumrandee C, Baimai V, Keokenchanh K, Samlane P, Roelants P *et al*: The insecticide resistance status of malaria vectors in the Mekong region. *Malar J* 2008, 7:102.

[24] Trung HD, Van Bortel W, Sochantha T, Keokenchanh K, Quang NT, Cong LD, Coosemans M: Malaria transmission and major malaria vectors in different geographical areas of Southeast Asia. *Trop Med Int Health* 2004, 9(2):230-237.

[25] Chareonviriyaphap T, Aum-aung B, Ratanatham S: Current insecticide resistance patterns in mosquito vectors in Thailand. *Southeast Asian J Trop Med Public Health* 1999, 30(1):184-194.

[26] Hamon J, Subra R, Sales S, Coz J: [Presence in the southwestern part of Upper Volta of a population of *Anopheles gambiae* "A" resistant to DDT]. *Med Trop (Mars)* 1968, 28(4):521-528.

[27] Carnevale P, Robert V: *Anopheles*: Biologie, transmission du *Plasmodium* et lutte antivectorielle. Bondy: IRD; 2009.

[28] Chandre F, Darriet F, Manguin S, Brengues C, Carnevale P, Guillet P: Pyrethroid cross resistance spectrum among populations of *Anopheles gambiae* s.s. from Cote d'Ivoire. *J Am Mosq Control Assoc* 1999, 15(1):53-59.

[29] Armstrong JA, Ramsdale CD, Ramakrishna V: Insecticide resistance in *Anopheles gambiae* Giles in Western Sokoto, Northern Nigeria. *Ann Trop Med Parasitol* 1958, 52(3):247-256.

[30] Hamon J, Garrett-Jones C: [Resistance to insecticides in the major malaria vectors and its operational importance]. *Bull World Health Organ* 1963, 28(1):1-24.

[31] Wondji CS, Dabire RK, Tukur Z, Irving H, Djouaka R, Morgan JC: Identification and distribution of a GABA receptor mutation conferring dieldrin resistance in the malaria vector *Anopheles funestus* in Africa. *Insect Biochem Mol Biol* 2011, 41(7):484-491.

[32] Mouchet J: Mini-Review : Agriculture and Vector Resistance. *Insect Sci Applic* 1988, 9(3):291-302.

[33] Mahande AM, Dusfour I, Matias JR, Kweka EJ: Knockdown Resistance, rdl Alleles, and the Annual Entomological Inoculation Rate of Wild Mosquito Populations from Lower Moshi, Northern Tanzania. *J Glob Infect Dis* 2012, 4(2):114-119.

[34] Brogdon WG, McAllister JC, Corwin AM, Cordon Rosales C: Oxidase-based DDT-pyrethroid cross-resistance in Guatemalan *Anopheles albimanus*. *Pesticide Biochemistry and Physiology* 1999, 64(2):101-111.

[35] Fonseca-Gonzalez I, Quinones ML, McAllister J, Brogdon WG: Mixed-function oxidases and esterases associated with cross-resistance between DDT and lambda-cyhalothrin in *Anopheles darlingi* Root 1926 populations from Colombia. *Mem Inst Oswaldo Cruz* 2009, 104(1):18-26.

[36] Raghavendra K, Verma V, Srivastava HC, Gunasekaran K, Sreehari U, Dash AP: Persistence of DDT, malathion & deltamethrin resistance in *Anopheles culicifacies* after their sequential withdrawal from indoor residual spraying in Surat district, India. *Indian J Med Res* 2010, 132:260-264.

[37] Tiwari S, Ghosh SK, Ojha VP, Dash AP, Raghavendra K: Reduced susceptibility to selected synthetic pyrethroids in urban malaria vector *Anopheles stephensi*: a case study in Mangalore city, South India. *Malar J* 2010, 9:179.

[38] Elissa N, Mouchet J, Riviere F, Meunier JY, Yao K: Resistance of *Anopheles gambiae* s.s. to pyrethroids in Cote d'Ivoire. *Ann Soc Belg Med Trop* 1993, 73(4):291-294.

[39] Hargreaves K, Koekemoer LL, Brooke BD, Hunt RH, Mthembu J, Coetzee M: *Anopheles funestus* resistant to pyrethroid insecticides in South Africa. *Medical and Veterinary Entomology* 2000, 14(2):181-189.

[40] Chareonviriyaphap T, Rongnoparut P, Juntarumporn P: Selection for pyrethroid resistance in a colony of *Anopheles minimus* species A, a malaria vector in Thailand. *J Vector Ecol* 2002, 27(2):222-229.

[41] Ayad H, Georghiou GP: Resistance to organophosphates and carbamates in *Anophe-les albimanus* based on reduced sensitivity of acetylcholinesterase. *Journal of Economic Entomology* 1975, 68(3):295-297.

[42] Hemingway J: Genetics of organophosphate and carbamate resistance in *Anopheles atroparvus* (Diptera: Culicidae). *J Econ Entomol* 1982, 75(6):1055-1058.

[43] Elissa N, Mouchet J, Riviere F, Meunier JY, Yao K: [Susceptibility of *Anopheles gambiae* to insecticides in the Ivory Coast]. *Sante* 1994, 4(2):95-99.

[44] N'Guessan R, Darriet F, Guillet P, Carnevale P, Traore-Lamizana M, Corbel V, Koffi AA, Chandre F: Resistance to carbosulfan in *Anopheles gambiae* from Ivory Coast, based on reduced sensitivity of acetylcholinesterase. *Med Vet Entomol* 2003, 17(1): 19-25.

[45] Dabire KR, Diabate A, Namontougou M, Djogbenou L, Kengne P, Simard F, Bass C, Baldet T: Distribution of insensitive acetylcholinesterase (ace-1R) in *Anopheles gambiae* s.l. populations from Burkina Faso (West Africa). *Trop Med Int Health* 2009, 14(4): 396-403.

[46] Djogbenou L, Dabire R, Diabate A, Kengne P, Akogbeto M, Hougard JM, Chandre F: Identification and geographic distribution of the ACE-1R mutation in the malaria vector *Anopheles gambiae* in south-western Burkina Faso, West Africa. *Am J Trop Med Hyg* 2008, 78(2):298-302.

[47] Djogbenou L, Pasteur N, Akogbeto M, Weill M, Chandre F: Insecticide resistance in the *Anopheles gambiae* complex in Benin: a nationwide survey. *Med Vet Entomol* 2011, 25(3):256-267.

[48] Oduola AO, Idowu ET, Oyebola MK, Adeogun AO, Olojede JB, Otubanjo OA, Awo-lola TS: Evidence of carbamate resistance in urban populations of *Anopheles gambiae* s.s. mosquitoes resistant to DDT and deltamethrin insecticides in Lagos, South-West-ern Nigeria. *Parasit Vectors* 2012, 5:116.

[49] USAID: The President's Malaria Initiative: fourth annual report. In. Washigton: U.S. Agency for International Development; 2010.

[50] Nkya TE, Akhouayri I, Kisinza W, David JP: Impact of environment on mosquito re-sponse to pyrethroid insecticides: Facts, evidences and prospects. *Insect Biochem Mol Biol* 2012.

[51] Despres L, David JP, Gallet C: The evolutionary ecology of insect resistance to plant chemicals. *Trends Ecol Evol* 2007, 22(6):298-307.

[52] Hemingway J, Hawkes NJ, McCarroll L, Ranson H: The molecular basis of insecticide resistance in mosquitoes. *Insect Biochem Mol Biol* 2004, 34(7):653-665.

[53] Guillemaud T, Makate N, Raymond M, Hirst B, Callaghan A: Esterase gene amplifi-cation in *Culex pipiens*. *Insect Molecular Biology* 1997, 6(4):319-327.

[54] Hawkes NJ, Hemingway J: Analysis of the promoters for the beta-esterase genes associated with insecticide resistance in the mosquito *Culex quinquefasciatus*. *Biochim Biophys Acta* 2002, 1574(1):51-62.

[55] Vaughan A, Hawkes N, Hemingway J: Co-amplification explains linkage disequilibrium of two mosquito esterase genes in insecticide-resistant *Culex quinquefasciatus*. *Biochem J* 1997, 325 (Pt 2):359-365.

[56] Herath PR, Miles SJ, Davidson G: Fenitrothion (OMS 43) resistance in the taxon *Anopheles culicifacies* Giles. *J Trop Med Hyg* 1981, 84(2):87-88.

[57] Hemingway J: The genetics of malathion resistance in *Anopheles stephensi* from Pakistan. *Trans R Soc Trop Med Hyg* 1983, 77(1):106-108.

[58] Vontas J, Blass C, Koutsos AC, David JP, Kafatos FC, Louis C, Hemingway J, Christophides GK, Ranson H: Gene expression in insecticide resistant and susceptible *Anopheles gambiae* strains constitutively or after insecticide exposure. *Insect Mol Biol* 2005, 14(5):509-521.

[59] Somwang P, Yanola J, Suwan W, Walton C, Lumjuan N, Prapanthadara LA, Somboon P: Enzymes-based resistant mechanism in pyrethroid resistant and susceptible *Aedes aegypti* strains from northern Thailand. *Parasitol Res* 2011, 109(3):531-537.

[60] Feyereisen R, Lawrence IG, Kostas I, Sarjeet SG: Insect Cytochrome P450. In: *Comprehensive Molecular Insect Science*. Amsterdam: Elsevier; 2005: 1-77.

[61] Holt RA, Subramanian GM, Halpern A, Sutton GG, Charlab R, Nusskern DR, Wincker P, Clark AG, Ribeiro JM, Wides R *et al*: The genome sequence of the malaria mosquito *Anopheles gambiae*. *Science* 2002, 298(5591):129-149.

[62] Ranson H, Nikou D, Hutchinson M, Wang X, Roth CW, Hemingway J, Collins FH: Molecular analysis of multiple cytochrome P450 genes from the malaria vector, *Anopheles gambiae*. *Insect Mol Biol* 2002, 11(5):409-418.

[63] Nikou D, Ranson H, Hemingway J: An adult-specific CYP6 P450 gene is overexpressed in a pyrethroid-resistant strain of the malaria vector, *Anopheles gambiae*. *Gene* 2003, 318:91-102.

[64] David JP, Strode C, Vontas J, Nikou D, Vaughan A, Pignatelli PM, Louis C, Hemingway J, Ranson H: The *Anopheles gambiae* detoxification chip: a highly specific microarray to study metabolic-based insecticide resistance in malaria vectors. *Proc Natl Acad Sci U S A* 2005, 102(11):4080-4084.

[65] Irving H, Riveron JM, Ibrahim SS, Lobo NF, Wondji CS: Positional cloning of rp2 QTL associates the P450 genes CYP6Z1, CYP6Z3 and CYP6M7 with pyrethroid resistance in the malaria vector *Anopheles funestus*. *Heredity (Edinb)* 2012, 109(6):383-392.

[66] Chiu TL, Wen Z, Rupasinghe SG, Schuler MA: Comparative molecular modeling of *Anopheles gambiae* CYP6Z1, a mosquito P450 capable of metabolizing DDT. *Proc Natl Acad Sci U S A* 2008, 105(26):8855-8860.

[67] McLaughlin LA, Niazi U, Bibby J, David JP, Vontas J, Hemingway J, Ranson H, Sutcliffe MJ, Paine MJ: Characterization of inhibitors and substrates of *Anopheles gambiae* CYP6Z2. *Insect Mol Biol* 2008, 17(2):125-135.

[68] Muller P, Chouaibou M, Pignatelli P, Etang J, Walker ED, Donnelly MJ, Simard F, Ranson H: Pyrethroid tolerance is associated with elevated expression of antioxidants and agricultural practice in *Anopheles arabiensis* sampled from an area of cotton fields in Northern Cameroon. *Mol Ecol* 2008, 17(4):1145-1155.

[69] Djouaka RF, Bakare AA, Coulibaly ON, Akogbeto MC, Ranson H, Hemingway J, Strode C: Expression of the cytochrome P450s, CYP6P3 and CYP6M2 are significantly elevated in multiple pyrethroid resistant populations of *Anopheles gambiae* s.s. from Southern Benin and Nigeria. *BMC Genomics* 2008, 9:538.

[70] Muller P, Donnelly MJ, Ranson H: Transcription profiling of a recently colonised pyrethroid resistant *Anopheles gambiae* strain from Ghana. *BMC Genomics* 2007, 8:36.

[71] Muller P, Warr E, Stevenson BJ, Pignatelli PM, Morgan JC, Steven A, Yawson AE, Mitchell SN, Ranson H, Hemingway J *et al*: Field-caught permethrin-resistant *Anopheles gambiae* overexpress CYP6P3, a P450 that metabolises pyrethroids. *PLoS Genet* 2008, 4(11):e1000286.

[72] Wondji CS, Irving H, Morgan J, Lobo NF, Collins FH, Hunt RH, Coetzee M, Hemingway J, Ranson H: Two duplicated P450 genes are associated with pyrethroid resistance in *Anopheles funestus*, a major malaria vector. *Genome Res* 2009, 19(3):452-459.

[73] Wondji CS, Morgan J, Coetzee M, Hunt RH, Steen K, Black WCt, Hemingway J, Ranson H: Mapping a quantitative trait locus (QTL) conferring pyrethroid resistance in the African malaria vector *Anopheles funestus*. *BMC Genomics* 2007, 8:34.

[74] Riveron JM, Irving H, Ndula M, Barnes KG, Ibrahim SS, Paine MJ, Wondji CS: Directionally selected cytochrome P450 alleles are driving the spread of pyrethroid resistance in the major malaria vector *Anopheles funestus*. *Proc Natl Acad Sci U S A* 2012, 110(1):252-257.

[75] Rongnoparut P, Boonsuepsakul S, Chareonviriyaphap T, Thanomsing N: Cloning of cytochrome P450, CYP6P5, and CYP6AA2 from *Anopheles minimus* resistant to deltamethrin. *J Vector Ecol* 2003, 28(2):150-158.

[76] Duangkaew P, Kaewpa D, Rongnoparut P: Protective efficacy of *Anopheles minimus* CYP6P7 and CYP6AA3 against cytotoxicity of pyrethroid insecticides in *Spodoptera frugiperda* (Sf9) insect cells. *Trop Biomed* 2011, 28(2):293-301.

[77] Duangkaew P, Pethuan S, Kaewpa D, Boonsuepsakul S, Sarapusit S, Rongnoparut P: Characterization of mosquito CYP6P7 and CYP6AA3: differences in substrate preference and kinetic properties. *Arch Insect Biochem Physiol* 2011, 76(4):236-248.

[78] Ranson H, Cornel AJ, Fournier D, Vaughan A, Collins FH, Hemingway J: Cloning and Localization of a Glutathione S-transferase Class I Gene from *Anopheles gambiae*. *J Biol Chem* 1997, 272(9):5464-5967.

[79] Ranson H, Hemingway J: Mosquito glutathione transferases. *Methods Enzymol* 2005, 401:226-241.

[80] Fournier D, Bride JM, Poirie M, Berge JB, Plapp FW, Jr.: Insect glutathione S-transferases. Biochemical characteristics of the major forms from houseflies susceptible and resistant to insecticides. *Journal of Biological Chemistry* 1992, 267(3):1840-1845.

[81] Ranson H, Rossiter L, Ortelli F, Jensen B, Wang XL, Roth CW, Collins FH, Hemingway J: Identification of a novel class of insect glutathione S-transferases involved in resistance to DDT in the malaria vector *Anopheles gambiae*. *Biochemical Journal* 2001, 359 Part 2:295-304.

[82] Gunasekaran K, Muthukumaravel S, Sahu SS, Vijayakumar T, Jambulingam P: Glutathione S transferase activity in Indian vectors of malaria: A defense mechanism against DDT. *J Med Entomol* 2011, 48(3):561-569.

[83] Prapanthadara LA, Ketterman AJ: Qualitative and quantitative changes in glutathione S-transferases in the mosquito *Anopheles gambiae* confer DDT-resistance. *Biochem Soc Trans* 1993, 21 (Pt 3)(3):304S.

[84] Ranson H, Jensen B, Wang X, Prapanthadara L, Hemingway J, Collins FH: Genetic mapping of two loci affecting DDT resistance in the malaria vector *Anopheles gambiae*. *Insect Mol Biol* 2000, 9(5):499-507.

[85] Vontas JG, Small GJ, Hemingway J: Glutathione S-transferases as antioxidant defence agents confer pyrethroid resistance in *Nilaparvata lugens*. *Biochem J* 2001, 357(Pt 1): 65-72.

[86] Kostaropoulos I, Papadopoulos AI, Metaxakis A, Boukouvala E, Papadopoulou-Mourkidou E: Glutathione S-transferase in the defence against pyrethroids in insects. *Insect Biochem Mol Biol* 2001, 31(4-5):313-319.

[87] Fournier D: Mutations of acetylcholinesterase which confer insecticide resistance in insect populations. *Chem Biol Interact* 2005.

[88] Weill M, Lutfalla G, Mogensen K, Chandre F, Berthomieu A, Berticat C, Pasteur N, Philips A, Fort P, Raymond M: Comparative genomics: Insecticide resistance in mosquito vectors. *Nature* 2003, 423(6936):136-137.

[89] Alout H, Labbe P, Berthomieu A, Pasteur N, Weill M: Multiple duplications of the rare ace-1 mutation F290V in *Culex pipiens* natural populations. *Insect Biochem Mol Biol* 2009.

[90] Weill M, Malcolm C, Chandre F, Mogensen K, Berthomieu A, Marquine M, Raymond M: The unique mutation in ace-1 giving high insecticide resistance is easily detectable in mosquito vectors. *Insect Mol Biol* 2004, 13(1):1-7.

[91] Djogbenou L, Chandre F, Berthomieu A, Dabire R, Koffi A, Alout H, Weill M: Evidence of introgression of the ace-1(R) mutation and of the ace-1 duplication in West African *Anopheles gambiae* s. s. *PLoS ONE* 2008, 3(5):e2172.

[92] Ffrench-Constant RH: The molecular and population genetics of cyclodiene insecticide resistance. *Insect Biochem Mol Biol* 1994, 24(4):335-345.

[93] Andreasen MH, Ffrench-Constant RH: In situ hybridization to the Rdl locus on polytene chromosome 3L of *Anopheles stephensi*. *Med Vet Entomol* 2002, 16(4):452-455.

[94] Du W, Awolola TS, Howell P, Koekemoer LL, Brooke BD, Benedict MQ, Coetzee M, Zheng L: Independent mutations in the Rdl locus confer dieldrin resistance to *Anopheles gambiae* and *An. arabiensis*. *Insect Mol Biol* 2005, 14(2):179-183.

[95] Davies TG, Field LM, Usherwood PN, Williamson MS: DDT, pyrethrins, pyrethroids and insect sodium channels. *IUBMB Life* 2007, 59(3):151-162.

[96] Donnelly MJ, Corbel V, Weetman D, Wilding CS, Williamson MS, Black WCt: Does *kdr* genotype predict insecticide-resistance phenotype in mosquitoes? *Trends Parasitol* 2009, 25(5):213-219.

[97] Martinez Torres D, Chandre F, Williamson MS, Darriet F, Berge JB, Devonshire AL, Guillet P, Pasteur N, Pauron D: Molecular characterization of pyrethroid knockdown resistance (*kdr*) in the major malaria vector *Anopheles gambiae* s.s. *Insect Molecular Biology* 1998, 7(2):179-184.

[98] Ranson H, Jensen B, Vulule JM, Wang X, Hemingway J, Collins FH: Identification of a point mutation in the voltage-gated sodium channel gene of Kenyan *Anopheles gambiae* associated with resistance to DDT and pyrethroids. *Insect Molecular Biology* 2000, 9(5):491-497.

[99] O'Reilly AO, Khambay BP, Williamson MS, Field LM, Wallace BA, Davies TG: Modelling insecticide-binding sites in the voltage-gated sodium channel. *Biochem J* 2006, 396(2):255-263.

[100] Jones CM, Liyanapathirana M, Agossa FR, Weetman D, Ranson H, Donnelly MJ, Wilding CS: Footprints of positive selection associated with a mutation (N1575Y) in the voltage-gated sodium channel of *Anopheles gambiae*. *Proc Natl Acad Sci U S A* 2012, 109(17):6614-6619.

[101] Plapp FW, Jr.: The genetic basis of insecticide resistance in the house fly: evidence that a single locus plays a major role in metabolic resistance to insecticides. *Pesticide Biochemistry and Physiology* 1984, 22(2):194-201.

[102] Georghiou GP, Ariaratnam V, Pasternak ME, Lin CS: Organophosphorus multiresistance in *Culex pipiens quinquefasciatus* in California. *Journal of Economic Entomology* 1975, 68(4):461-467.

[103] Vontas J, David JP, Nikou D, Hemingway J, Christophides GK, Louis C, Ranson H: Transcriptional analysis of insecticide resistance in *Anopheles stephensi* using cross-species microarray hybridization. *Insect Mol Biol* 2007, 16(3):315-324.

[104] Awolola TS, Oduola OA, Strode C, Koekemoer LL, Brooke B, Ranson H: Evidence of multiple pyrethroid resistance mechanisms in the malaria vector *Anopheles gambiae* sensu stricto from Nigeria. *Trans R Soc Trop Med Hyg* 2009, 103(11):1139-1145.

[105] Wood O, Hanrahan S, Coetzee M, Koekemoer L, Brooke B: Cuticle thickening associated with pyrethroid resistance in the major malaria vector *Anopheles funestus*. *Parasit Vectors* 2010, 3:67.

[106] Roberts DR, Chareonviriyaphap T, Harlan HH, Hshieh P: Methods of testing and analyzing excito-repellency responses of malaria vectors to insecticides. *J Am Mosq Control Assoc* 1997, 13(1):13-17.

[107] Chandre F, Darriet F, Duchon S, Finot L, Manguin S, Carnevale P, Guillet P: Modifications of pyrethroid effects associated with *kdr* mutation in *Anopheles gambiae*. *Medical and Veterinary Entomology* 2000, 14(1):81-88.

[108] Gahan JB, Lindquist AW: DDT residual sprays applied in buildings to control *Anopheles quadrimaculatus*. *Journal of Economic Entomology* 1945, 38 (2):223-230.

[109] Chareonviriyaphap T, Roberts DR, Andre RG, Harlan HJ, Manguin S, Bangs MJ: Pesticide avoidance behavior in *Anopheles albimanus*, a malaria vector in the Americas. *J Am Mosq Control Assoc* 1997, 13(2):171-183.

[110] Garros C, Marchand RP, Quang NT, Hai NS, Manguin S: First record of *Anopheles minimus* C and significant decrease of *An. minimus* A in central Vietnam. *J Am Mosq Control Assoc* 2005, 21(2):139-143.

[111] Russell TL, Govella NJ, Azizi S, Drakeley CJ, Kachur SP, Killeen GF: Increased proportions of outdoor feeding among residual malaria vector populations following increased use of insecticide-treated nets in rural Tanzania. *Malar J* 2011, 10:80.

[112] Moiroux N, Gomez MB, Pennetier C, Elanga E, Djenontin A, Chandre F, Djegbe I, Guis H, Corbel V: Changes in *Anopheles funestus* Biting Behavior Following Universal Coverage of Long-Lasting Insecticidal Nets in Benin. *J Infect Dis* 2012, 206(10): 1622-1629.

[113] WHO: Guidelines for testing mosquito adulticides intended for Indoor Residual Spraying (IRS) and Insecticide Treated Nets (ITNs). 2006, WHO/CDS/NTD/WHOPES/GCDDP/2006.3.

[114] WHO: Report of the WHO Informal Consultation Tests procedures for insecticide resistance monitoring in malaria vectors, bio-efficacy and persistence of insecticides on treated surfaces. In. Geneva: World Health Organization: Parasitic Diseases and Vector Control (PVC)/Communicable Disease Control, Prevention and Eradication (CPE); 1998: 43.

[115] Williams J, Pinto J: Training Manual on Malaria Entomology; For Entomology and Vector Control Technicians (Basic Level) In. Edited by USAID. Washington, D.C.; 2012: 78.

[116] Ranson H, Abdallah H, Badolo A, Guelbeogo WM, Kerah-Hinzoumbe C, Yangalbe-Kalnone E, Sagnon N, Simard F, Coetzee M: Insecticide resistance in *Anopheles gambiae*: data from the first year of a multi-country study highlight the extent of the problem. *Malar J* 2009, 8(1):299.

[117] Skovmand O, Bonnet J, Pigeon O, Corbel V: Median knock-down time as a new method for evaluating insecticide-treated textiles for mosquito control. *Malar J* 2008, 7:114.

[118] Brogdon WG, McAllister JC: Simplification of adult mosquito bioassays through use of time-mortality determinations in glass bottles. *J Am Mosq Control Assoc* 1998, 14(2): 159-164.

[119] World Health Organization: Techniques to detect insecticide resistance mechanisms (field and laboratory manual). In. Edited by WHO/CDS/CPC/MAL/98.6 WHO. Geneva: World Health Organization; 1998.

[120] Munhenga G, Masendu HT, Brooke BD, Hunt RH, Koekemoer LK: Pyrethroid resistance in the major malaria vector *Anopheles arabiensis* from Gwave, a malaria-endemic area in Zimbabwe. *Malar J* 2008, 7:247.

[121] Okoye PN, Brooke BD, Koekemoer LL, Hunt RH, Coetzee M: Characterisation of DDT, pyrethroid and carbamate resistance in *Anopheles funestus* from Obuasi, Ghana. *Trans R Soc Trop Med Hyg* 2008, 102(6):591-598.

[122] Kelly-Hope L, Ranson H, Hemingway J: Lessons from the past: managing insecticide resistance in malaria control and eradication programmes. *Lancet Infect Dis* 2008.

[123] Chouaibou M, Etang J, Brevault T, Nwane P, Hinzoumbe CK, Mimpfoundi R, Simard F: Dynamics of insecticide resistance in the malaria vector *Anopheles gambiae* s.l. from an area of extensive cotton cultivation in Northern Cameroon. *Trop Med Int Health* 2008, 13(4):476-486.

[124] Djegbe I, Boussari O, Sidick A, Martin T, Ranson H, Chandre F, Akogbeto M, Corbel V: Dynamics of insecticide resistance in malaria vectors in Benin: first evidence of the

presence of L1014S *kdr* mutation in *Anopheles gambiae* from West Africa. *Malaria Journal* 2011, 10(1):261.

[125] Dabire KR, Diabate A, Pare-Toe L, Rouamba J, Ouari A, Fontenille D, Baldet T: Year to year and seasonal variations in vector bionomics and malaria transmission in a humid savannah village in west Burkina Faso. *J Vector Ecol* 2008, 33(1):70-75.

[126] Bass C, Nikou D, Donnelly MJ, Williamson MS, Ranson H, Ball A, Vontas J, Field LM: Detection of knockdown resistance (*kdr*) mutations in *Anopheles gambiae*: a comparison of two new high-throughput assays with existing methods. *Malar J* 2007, 6:111.

[127] Corbel V, N'Guessan R, Brengues C, Chandre F, Djogbenou L, Martin T, Akogbeto M, Hougard JM, Rowland M: Multiple insecticide resistance mechanisms in *Anopheles gambiae* and *Culex quinquefasciatus* from Benin, West Africa. *Acta Trop* 2007, 101(3): 207-216.

[128] Diabate A: The Role of Agricultural Uses of Insecticides in Resistance to Pyrethroids in *Anopheles gambiae* S.L. in Burkina Faso. *Am J Trop Med Hyg* 2002, 67(6):617-622.

[129] Carnevale P, Toto JC, Guibert P, Keita M, Manguin S: Entomological survey and report of a knockdown resistance mutation in the malaria vector *Anopheles gambiae* from the Republic of Guinea. *Trans R Soc Trop Med Hyg*, 104(7):484-489.

[130] Yawson AE, McCall PJ, Wilson MD, Donnelly MJ: Species abundance and insecticide resistance of *Anopheles gambiae* in selected areas of Ghana and Burkina Faso. *Med Vet Entomol* 2004, 18(4):372-377.

[131] C. Fanello VP, A. della Torre, F. Santolamazza, G. Dolo, M. Coulibaly, A. Alloueche, C. F. Curtis, Y. T. Touré and M. Coluzzi: The pyrethroid knock-down resistance gene in the *Anopheles gambiae* complex in Mali and further indication of incipient speciation within *An. gambiae* s.s. *Insect Molecular Biology* 2003, 12(3):241-245.

[132] Czeher C, Labbo R, Arzika I, Duchemin J-B: Evidence of increasing Leu-Phe knockdown resistance mutation in *Anopheles gambiae* from Niger following a nationwide long-lasting insecticide-treated nets implementation. *Malaria Journal* 2008, 7(1):189.

[133] Awolola TS, Brooke BD, Hunt RH, Coetze M: Resistance of the malaria vector *Anopheles gambiae* s.s. to pyrethroid insecticides, in south-western Nigeria. *Annals of Tropical Medicine and Parasitology* 2002, 96(8):849-852.

[134] Koffi AA, Alou LP, Adja MA, Kone M, Chandre F, N'Guessan R: Update on resistance status of *Anopheles gambiae* s.s. to conventional insecticides at a previous WHOPES field site, "Yaokoffikro", 6 years after the political crisis in Cote d'Ivoire. *Parasit Vectors* 2012, 5:68.

[135] Dabire KR, Diabate A, Agostinho F, Alves F, Manga L, Faye O, Baldet T: Distribution of the members of *Anopheles gambiae* and pyrethroid knock-down resistance gene (*kdr*) in Guinea-Bissau, West Africa. *Bull Soc Pathol Exot* 2008, 101(2):119-123.

[136] Etang J, Fondjo E, Chandre F, Morlais I, Brengues C, Nwane P, Chouaibou M, Ndjemai H, Simard F: First report of knockdown mutations in the malaria vector *Anopheles gambiae* from Cameroon. *Am J Trop Med Hyg* 2006, 74(5):795-797.

[137] Ndjemai HN, Patchoke S, Atangana J, Etang J, Simard F, Bilong CF, Reimer L, Cornel
A, Lanzaro GC, Fondjo E: The distribution of insecticide resistance in *Anopheles gambiae* s.l. populations from Cameroon: an update. *Trans R Soc Trop Med Hyg* 2009.

[138] Nwane P, Etang J, Chouaibou M, Toto JC, Kerah-Hinzoumbe C, Mimpfoundi R,
Awono-Ambene HP, Simard F: Trends in DDT and pyrethroid resistance in *Anopheles gambiae* s.s. populations from urban and agro-industrial settings in southern Cameroon. *BMC Infect Dis* 2009, 9:163.

[139] Kerah-Hinzoumbe C, Peka M, Nwane P, Donan-Gouni I, Etang J, Same-Ekobo A, Simard F: Insecticide resistance in *Anopheles gambiae* from south-western Chad, Central
Africa. *Malar J* 2008, 7:192.

[140] Janeira F, Vicente JL, Kanganje Y, Moreno M, Do Rosario VE, Cravo P, Pinto J: A pri-
mer-introduced restriction analysis-polymerase chain reaction method to detect
knockdown resistance mutations in *Anopheles gambiae*. *J Med Entomol* 2008, 45(2):
237-241.

[141] Mourou JR, Coffinet T, Jarjaval F, Pradines B, Amalvict R, Rogier C, Kombila M, Pages F: Malaria transmission and insecticide resistance of *Anopheles gambiae* in Libreville and Port-Gentil, Gabon. *Malar J* 2010, 9:321.

[142] Himeidan YE, Chen H, Chandre F, Donnelly MJ, Yan G: Short report: permethrin
and DDT resistance in the malaria vector *Anopheles arabiensis* from eastern Sudan. *Am
J Trop Med Hyg* 2007, 77(6):1066-1068.

[143] Abdalla H, Matambo TS, Koekemoer LL, Mnzava AP, Hunt RH, Coetzee M: Insecticide susceptibility and vector status of natural populations of *Anopheles arabiensis*
from Sudan. *Transactions of the Royal Society of Tropical Medicine and Hygiene* 2008,
102(3):263-271.

[144] Costantini C, Ayala D, Guelbeogo WM, Pombi M, Some CY, Bassole IH, Ose K, Fots-
ing JM, Sagnon N, Fontenille D *et al*: Living at the edge: biogeographic patterns of
habitat segregation conform to speciation by niche expansion in *Anopheles gambiae*.
BMC Ecol 2009, 9(1):16.

[145] Kulkarni MA, Malima R, Mosha FW, Msangi S, Mrema E, Kabula B, Lawrence B, Ki-
nung'hi S, Swilla J, Kisinza W *et al*: Efficacy of pyrethroid-treated nets against malaria
vectors and nuisance-biting mosquitoes in Tanzania in areas with long-term insecticide-treated net use. *Trop Med Int Health* 2007, 12(9):1061-1073.

[146] Kabula B, Tungu P, Matowo J, Kitau J, Mweya C, Emidi B, Masue D, Sindato C, Malima R, Minja J *et al*: Susceptibility status of malaria vectors to insecticides commonly
used for malaria control in Tanzania. *Trop Med Int Health* 2012, 17(6):742-750.

[147] Coleman M, Casimiro S, Hemingway J, Sharp B: Operational impact of DDT reintro-
       duction for malaria control on *Anopheles arabiensis* in Mozambique. *J Med Entomol*
       2008, 45(5):885-890.

[148] Ratovonjato J, Le Goff G, Rajaonarivelo E, Rakotondraibe EM, Robert V: [Recent ob-
       servations on the sensitivity to pyrethroids and DDT of *Anopheles arabiensis* and
       Anopheles funestus in the central Highlands of Madagascar; preliminary results on the
       absence of the *kdr* mutation in *An. arabiensis*]. *Arch Inst Pasteur Madagascar* 2003,
       69(1-2):63-69.

[149] Ramphul U, Boase T, Bass C, Okedi LM, Donnelly MJ, Muller P: Insecticide resist-
       ance and its association with target-site mutations in natural populations of *Anopheles
       gambiae* from eastern Uganda. *Trans R Soc Trop Med Hyg* 2009.

[150] Verhaeghen K, Bortel WV, Roelants P, Okello PE, Talisuna A, Coosemans M: Spatio-
       temporal patterns in *kdr* frequency in permethrin and DDT resistant *Anopheles gam-
       biae* s.s. from Uganda. *Am J Trop Med Hyg* 2010, 82(4):566-573.

[151] Abate A, Hadis M: Susceptibility of *Anopheles gambiae* s.l. to DDT, malathion, perme-
       thrin and deltamethrin in Ethiopia. *Trop Med Int Health* 2011, 16(4):486-491.

[152] Ochomo E, Bayoh MN, Brogdon WG, Gimnig JE, Ouma C, Vulule JM, Walker ED:
       Pyrethroid resistance in *Anopheles gambiae* s.s. and *Anopheles arabiensis* in western
       Kenya: phenotypic, metabolic and target site characterizations of three populations.
       Med Vet Entomol 2012.

[153] Mathias DK, Ochomo E, Atieli F, Ombok M, Bayoh MN, Olang G, Muhia D, Kamau
       L, Vulule JM, Hamel MJ *et al*: Spatial and temporal variation in the *kdr* allele L1014S
       in *Anopheles gambiae* s.s. and phenotypic variability in susceptibility to insecticides in
       Western Kenya. *Malar J* 2011, 10:10.

[154] Chanda E, Hemingway J, Kleinschmidt I, Rehman AM, Ramdeen V, Phiri FN, Coet-
       zer S, Mthembu D, Shinondo CJ, Chizema-Kawesha E *et al*: Insecticide resistance and
       the future of malaria control in Zambia. *PLoS ONE* 2011, 6(9):e24336.

[155] Mouatcho JC, Munhenga G, Hargreaves K, Brooke BD, Coetzee M, Koekemoer LL:
       Pyrethroid resistance in a major African malaria vector *Anopheles arabiensis* from
       Mamfene, northern KwaZulu-Natal, South Africa. *South African Journal of Science*
       2009, 105(3-4):127-131.

[156] Mouatcho JC, Hargreaves K, Koekemoer LL, Brooke BD, Oliver SV, Hunt RH, Coet-
       zee M: Indoor collections of the *Anopheles funestus* group (Diptera: Culicidae) in
       sprayed houses in northern KwaZulu-Natal, South Africa. *Malar J* 2007, 6:30.

[157] Brooke BD, Kloke G, Hunt RH, Koekemoer LL, Temu EA, Taylor ME, Small G, Hem-
       ingway J, Coetzee M: Bioassay and biochemical analyses of insecticide resistance in
       southern African *Anopheles funestus* (Diptera: Culicidae). *Bulletin of Entomological Re-
       search* 2001, 91(4):265-272.

[158] Cuamba N, Morgan JC, Irving H, Steven A, Wondji CS: High level of pyrethroid resistance in an *Anopheles funestus* population of the Chokwe District in Mozambique. *PLoS ONE* 2010, 5(6):e11010.

[159] Kloke RG, Nhamahanga E, Hunt RH, Coetzee M: Vectorial status and insecticide resistance of *Anopheles funestus* from a sugar estate in southern Mozambique. *Parasit Vectors* 2011, 4:16.

[160] Hunt R, Edwardes M, Coetzee M: Pyrethroid resistance in southern African *Anopheles funestus* extends to Likoma Island in Lake Malawi. *Parasit Vectors* 2010, 3:122.

[161] Wondji CS, Coleman M, Kleinschmidt I, Mzilahowa T, Irving H, Ndula M, Rehman A, Morgan J, Barnes KG, Hemingway J: Impact of pyrethroid resistance on operational malaria control in Malawi. *Proc Natl Acad Sci U S A* 2012, 109(47):19063-19070.

[162] Anto F, Asoala V, Anyorigiya T, Oduro A, Adjuik M, Owusu-Agyei S, Dery D, Bimi L, Hodgson A: Insecticide resistance profiles for malaria vectors in the Kassena-Nankana district of Ghana. *Malaria Journal* 2009, 8(1):81.

[163] Djouaka R, Irving H, Tukur Z, Wondji CS: Exploring mechanisms of multiple insecticide resistance in a population of the malaria vector *Anopheles funestus* in Benin. *PLoS ONE* 2011, 6(11):e27760.

[164] Dabire KR, Baldet T, Diabate A, Dia I, Costantini C, Cohuet A, Guiguemde TR, Fontenille D: *Anopheles funestus* (Diptera: Culicidae) in a humid savannah area of western Burkina Faso: bionomics, insecticide resistance status, and role in malaria transmission. *J Med Entomol* 2007, 44(6):990-997.

[165] Faraj C, Adlaoui E, Brengues C, Fontenille D, Lyagoubi M: [Resistance of *Anopheles labranchiae* to DDT in Morocco: identification of the mechanisms and choice of replacement insecticide]. *Eastern Mediterranean health journal = La revue de sante de la Mediterranee orientale = al-Majallah al-sihhiyah li-sharq al-mutawassit* 2008, 14(4):776-783.

[166] Mostafa AA, Allam KA: Studies on the present status of insecticides resistance on mosquitoes using the diagnostic dosages in El-Fayium Governorate, a spot area of malaria in Egypt. *J Egypt Soc Parasitol* 2001, 31(1):177-186.

[167] Balkew M, Elhassan I, Ibrahim M, GebreMichael T, Engers H: Very high DDT-resistant population of *Anopheles pharoensis* Theobald (Diptera: Culicidae) from Gorgora, northern Ethiopia. *Parasite* 2006, 13(4):327-239.

[168] Yadouleton AW, Padonou G, Asidi A, Moiroux N, Bio-Banganna S, Corbel V, N'Guessan R, Gbenou D, Yacoubou I, Gazard K *et al*: Insecticide resistance status in *Anopheles gambiae* in southern Benin. *Malar J* 2010, 9:83.

[169] Pinto J, Lynd A, Vicente JL, Santolamazza F, Randle NP, Gentile G, Moreno M, Simard F, Charlwood JD, do Rosario VE *et al*: Multiple Origins of Knockdown Resistance Mutations in the Afrotropical Mosquito Vector *Anopheles gambiae*. *PLoS ONE* 2007, 2(11):e1243.

[170] della Torre A, Fanello C, Akogbeto M, Dossou-yovo J, Favia G, Petrarca V, Coluzzi M: Molecular evidence of incipient speciation within *Anopheles gambiae* s.s. in West Africa. *Insect Mol Biol* 2001, 10(1):9-18.

[171] Weill M, Chandre F, Brengues C, Manguin S, Akogbeto M, Pasteur N, Guillet P, Raymond M: The *kdr* mutation occurs in the Mopti form of *Anopheles gambiae* s.s. through introgression. *Insect Molecular Biology* 2000, 9(5):451-455.

[172] Reimer LJ, Tripet F, Slotman M, Spielman A, Fondjo E, Lanzaro GC: An unusual distribution of the *kdr* gene among populations of *Anopheles gambiae* on the island of Bioko, Equatorial Guinea. *Insect Mol Biol* 2005, 14(6):683-688.

[173] Protopopoff N, Verhaeghen K, Van Bortel W, Roelants P, Marcotty T, Baza D, D'Alessandro U, Coosemans M: A significant increase in *kdr* in *Anopheles gambiae* is associated with an intensive vector control intervention in Burundi highlands. *Trop Med Int Health* 2008, 13(12):1479-1487.

[174] Pinto J, Lynd A, Elissa N, Donnelly MJ, Costa C, Gentile G, Caccone A, do Rosario VE: Co-occurrence of East and West African *kdr* mutations suggests high levels of resistance to pyrethroid insecticides in *Anopheles gambiae* from Libreville, Gabon. *Med Vet Entomol* 2006, 20(1):27-32.

[175] Moreno M, Vicente JL, Cano J, Berzosa PJ, de Lucio A, Nzambo S, Bobuakasi L, Buatiche JN, Ondo M, Micha F *et al*: Knockdown resistance mutations (*kdr*) and insecticide susceptibility to DDT and pyrethroids in *Anopheles gambiae* from Equatorial Guinea. *Trop Med Int Health* 2008, 13(3):430-433.

[176] Verhaeghen K, Van Bortel W, Roelants P, Backeljau T, Coosemans M: Detection of the East and West African *kdr* mutation in *Anopheles gambiae* and *Anopheles arabiensis* from Uganda using a new assay based on FRET/Melt Curve analysis. *Malaria Journal* 2006, 5(1):16.

[177] Koekemoer LL, Spillings BL, Christian RN, Lo TC, Kaiser ML, Norton RA, Oliver SV, Choi KS, Brooke BD, Hunt RH *et al*: Multiple insecticide resistance in *Anopheles gambiae* (Diptera: Culicidae) from Pointe Noire, Republic of the Congo. *Vector Borne Zoonotic Dis* 2011, 11(8):1193-1200.

[178] Reimer L, Fondjo E, Patchoke S, Diallo B, Lee Y, Ng A, Ndjemai HM, Atangana J, Traore SF, Lanzaro G *et al*: Relationship between *kdr* mutation and resistance to pyrethroid and DDT insecticides in natural populations of *Anopheles gambiae*. *J Med Entomol* 2008, 45(2):260-266.

[179] Badolo A, Traore A, Jones CM, Sanou A, Flood L, Guelbeogo WM, Ranson H, Sagnon N: Three years of insecticide resistance monitoring in *Anopheles gambiae* in Burkina Faso: resistance on the rise? *Malar J* 2012, 11:232.

[180] Santolamazza F, Calzetta M, Etang J, Barrese E, Dia I, Caccone A, Donnelly MJ, Petrarca V, Simard F, Pinto J *et al*: Distribution of knock-down resistance mutations in

Anopheles gambiae molecular forms in west and west-central Africa. *Malar J* 2008, 7(1): 74.

[181] Ridl F, Bass C, Torrez M, Govender D, Ramdeen V, Yellot L, Edu A, Schwabe C, Mohloai P, Maharaj R *et al*: A pre-intervention study of malaria vector abundance in Rio Muni, Equatorial Guinea: Their role in malaria transmission and the incidence of insecticide resistance alleles. *Malaria Journal* 2008, 7(1):194.

[182] Reimer L, Fondjo E, Patchok, Salomon, Diallo B, Lee Y, Ng A, Ndjemai HM, Atangana J, Traore SF *et al*: Relationship Between *kdr* Mutation and Resistance to Pyrethroid and DDT Insecticides in Natural Populations of *Anopheles gambiae*. *Journal of Medical Entomology* 2008, 45:260-266.

[183] Matambo TS, Abdalla H, Brooke BD, Koekemoer LL, Mnzava A, Hunt RH, Coetzee M: Insecticide resistance in the malarial mosquito *Anopheles arabiensis* and association with the *kdr* mutation. *Medical and Veterinary Entomology* 2007, 21(1):97-102.

[184] Kulkarni M, Rowland M, Alifrangis M, Mosha F, Matowo J, Malima R, Peter J, Kweka E, Lyimo I, Magesa S *et al*: Occurrence of the leucine-to-phenylalanine knockdown resistance (*kdr*) mutation in *Anopheles arabiensis* populations in Tanzania, detected by a simplified high-throughput SSOP-ELISA method. *Malaria Journal* 2006, 5(1):56.

[185] Chen H, Githeko AK, Githure JI, Mutunga J, Zhou G, Yan G: Monooxygenase Levels and Knockdown Resistance (*kdr*) Allele Frequencies in *Anopheles gambiae* and *Anopheles arabiensis* in Kenya. *Journal of Medical Entomology* 2008, 45:242-250.

[186] Etang J, Manga L, Toto JC, Guillet P, Fondjo E, Chandre F: Spectrum of metabolic-based resistance to DDT and pyrethroids in *Anopheles gambiae* s.l. populations from Cameroon. *J Vector Ecol* 2007, 32(1):123-133.

[187] Hargreaves K, Hunt RH, Brooke BD, Mthembu J, Weeto MM, Awolola TS, Coetzee M: *Anopheles arabiensis* and *An. quadriannulatus* resistance to DDT in South Africa. *Med Vet Entomol* 2003, 17(4):417-422.

[188] Amenya DA, Naguran R, Lo TC, Ranson H, Spillings BL, Wood OR, Brooke BD, Coetzee M, Koekemoer LL: Over expression of a cytochrome P450 (CYP6P9) in a major African malaria vector, *Anopheles funestus*, resistant to pyrethroids. *Insect Mol Biol* 2008, 17(1):19-25.

[189] Somboon P, Prapanthadara LA, Suwonkerd W: Insecticide susceptibility tests of *Anopheles minimus* s.l., *Aedes aegypti*, *Aedes albopictus*, and *Culex quinquefasciatus* in northern Thailand. *Southeast Asian J Trop Med Public Health* 2003, 34(1):87-93.

[190] Verhaeghen K, Van Bortel W, Trung HD, Sochantha T, Coosemans M: Absence of knockdown resistance suggests metabolic resistance in the main malaria vectors of the Mekong region. *Malar J* 2009, 8:84.

[191] Chareonviriyaphap T, Rongnoparut P, Chantarumporn P, Bangs MJ: Biochemical detection of pyrethroid resistance mechanisms in *Anopheles minimus* in Thailand. *J Vector Ecol* 2003, 28(1):108-116.

[192] Rodpradit P, Boonsuepsakul S, Chareonviriyaphap T, Bangs MJ, Rongnoparut P: Cytochrome P450 genes: molecular cloning and overexpression in a pyrethroid-resistant strain of *Anopheles minimus* mosquito. *J Am Mosq Control Assoc* 2005, 21(1):71-79.

[193] Verhaeghen K, Van Bortel W, Trung HD, Sochantha T, Keokenchanh K, Coosemans M: Knockdown resistance in *Anopheles vagus, An. sinensis, An. paraliae* and *An. peditaeniatus* populations of the Mekong region. *Parasit Vectors* 2011, 3(1):59.

[194] Kang S, Jung J, Lee S, Hwang H, Kim W: The polymorphism and the geographical distribution of the knockdown resistance (*kdr*) of *Anopheles sinensis* in the Republic of Korea. *Malar J* 2012, 11:151.

[195] Tan WL, Wang ZM, Li CX, Chu HL, Xu Y, Dong YD, Wang ZC, Chen DY, Liu H, Liu DP *et al*: First report on co-occurrence knockdown resistance mutations and susceptibility to beta-cypermethrin in *Anopheles sinensis* from Jiangsu Province, China. *PLoS ONE* 2012, 7(1):e29242.

[196] Syafruddin D, Hidayati AP, Asih PB, Hawley WA, Sukowati S, Lobo NF: Detection of 1014F *kdr* mutation in four major Anopheline malaria vectors in Indonesia. *Malar J* 2010, 9:315.

[197] Singh OP, Dykes CL, Das MK, Pradhan S, Bhatt RM, Agrawal OP, Adak T: Presence of two alternative *kdr*-like mutations, L1014F and L1014S, and a novel mutation, V1010L, in the voltage gated Na+ channel of *Anopheles culicifacies* from Orissa, India. *Malar J* 2010, 9:146.

[198] Mishra AK, Chand SK, Barik TK, Dua VK, Raghavendra K: Insecticide resistance status in *Anopheles culicifacies* in Madhya Pradesh, central India. *J Vector Borne Dis* 2012, 49(1):39-41.

[199] Sharma SN, Shukla RP, Raghavendra K: Susceptibility status of *An. fluviatilis* and *An. culicifacies* to DDT, deltamethrin and lambdacyhalothrin in District Nainital, Uttar Pradesh. *Indian J Malariol* 1999, 36(3-4):90-93.

[200] Singh OP, Dykes CL, Lather M, Agrawal OP, Adak T: Knockdown resistance (*kdr*)-like mutations in the voltage-gated sodium channel of a malaria vector *Anopheles stephensi* and PCR assays for their detection. *Malar J* 2011, 10:59.

[201] Tikar SN, Mendki MJ, Sharma AK, Sukumaran D, Veer V, Prakash S, Parashar BD: Resistance status of the malaria vector mosquitoes, *Anopheles stephensi* and *Anopheles subpictus* towards adulticides and larvicides in arid and semi-arid areas of India. *J Insect Sci* 2011, 11:85.

[202] Baruah K, Lal S: A report on the susceptibility status of *Anopheles minimus* (Theobald) against DDT and deltamethrin in three districts of Assam. *J Vector Borne Dis* 2004, 41(1-2):42-44.

[203] Karunaratne SH, Hemingway J: Malathion resistance and prevalence of the malathion carboxylesterase mechanism in populations of mosquito vectors of disease in Sri Lanka. *Bull World Health Organ* 2001, 79(11):1060-1064.

[204] Kelly-Hope LA, Yapabandara AM, Wickramasinghe MB, Perera MD, Karunaratne SH, Fernando WP, Abeyasinghe RR, Siyambalagoda RR, Herath PR, Galappaththy GN *et al*: Spatiotemporal distribution of insecticide resistance in *Anopheles culicifacies* and *Anopheles subpictus* in Sri Lanka. *Trans R Soc Trop Med Hyg* 2005, 99(10):751-761.

[205] Perera MD, Hemingway J, Karunaratne SP: Multiple insecticide resistance mechanisms involving metabolic changes and insensitive target sites selected in anopheline vectors of malaria in Sri Lanka. *Malar J* 2008, 7:168.

[206] Surendran SN, Jude PJ, Weerarathne TC, Parakrama Karunaratne SH, Ramasamy R: Variations in susceptibility to common insecticides and resistance mechanisms among morphologically identified sibling species of the malaria vector *Anopheles subpictus* in Sri Lanka. *Parasit Vectors* 2012, 5:34.

[207] Mittal PK, Wijeyaratne P, Pandey S: Status of Insecticide Resistance of Malaria, Kala-azar and Japanese Encephalitis Vectors in Bangladesh, Bhutan, India and Nepal (BBIN). In. Edited by Project EH. Washington 2004.

[208] Rowland M: Location of the gene for malathion resistance in *Anopheles stephensi* (Diptera: Culicidae) from Pakistan. *J Med Entomol* 1985, 22(4):373-380.

[209] Abai MR, Mehravaran A, Vatandoost H, Oshaghi MA, Javadian E, Mashayekhi M, Moslemimia A, Piyazak N, Edallat H, Mohtarami F *et al*: Comparative performance of imagicides on *Anopheles stephensi*, main malaria vector in a malarious area, southern Iran. *J Vector Borne Dis* 2008, 45(4):307-312.

[210] Lak SH, vatandoost H, Entezarmahdi MR, Ashraf H, Abai MR, Nazari M: Monitoring of Insecticide Resistance in *Anopheles sacharovi* (Favre, 1903) in Borderline of Iran, Armenia, Naxcivan and Turkey, 2001. *Iranian J Publ Health* 2002, 31(3-4):96-99.

[211] Vatandoost H, Mashayekhi M, Abaie MR, Aflatoonian MR, Hanafi-Bojd AA, Sharifi I: Monitoring of insecticides resistance in main malaria vectors in a malarious area of Kahnooj district, Kerman province, southeastern Iran. *J Vector Borne Dis* 2005, 42(3): 100-108.

[212] Malcolm CA: Current status of pyrethroid resistance in anophelines. *Parasitol Today* 1988, 4(7):S13-15.

[213] Quinones ML, Suarez MF: Irritability to DDT of natural populations of the primary malaria vectors in Colombia. *J Am Mosq Control Assoc* 1989, 5(1):56-59.

[214] Suarez MF, Quinones ML, Palacios JD, Carrillo A: First record of DDT resistance in *Anopheles darlingi. J Am Mosq Control Assoc* 1990, 6(1):72-74.

[215] Fonseca-Gonzalez I: Estatus de la resistencia a insecticidas de los vectores primarios de malaria y dengue en Antioquia, Chocó, Norte de Santander y Putumayo, Colombia. Universidad de Antioquia, Colombia; 2008.

[216] Fonseca-Gonzalez I, Cardenas R, Quinones ML, McAllister J, Brogdon WG: Pyrethroid and organophosphates resistance in *Anopheles (N.) nuneztovari* Gabaldon populations from malaria endemic areas in Colombia. *Parasitol Res* 2009, 105(5):1399-1409.

[217] Chareonviriyaphap T, Golenda CF, Roberts DR, Andre RG: Identification of Elevated Esterase Activity in a Pyrethroid-Resistant Population of *Anopheles albimanus* Wiedemann. *ScienceAsia* 1999, 25 153-156.

[218] Brogdon WG, McAllister JC, Corwin AM, Cordon Rosales C: Independent selection of multiple mechanisms for pyrethroid resistance in Guatemalan *Anopheles albimanus* (Diptera: Culicidae). *Journal of Economic Entomology* 1999, 92(2):298-302.

[219] Zamora Perea E, Balta Leon R, Palomino Salcedo M, Brogdon WG, Devine GJ: Adaptation and evaluation of the bottle assay for monitoring insecticide resistance in disease vector mosquitoes in the Peruvian Amazon. *Malar J* 2009, 8:208.

[220] Hemingway J, Penilla RP, Rodriguez AD, James BM, Edge W, Rogers H, Rodriguez MH: Resistance management strategies in malaria vector mosquito control. A large-scale field trial in Southern Mexico. *Pesticide Science* 1997, 51(3):375-382.

[221] Dzul FA, Patricia Penilla R, Rodriguez AD: [Susceptibility and insecticide resistance mechanisms in *Anopheles albimanus* from the southern Yucatan Peninsula, Mexico]. *Salud Publica Mex* 2007, 49(4):302-311.

[222] South Africa Department of Health: Malaria Updates. In. Pretoria, S.A: S.A.D.H.; 2003.

[223] Maharaj R, Mthembu DJ, Sharp BL: Impact of DDT re-introduction on malaria transmission in KwaZulu-Natal. *S Afr Med J* 2005, 95(11):871-874.

[224] Roberts DR, Manguin S, Mouchet J: DDT house spraying and re-emerging malaria. *Lancet* 2000, 356(9226):330-332.

[225] Protopopoff N, Van Bortel W, Marcotty T, Van Herp M, Maes P, Baza D, D'Alessandro U, Coosemans M: Spatial targeted vector control in the highlands of Burundi and its impact on malaria transmission. *Malar J* 2007, 6:158.

[226] Trape J-F, Tall A, Diagne N, Ndiath O, Ly AB, Faye J, Dieye-Ba F, Roucher C, Bouganali C, Badiane A *et al*: Malaria morbidity and pyrethroid resistance after the introduction of insecticide-treated bednets and artemisinin-based combination therapies: a longitudinal study. *The Lancet Infectious Diseases* 2011.

[227]   Lengeler C: Insecticide-treated bed nets and curtains for preventing malaria. *Cochrane Database of Systematic reviews* 2009(2):1-58.

[228]   Kitau J, Oxborough RM, Tungu PK, Matowo J, Malima RC, Magesa SM, Bruce J, Mosha FW, Rowland MW: Species shifts in the *Anopheles gambiae* complex: do LLINs successfully control *Anopheles arabiensis*? *PLoS ONE* 2012, 7(3):e31481.

[229]   Bradley J, Matias A, Schwabe C, Vargas D, Monti F, Nseng G, Kleinschmidt I: Increased risks of malaria due to limited residual life of insecticide and outdoor biting versus protection by combined use of nets and indoor residual spraying on Bioko Island, Equatorial Guinea. *Malar J* 2012, 11:242.

[230]   Henry MC, Assi SB, Rogier C, Dossou-Yovo J, Chandre F, Guillet P, Carnevale P: Protective efficacy of lambda-cyhalothrin treated nets in *Anopheles gambiae* pyrethroid resistance areas of Cote d'Ivoire. *Am J Trop Med Hyg* 2005, 73(5):859-864.

[231]   Corbel V, Akogbeto M, Damien GB, Djenontin A, Chandre F, Rogier C, Moiroux N, Chabi J, Banganna B, Padonou GG *et al*: Combination of malaria vector control interventions in pyrethroid resistance area in Benin: a cluster randomised controlled trial. *Lancet Infect Dis* 2012, 12(8):617-626.

[232]   Darriet F, N' Guessan R, Koffi AA, Konan L, Doannio JMC, Chandre F, Carnevale P: Impact of the resistance to pyrethroids on the efficacy of impregnated bednets used as a means of prevention against malaria: results of the evaluation carried out with deltamethrin SC in experimental huts. *Bulletin de la Société de Pathologie Exotique* 2000, 93(2):131-134.

[233]   Corbel V, Chandre F, Brengues C, Akogbeto M, Lardeux F, Hougard JM, Guillet P: Dosage-dependent effects of permethrin-treated nets on the behaviour of *Anopheles gambiae* and the selection of pyrethroid resistance. *Malar J* 2004, 3(1):22.

[234]   N'Guessan R, Corbel V, Akogbeto M, Rowland M: Reduced efficacy of insecticide-treated nets and indoor residual spraying for malaria control in pyrethroid resistance area, Benin. *Emerg Infect Dis* 2007, 13(2):199-206.

[235]   N'Guessan R, Asidi A, Boko P, Odjo A, Akogbeto M, Pigeon O, Rowland M: An experimental hut evaluation of PermaNet(R) 3.0, a deltamethrin-piperonyl butoxide combination net, against pyrethroid-resistant *Anopheles gambiae* and *Culex quinquefasciatus* mosquitoes in southern Benin. *Trans R Soc Trop Med Hyg* 2010, 104(12):758-765.

[236]   Asidi A, N'Guessan R, Akogbeto M, Curtis C, Rowland M: Loss of household protection from use of insecticide-treated nets against pyrethroid-resistant mosquitoes, Benin. *Emerg Infect Dis* 2012, 18(7):1101-1106.

[237]   Osse R, Gnanguenon V, Sezonlin M, Aikpon R, Padonou G, Yadouleton A, Akogbeto M: Relationship between the presence of *kdr* and Ace-1 mutations and the infection with *Plasmodium falciparum* in *Anopheles gambiae* s.s. in Benin. *Journal of Parassitology & Vector Biology* 2012, 4(3):31-39.

[238] Moiroux N, Boussari O, Djenontin A, Damien G, Cottrell G, Henry MC, Guis H, Cor-
       bel V: Dry season determinants of malaria disease and net use in Benin, West Africa.
       PLoS ONE 2012, 7(1):e30558.

[239] Poupardin R, Reynaud S, Strode C, Ranson H, Vontas J, David JP: Cross-induction of
       detoxification genes by environmental xenobiotics and insecticides in the mosquito
       Aedes aegypti: impact on larval tolerance to chemical insecticides. *Insect Biochem Mol
       Biol* 2008, 38(5):540-551.

[240] IRAC: Prevention and Management of Insecticide Resistance in Vectors of Public
       Health Importance In: *Resistance Management for Sustainable Agriculture and Improved
       Public Health : Second Edition 2010* Insecticide Resistance Action Commitee; 2010:
       72pp.

[241] Georghiou GP, Taylor CE: Genetic and biological influences in the evolution of insec-
       ticide resistance. *Journal of Economic Entomology* 1977, 70(3):319-323.

[242] Denholm I, Rowland MW: Tactics for managing pesticide resistance in arthropods:
       theory and practice. *Annu Rev Entomol* 1992, 37:91-112.

[243] Djogbenou L, Weill M, Hougard JM, Raymond M, Akogbeto M, Chandre F: Charac-
       terization of insensitive acetylcholinesterase (ace-1R) in *Anopheles gambiae* (Diptera:
       Culicidae): resistance levels and dominance. *J Med Entomol* 2007, 44(5):805-810.

[244] Berticat C, Bonnet J, Duchon S, Agnew P, Weill M, Corbel V: Costs and benefits of
       multiple resistance to insecticides for *Culex quinquefasciatus* mosquitoes. *BMC Evol Bi-
       ol* 2008, 8:104.

[245] Moore JH, Williams SM: Traversing the conceptual divide between biological and
       statistical epistasis: systems biology and a more modern synthesis. *Bioessays* 2005,
       27(6):637-646.

[246] Shono T, Zhang L, Scott JG: Indoxacarb resistance in the house fly, *Musca domestica*.
       Pesticide Biochemistry and Physiology 2004, 80(2):106-112.

[247] Shono T, Kasai S, Kamiya E, Kono Y, Scott JG: Genetics and mechanisms of perme-
       thrin resistance in the YPER strain of house fly. *Pesticide Biochemistry and Physiology*
       2002, 73(1):27-36.

[248] Scott JG, Shono T, Georghiou GP: Genetic analysis of permethrin resistance in the
       house fly, *Musca domestica* L. *Experientia* 1984, 40(12):1416-1418.

[249] Hardstone MC, Leichter CA, Scott JG: Multiplicative interaction between the two
       major mechanisms of permethrin resistance, *kdr* and cytochrome P450-monooxyge-
       nase detoxification, in mosquitoes. *J Evol Biol* 2009, 22(2):416-423.

[250] Berticat C, Boquien G, Raymond M, Chevillon C: Insecticide resistance genes induce
       a mating competition cost in *Culex pipiens* mosquitoes. *Genet Res* 2002, 79(1):41-47.

[251] Agnew P, Berticat C, Bedhomme S, Sidobre C, Michalakis Y: Parasitism increases and decreases the costs of insecticide resistance in mosquitoes. *Evolution Int J Org Evolution* 2004, 58(3):579-586.

[252] Foster SP, Harrington R, Devonshire AL, Denholm I, Devine GJ, Kenward MG: Comparative survival of insecticide-susceptible and resistant peach-potato aphids, *Myzus persicae* (Sulzer) (Hemiptera: Aphididae), in low temperature field trials. *Bull Ent Res* 1996, 86:17-27.

[253] Shi MA, Lougarre A, Alies C, Fremaux I, Tang ZH, Stojan J, Fournier D: Acetylcholinesterase alterations reveal the fitness cost of mutations conferring insecticide resistance. *BMC Evol Biol* 2004, 4:5.

[254] Djogbenou L, Noel V, Agnew P: Costs of insensitive acetylcholinesterase insecticide resistance for the malaria vector *Anopheles gambiae* homozygous for the G119S mutation. *Malar J* 2010, 9(1):12.

[255] Brogdon WG, McAllister JC: Insecticide resistance and vector control. *Emerg Infect Dis* 1998, 4(4):605-613.

[256] Diabate A, Baldet T, Chandre F, Akoobeto M, Guiguemde TR, Darriet F, Brengues C, Guillet P, Hemingway J, Small GJ *et al*: The role of agricultural use of insecticides in resistance to pyrethroids in *Anopheles gambiae* s.l. in Burkina Faso. *Am J Trop Med Hyg* 2002, 67(6):617-622.

[257] Yadouleton A, Martin T, Padonou G, Chandre F, Asidi A, Djogbenou L, Dabire R, Aikpon R, Boko M, Glitho I *et al*: Cotton pest management practices and the selection of pyrethroid resistance in *Anopheles gambiae* population in northern Benin. *Parasit Vectors* 2011, 4:60.

[258] Harrison G: Mosquitoes, malaria and man: A history of hostilities since 1880.; 1978.

[259] Read AF, Lynch PA, Thomas MB: How to make evolution-proof insecticides for malaria control. *PLoS Biol* 2009, 7(4):e1000058.

[260] Roush RT, Hoy CW, Ferro DN, Tingey WM: Insecticide resistance in the Colorado potato beetle (Coleoptera: Chrysomelidae): influence of crop rotation and insecticide use. *Journal of Economic Entomology* 1990, 83(2):315-319.

[261] Georghiou GP: Insecticide resistance and prospects for its management. *Residue Reviews* 1980, 76:131-145.

[262] Tabashnik BE: Managing resistance with multiple pesticide tactics: theory, evidence, and recommendations. *J Econ Entomol* 1989, 82(5):1263-1269.

[263] Chitnis N, Schapira A, Smith T, Steketee R: Comparing the effectiveness of malaria vector-control interventions through a mathematical model. *Am J Trop Med Hyg* 2010, 83(2):230-240.

[264] Yakob L, Dunning R, Yan G: Indoor residual spray and insecticide-treated bednets for malaria control: theoretical synergisms and antagonisms. *J R Soc Interface* 2011, 8(59):799-806.

[265] World Health Organization: Global strategic framework for integrated vector management. Geneva; 2004.

[266] Curtis CF: Theoretical models of the use of insecticide mixtures for management of resistance. *Bull Ent Res* 1985, 75: 259-265.

[267] Hougard JM, Poudiougo P, Guillet P, Back C, Akpoboua LK, Quillevere D: Criteria for the selection of larvicides by the Onchocerciasis Control Programme in west Africa. *Ann Trop Med Parasitol* 1993, 87(5):435-442.

[268] WHO: Pesticides and their application for the control of vectors and pests of public health importance; Sixth edition. In. Edited by WHO/CDS/NTD/WHOPES/GCDPP/2006.1 WHO, Geneva; 2006: 1-125.

[269] Corbel V, Chabi J, Dabire RK, Etang J, Nwane P, Pigeon O, Akogbeto M, Hougard JM: Field efficacy of a new mosaic long-lasting mosquito net (PermaNet 3.0) against pyrethroid-resistant malaria vectors: a multi centre study in Western and Central Africa. *Malar J* 2010, 9:113.

[270] Killeen GF, Okumu FO, N'Guessan R, Coosemans M, Adeogun A, Awolola S, Etang J, Dabire RK, Corbel V: The importance of considering community-level effects when selecting insecticidal malaria vector products. *Parasit Vectors* 2011, 4:160.

[271] Mani GS: Evolution of resistance in the presence of two insecticides. *Genetics* 1985, 109(4):761-783.

[272] Roush RT: Designing resistance management programs: how can you choose? *Pesticide Science* 1989, 26(4):423-441.

[273] Hougard JM, Corbel V, N'Guessan R, Darriet F, Chandre F, Akogbeto M, Baldet T, Guillet P, Carnevale P, Traore-Lamizana M: Efficacy of mosquito nets treated with insecticide mixtures or mosaics against insecticide resistant *Anopheles gambiae* and *Culex quinquefasciatus* (Diptera: Culicidae) in Cote d'Ivoire. *Bull Entomol Res* 2003, 93(6):491-498.

[274] Asidi AN, N'Guessan R, Koffi AA, Curtis CF, Hougard JM, Chandre F, Corbel V, Darriet F, Zaim M, Rowland MW: Experimental hut evaluation of bednets treated with an organophosphate (chlorpyrifos-methyl) or a pyrethroid (lambdacyhalothrin) alone and in combination against insecticide-resistant *Anopheles gambiae* and *Culex quinquefasciatus* mosquitoes. *Malar J* 2005, 4(1):25.

[275] Ohashi K, Nakada K, Ishiwatari T, Miyaguchi J, Shono Y, Lucas JR, Mito N: Efficacy of pyriproxyfen-treated nets in sterilizing and shortening the longevity of *Anopheles gambiae* (Diptera: Culicidae). *J Med Entomol* 2012, 49(5):1052-1058.

[276] Mosqueira B, Duchon S, Chandre F, Hougard JM, Carnevale P, Mas-Coma S: Efficacy of an insecticide paint against insecticide-susceptible and resistant mosquitoes - part 1: laboratory evaluation. *Malar J* 2010, 9:340.

[277] Ngufor C, N'Guessan R, Boko P, Odjo A, Vigninou E, Asidi A, Akogbeto M, Rowland M: Combining indoor residual spraying with chlorfenapyr and long-lasting insecticidal bed nets for improved control of pyrethroid-resistant *Anopheles gambiae*: an experimental hut trial in Benin. *Malar J* 2011, 10:343.

[278] Kleinschmidt I, Schwabe C, Shiva M, Segura JL, Sima V, Mabunda SJ, Coleman M: Combining indoor residual spraying and insecticide-treated net interventions. *Am J Trop Med Hyg* 2009, 81(3):519-524.

[279] Okumu FO, Moore SJ: Combining indoor residual spraying and insecticide-treated nets for malaria control in Africa: a review of possible outcomes and an outline of suggestions for the future. *Malar J* 2011, 10:208.

[280] Brosseau L, Drame PM, Besnard P, Toto JC, Foumane V, Le Mire J, Mouchet F, Remoue F, Allan R, Fortes F *et al*: Human antibody response to *Anopheles saliva* for comparing the efficacy of three malaria vector control methods in Balombo, Angola. *PLoS ONE* 2012, 7(9):e44189.

[281] Bill_&_Melinda_Gates_Fondation, Boston_Consulting_Group: Market Assessment for Public Health Pesticide Products. In.; 2007.

Chapter 6

Residual Transmission of Malaria:
An Old Issue for New Approaches

Lies Durnez and Marc Coosemans

Additional information is available at the end of the chapter

1. Introduction

Malaria is one of the most serious vector-borne diseases, affecting millions of people mainly in the tropics. Recently, a substantial decline in malaria incidence has been observed all over the world. Vector control is one of the key elements in achieving this world-wide malaria decline, with scaling up of Insecticide Treated Nets (ITNs) and the expansion of Indoor Residual Spraying (IRS) programmes contributing significantly. Besides the personal protection, ITNs confer a community protection when wide coverage is assured, meaning that unprotected persons benefit from the large scale intervention [1]. IRS is only meaningful when applied at a large coverage. In the 2011 World Malaria Report [2], the percentage of households owning at least one ITN in sub-Saharan Africa is estimated to have risen from 3% in 2000 to 50% in 2011 while the percentage protected by indoor residual spraying (IRS) rose from less than 5% in 2005 to 11% in 2010. Household surveys indicate that 96% of persons with access to an ITN within the household actually use it [2]. Although these numbers might overestimate the real ITN use, they show that in recent years, several vector control measures were scaled up substantially. Despite these large increases in coverage, a widely held view is that with the currently available tools, namely vector control tools, intermittent preventive treatment, and early diagnosis and treatment, much greater gains could be achieved, including elimination from a number of countries and regions [3].

When considering vector control tools, even when hypothesizing a full coverage of ITNs and IRS, malaria transmission may still continue. Indeed, IRS only affects endophilic[1] mosquitoes and ITNs only target night biting mosquitoes. Moreover both intervention methods will mainly affect anthropophilic[2] mosquitoes that are endophagic[3]. This leaves ample opportunity

---

1 Endophily is the tendency for mosquitoes to prefer resting indoors

for more exophilic[4], zoophilic[5] and/or exophagic[6] vectors to escape from contact with insecticide treated surfaces and to maintain a certain level of transmission. Independently of the ITN and/or IRS coverage, outdoor and early malaria transmission occurs in many malaria endemic regions. In the west of Eritrea for example over a two year sampling period 36.4% of infective bites were acquired outdoors [4], in southern Tanzania this was 10% for non ITN users [5]. A study in northeastern Tanzania showed that 12% of the malaria transmission occurred before sleeping time [6]. In Uganda, in 6 sentinel sites throughout the country, up to 36% of indoor transmission and 49 % of outdoor transmission occurred before sleeping time, with the highest proportion of early in- and outdoor transmission in the suburban area of Jinja where *An. gambiae*[7] was the main vector [7]. In central Vietnam, where ITNs are used at large scale, 69% of the infective bites in forest plots were acquired before sleeping time [8]. In a study conducted in the east and west of Cambodia before widespread ITN use, 29% of the bites occurred before sleeping time in villages and forest plots [9]. In North-East India, 21% of the indoor infective bites occurred before 21h [10]. Also in Nicaragua, in an area with mainly Vivax malaria, 50% of the infective bites were acquired before sleeping time [11]. This part of the malaria transmission has the possibility to continue despite high coverage of ITNs and IRS, and is defined for the purpose of this review as 'residual transmission'.

Controlling residual transmission requires a different approach as compared to the currently used vector control measures. This is not new and was already perceived as a major obstacle in the previous malaria eradication era [12]. In 2007 malaria eradication was put as the ultimate goal [3] and renewed attention was given to residual transmission, with vector control models also incorporating outdoor and zoophilic malaria vectors. Recently, an established mathematical model adjusted for human in- and outdoor movements was used to illustrate that even with 50% outdoor biting vectors, transmission suppression can be achieved by a large ITN coverage [13]. However the authors assumed a uniform exposure so that the ITN induced mortality affects equally in- and outdoor biting vectors. When assuming a uniform exposure all individuals of the vector population (belonging to the same or to different species), will exhibit at each gonotrophic cycle a random behaviour (e.g. exo- or endophily, exo-or endophagy, anthropo- or zoophily, early- or late-biting), so that all individual mosquitoes are equally affected by indoor-based vector control measures. In case of non-uniform exposure, two or more subpopulations of vectors (belonging to the same or to different species) are assumed, each exhibiting a specific behaviour. Therefore, each of these subpopulations is affected differently by indoor-based vector control measures [14]. As a result, a fraction of vectors will persist in the presence of these control measures and can be responsible for residual transmission. It was shown that pre-intervention variables reflecting behavior, such as the degree

---

2 Anthropophily is the tendency for mosquitoes to prefer feeding on human hosts

3 Endophagy is the tendency for mosquitoes to prefer biting indoors

4 Exophily is the tendency for mosquitoes to prefer resting outdoors

5 Zoophily is the tendency for mosquitoes to prefer feeding on animal hosts

6 Exophagy is the tendency for mosquitoes to prefer biting outdoors

7 In this paper, s.l. (sensu lato) is added to the species name when referred to the species complex *(An. gambiae s.l., An. minimus s.l., An. dirus s.l.)*. In the absence of s.l., the species is concerned *(e.g. An. gambiae, An. minimus, An. dirus)*.

of exophily, may predict the efficacy of a specific intervention [15,16]. Assuming non-uniform exposure, the exophagic fractions of vectors will be less exposed to ITNs, the probability of survival and the vectorial capacity of this subpopulation will be weakly affected, and malaria transmission cannot be reduced further. The model developed in [17] takes into account the non-uniform exposure of the different anopheline species, i.e., the anthropo-endophilic vector species *An. gambiae* and *An. funestus*, and the more zoo-exophilic vector *An. arabiensis*. As would be intuitively expected, this model predicts that even the combination of very effective ITN distribution, twice yearly mass screening and treatment campaigns, and IRS will not succeed in getting the parasite prevalence rate below the 1% threshold if the zoo-exophilic *An. arabiensis* is present. When only *An. gambiae* or *An. funestus* are present, the same combination of interventions are successful in this model [17]. Moreover even within a well-defined species different subpopulations may occur exhibiting different behavioural patterns, resulting in non-uniform exposure within a species.

Therefore, when designing and applying vector control strategies it would be essential to have a good knowledge of the vector behavioural traits particularly those relevant to the chosen control method. However, entomological findings for one region or one anopheline species do not necessarily hold true for the same or different anopheline species encountered in the same or different malaria-endemic regions. In this chapter we will show that even before widespread use of vector control measures, a heterogeneity in behaviour between and within species was present. Because of the heterogeneity in behaviour, mosquitoes have different opportunities to escape from the killing or excito-repellent actions of insecticides used in ITNs or IRS. We will give examples of species shifts, shifts to outdoor- or early biting, shifts to zoophily or to exophily from different malaria endemic regions linked to the use of ITNs and IRS. Although the causes and mechanisms behind these shifts are not yet well understood, we will argue that ITNs and IRS may select for vector populations that predominantly feed early or outdoors, rest outdoors, or that are able to change their behaviour in response to the presence of these insecticides. Therefore, residual transmission will be dominated by vectors that bite outdoors, early or on animals, and that rest outdoors. These vectors require different control strategies, which might also be based on reducing host-vector contact, or target other key environmental resources.

The concept of uniform versus non-uniform exposure is illustrated in Figure 1.

2. Heterogeneity in anopheline behaviour

Heterogeneity in behaviour of anopheline mosquitoes between and within species is present in all malaria endemic regions. In Africa, the two most efficient malaria vector species, *An. gambiae* and *An. funestus*, are very anthropophilic, endophilic, endophagic, and late-night biting [18]. In contrast, *An. arabiensis*, a species belonging to the same complex as *An. gambiae*, is more plastic in its behaviour, exhibiting more often zoophily, exophily, exophagy, and early-night biting as compared to *An. gambiae* and *An. funestus*. However, different factors can influence the behaviour of the anophelines. Host availability for example plays an important

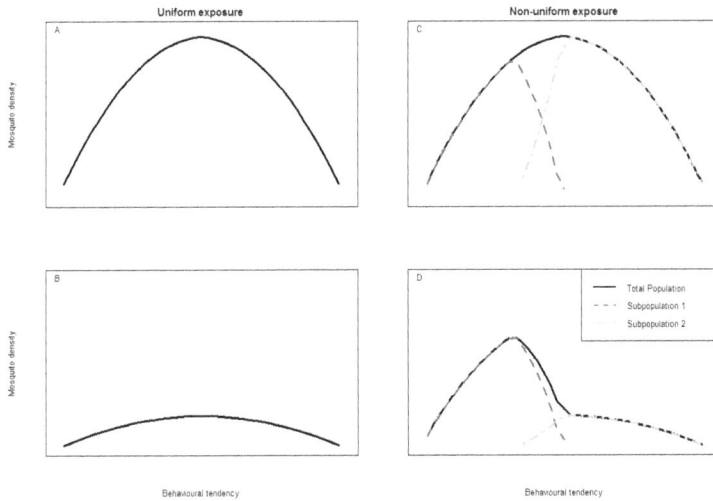

Figure 1. Effect of control measures on mosquito populations in the assumption of uniform exposure and non-uniform exposure. The density of a uniform population (belonging to the same or to different species) A. before applying the control measure. B. after applying the control measure. The control measure reduces the density of the whole population by 80%. The density of a non-uniform population C. before applying the control measure. D. after applying the control measure. The population consists of two subpopulations (Subpopulations 1 and 2, belonging to the same or to different species) each with a different behavioural tendency. Limited contact with the insecticide due to its behavioural tendency makes that Subpopulation 1 is reduced by 20% only, while Subpopulation 2 is reduced by 80% of its initial density. As a result, a fraction of vectors will persist in the presence of these control measures and can be responsible for malaria transmission.

factor in the final host choice of the vector. This has been shown for *An. gambiae* in several study sites. In Burkina Faso for example, a double choice experiment shows that 88% of the *An. gambiae* choose for a human odour baited trap and only 12 % for a cattle odour trap. In contrast, the human blood index of indoor-resting *An. gambiae* collected in the same locality was only 40% [19], showing that this population of *An. gambiae* will adapt its host choice in case of a lower availability of human hosts. *An. gambiae* in São Tomé feeds more on dogs and was observed to be extremely exophagic most probably due to a combination of preference and the ease to reach the dogs sleeping outside under pillar houses [20]. On the Bioko Island (Equatorial Guinea), *An. gambiae* was also observed to be partly exophagic and early-biting [21]. This means that when humans are not available inside, e.g. because of a high bed net use, some populations of *An. gambiae* are observed to feed outside or on animal hosts. In those cases, the frequency of human-vector contact will be lowered although humans will still be bitten in the evening. As a consequence, the longevity of these exophagic or zoophilic vectors will slightly, or not, be affected by ITNs, meaning that the vectorial capacity is not affected and malaria transmission continues.

Also in South-East Asia, heterogeneity of behaviour is observed for the primary and secondary vector species [22]: *An. dirus* is for example very anthropophilic, whereas *An. minimus*, depending on the geographical region, has both anthropophilic and zoophilic tendencies. *An. maculatus* has a high tendency for early biting as compared to *An. dirus* or *An. minimus*, but there are large differences between localities. Different populations of *An. minimus* observed in various localities also differ in their endophilic and endophagic tendencies [22]. Whereas *An. dirus* is generally observed to be very exophagic and exophilic, populations in Lao PDR have shown highly endophilic and endophagic trends [23]. Moreover, as reviewed in [24], *An. dirus* s.l. can even take blood-meals during daylight in the jungle.

In Latin-America, one of the most efficient vectors, *An. darlingi* is mainly anthropophilic, whereas the other dominant vectors, such as *An. albimanus*, *An. nuneztovari*, and *An. aquasalis* also have zoophilic tendencies or are more opportunistic. Most of the vectors in Latin America are mainly exophilic, but within each species, the degree of exophily can vary between geographical regions. *An. albimanus* for example is predominantly exophagic and exophilic, as observed in the Dominican Republic, Colombia, and Haiti. However, in Mexico and Central America, 80% of the *An. albimanus* was observed to have an endophilic resting behaviour [25]. Also the time and place of biting differs between sites for most of the species. In some localities for example, *An. darlingi* bites mostly during sleeping hours, or early in the morning [26], whereas in other localities, the main biting peak is early in the evening [27]. In French Guiana, *An. darlingi* was endo-exophagous with a clear predilection for biting outdoors [28].

3. How can the indoor use of insecticides select for exophilic, exophagic, zoophilic and/or early biting mosquito populations?

Insecticides can elicit different actions with different results on mosquitoes [29–31]. These various modes of action are important when talking about selection of 'insecticide avoiding' mosquitoes. Toxic or cidal actions result in knockdown or death after contact with the insecticide. Excito-repellent actions, including contact irritancy and non-contact repellency, result in above-normal levels of undirected movements coupled with loss of responsiveness to host cues. The insecticidal actions and their results depend among others on the insecticidal product used and on the mosquito species present. Large differences in actions of insecticides used in IRS have been observed: dieldrin for example only elicits a cidal action, while alpha-cypermethrin has both contact-irritant and killing actions, and DDT elicits mainly a repellent effect and secondarily a toxic action. [30]. Pyrethroids, the only family of insecticides used on ITNs, have well-documented excito-repellent actions [21] which are dose-dependent, but with for example higher toxic actions of alphacypermethrin as compared to deltamethrin and permethrin [31].

The general concepts of stress-induced variation in evolution [32] can be applied to the effect of insecticides on mosquito populations. Indoor use of insecticides will pose a stress on the female anopheline population, but only when the insecticides present a barrier for indoor feeding or indoor resting. At least three processes can be at the origin of perceived shifts in mosquito behaviour by insecticides:

1. A first protective mechanism can be behavioural plasticity in response to the presence of the insecticide. The ability to actively remove from the insecticide by either relocation or avoidance requires an ability to detect (either by contact or non-contact) or anticipate the presence of the insecticide and the ability to exhibit insecticide avoidance strategies or adjustments [32]. The insecticide, or the unavailability of the host, can then trigger the expression of gene variants that have been accumulated, but were phenotypically neutral under a normal range of environments [32]. Many mosquitoes indeed naturally possess a high degree of irritability or repellency which is evident at the very first exposure of the population to residual insecticides [29]. Where this irritation is such that mosquitoes settling on the insecticide deposit are activated before they have absorbed a lethal dose of insecticide, and are able to avoid further contact and to escape unharmed, the term "protective avoidance" has been suggested. In the presence of a high coverage of IRS or ITNs, mosquitoes exhibiting this protective avoidance should then be able to redirect their behaviour to low-risk behaviour which also can lower their survival. For example, for a species that is normally endophilic changing its behaviour to resting outdoors, the external environment may be unfavourable to the survival of the species [12].

2. A second protective mechanism for the mosquito is a consistent "protective behaviour" [29] such as exophily, exophagy, zoophily or early-biting resulting in a minimal contact with the insecticides used indoors. As mentioned above, some mosquito populations naturally exhibit this kind of protective behaviour, which is probably genetically determined (see further). Also differences in responses to the insecticides can result in diverse exposure rates of different species or subpopulations to the insecticide. *An. minimus* for example, shows very strong repellency responses to several insecticides and would have a higher survival chance in the presence of insecticides as compared to *An. harrisoni* which shows a much lower repellency response [33]. In this case, insecticides will favour the (sub) populations of mosquitoes that have this innate preference for protective behaviour or for avoidant strategies by which they will escape the exposure to the insecticide. This is probably the mechanism that is occurring for many of the perceived species shifts that are illustrated below.

3. Where these phenomena of protective avoidance or protective behaviour are not evident at the very first exposure of the population to the insecticides, but develop only gradually, perhaps over several years under continued insecticide pressure, the term "behaviouristic resistance" is employed [29]. The presence of the insecticide will in that case result in the selection of mutations and recombination that favour the survival of the mosquito in the presence of the insecticide, eventually leading to a directional selection. This can be compared to the development of insecticide resistance, although selections of many mutations will probably be required before an appropriate behavioural change may occur. Classification as "behaviouristic resistance" is only valid on the basis of accurate comparisons made before and subsequent to the widespread use of residual insecticides in any particular area. As shown below, very few behaviour shifts observed so far, would fit this definition of behaviouristic resistance.

4. Shifts observed in the presence of indoor insecticidal pressure

In the following paragraphs we will review the shifts that were observed in the presence of IRS and ITNs. For the purpose of this review, a 'shift' means an observed change, including relative changes, with a reasonable link to the indoor use of insecticides (ITNs or IRS). A distinction is made between different kinds of shifts: species shifts describe changes in the species composition which can also be within species complexes, whereas shifts to early biting, exophagy, zoophily or exophily describe changes in biting time, biting place, host, or resting place within a species, or within a species complex if no species information was available. Because a large part of the shifts in literature are described in the Afrotropical region, this region will be handled separately.

5. Afrotropical region

5.1. Species shifts

An IRS campaign resulted in the elimination of *An. funestus* from the South Pare District (at the Tanzania-Kenya border), at the same time reducing the numbers of indoor-resting *An. gambiae* s.l. [34]. In the years immediately following this IRS campaign, populations of endophilic *An. gambiae* s.l. slowly regained their former levels, whereas gradual resurgence of *An. funestus* was not observed until almost 10 years after the campaign was abandoned. IRS campaigns in two Kenyan villages resulted in a large decrease (up to total disappearance) of *An. funestus*, with an increase in the more exophagic *An. rivulorum* [35] or *An. parensis* [36], both not considered as malaria vectors in the study sites. In Niger, nation-wide Long-lasting insecticidal net (LLIN) distribution caused a marked decrease of *An. funestus*, without effect on *An. gambiae* s.l. abundance [37]. Following an IRS campaign, *An. gambiae* was completely eliminated from Pemba Island (Tanzania), leaving the salt-water breeding *An. merus*, an exophilic mosquito with a preference for cattle [38]. In Kenya and Tanzania, large scale ITN use significantly decreased the proportion of indoor-resting *An. funestus* [39] and *An. gambiae* [39–42] while the proportion of *An. arabiensis* increased. The shift from *An. gambiae* to *An. arabiensis* was also observed in the larval collections [40,41]. As larvae of *An. gambiae* and *An. arabiensis* show no habitat segregation, larval sampling reflects true proportions of the two species. The change from sub-populations dominated by *An. gambiae* to those dominated by *An. arabiensis* took about a decade, as would be expected if caused by a constant ITN selection pressure [43].

In contrast, in Kenya and on the Bioko Island (Equatorial Guinea), the same species compositions were observed regardless of the use of ITNs or IRS [21,44]. Moreover, in the north-east of Tanzania, a species shift has been observed in the absence of insecticide selective pressure, in a region without organized vector control activities reported [45]: *An. gambiae*, the most dominant in the past, was replaced by *An. arabiensis* without any known reason.

5.2. Shifts to early-evening or early-morning biting

Studies have shown that widespread ITN use increases the proportion of early bites by *An. gambiae* [46] and *An. funestus* [42,46] in Tanzania. Such shift was not observed for *Culex quinquefasciatus* which is highly resistant against pyrethroids [46]. According to the authors [46], this suggests that for anophelines, where there is considerable killing by contact with ITNs, several years of selection has begun to produce an upward shift in the proportions of insects biting at a time when people are accessible. Also in southern Benin, a significant change in host seeking behaviour of *An. funestus* was observed after achieving a universal coverage of ITNs. The shift in biting time was here not to the early evening but to the early morning. Moreover in one locality about 26% of the *An. funestus* bites were observed after sunrise [47].

The use of ITNs resulted in a shift towards earlier biting of *An. gambiae* s.l. in Kenya [48] and Tanzania [42,49], possibly [48,49] or certainly [42] related to a species shift from *An. gambiae* to *An. arabiensis*.

In other studies however, no evidence for a shift in biting time after the introduction of ITNs or IRS was obtained for *An. gambiae* s.l. in Tanzania, Kenya, The Gambia and Nigeria [44,50–52], for *An. gambiae* the Bioko Island (Equatorial Guinea) [21], or for *An. funestus* in Kenya [44]. Widespread use of mostly untreated bed nets did not result in more early biting of *An. gambiae* [5].

Country	Vector control measure [a]	Insecticide [b]	Collection methods [c]	Species shift [d]	Shift to early-biting [d]	Shift to exophagy [d]	Shift to zoophily [d]	Reference
Benin	ITN	Deltamethrin	Indoor/ outdoor HLC	ND	Yes	Yes	ND	[47]
Burkina Faso	ITC	Permethrin	Indoor/ outdoor CDC LT	ND	ND	Not observed	Not observed	[53]
Burkina Faso	ITN	Unspecified	IRC, Odour-baited traps	ND	ND	ND	Yes	[19]
Equatorial Guinea	IRS ITN	Deltamethrin, alpha cypermethrin, bendiocarb. Unspecified LLIN	Indoor/ outdoor HLC	Not observed	Not observed	Yes	ND	[21]
Kenya	IRS	Dieldrin	ORC, IRC, LD, HLC	Yes	ND	ND	ND	[35]
Kenya	IRS	DDT	Indoor/ outdoor HLC	Yes	ND	ND	ND	[36]
Kenya	IRS	Dieldrin	IRC, ORC	Yes	ND	ND	Not observed,	[34]
Kenya	ITN	Permethrin	IRC, indoor and outdoor HLC	ND	Yes	Yes	Yes, but not significant	[48]
Kenya	ITN	Permethrin	IRC, ORC	ND	ND	ND	Yes	[54]
Kenya	ITN	Permethrin	WET, IRC, outdoor bed net traps	Not observed	Not observed	ND	ND	[44]
Kenya	ITN	Permethrin,	IRC	Yes	ND	ND	ND	[39]
Kenya	ITN	Permethrin, alpha cypermethrin, Unspecified LLINs	IRC, LD	Yes	ND	ND	Not observed	[41]

Country	Vector control measure[a]	Insecticide[b]	Collection methods[c]	Species shift[d]	Shift to early-biting[d]	Shift to exophagy[d]	Shift to zoophily[d]	Reference
Kenya	ITN, ITC	Permethrin, alpha cypermethrin, deltamethrin	Bed net traps, IRC, LD	Yes	ND	ND	ND	[43]
Kenya	ITN	Unspecified	IRC, ORC, LD	Yes	ND	ND	Yes, but not significant	[40]
Niger	ITN	Unspecified LLINs	IRC, indoor/outdoor HLC, indoor/outdoor CDC LT	ND	ND	Yes	ND	[37]
Nigeria	IRS	Propoxur	Indoor/outdoor HLC, IRC	ND	ND	Yes	ND	[14]
Nigeria	IRS	Propoxur	Indoor/outdoor HLC, IRC, ORC, WET	Not observed	Not observed	Yes	Not observed	[52]
Tanzania (Pemba)	IRS	Dieldrin	IRC, ORC, indoor & outdoor HLC	Yes	ND	Not clear	Not clear	[38]
Tanzania	ITN+IRS	Permethrin or lambda cyhalothrin, DDT	Indoor CDC LT, outdoor HLC, IRC, ORC	ND	Inconclusive	Not observed	Inconclusive	[50]
Tanzania	ITN	Lambda cyhalothrin, deltamethrin	IRC, WET, indoor HLC	ND	Yes	ND	ND	[49]
Tanzania	ITN	Majority untreated nets	Indoor/outdoor HLC	ND	Not observed	Not observed	ND	[5]
Tanzania	ITN	Unspecified	Indoor CDC LTs, Mbita traps	ND	Yes	ND	ND	[46]
Tanzania	ITN	Unspecified	Indoor/Outdoor HLC	Yes	Yes	Yes	ND	[42]
The Gambia	ITN	Permethrin	Outdoor HLC, IRC, indoor CDC LT, bed net searches	ND	ND	Yes	Not observed	[55]
The Gambia	ITN	Permethrin	Indoor/outdoor HLC, IRC, WET	ND	Not observed	Not observed	Yes, but not significant	[51]

[a] ITN: Insecticide treated nets; IRC: Indoor residual spraying; ITC: Insecticide treated curtains
[b] LLINs: Long lasting insecticidal nets
[c] IRS: Indoor resting collection; ORC: Outdoor resting collection; CDC LT: Center for Disease Control light trap; HLC: Human landing collection; WET: Window exit trap; LD: Larval dipping; CMR: Capture-Mark-Recapture
[d] ND: Not done

Table 1. Review of the effect of insecticide based indoor vector control measures on malaria vectors in the Afrotropical region

5.3. Shifts to exophagy

In Nigeria, IRS resulted in a threefold increase of the proportion of *An. gambiae* s.l. biting outdoors [14,52]. Several years of vector control by IRS and later ITNs in the Bioko Island, increased the trend for outdoor biting of *An. gambiae* [21] as compared to historical data in the same region of preferred behaviour for indoor biting. Also in Tanzania, high ITN-use resulted in an increased outdoor biting for *An. funestus* [42]. In the latter study the proportion of indoor contact with *An. funestus* bites had dropped to only half of the indoor contact before wide-spread ITN-use. In southern Benin as well, after achieving universal ITN coverage, a higher proportion of outdoor biting was observed for *An. funestus* [47], although this was only observed in one out of two localities that were studied.

Some studies have shown that distribution of ITNs in Niger, Kenya, and The Gambia decreased the endophagic rate of *An. gambiae* s.l. [37,48,55], and to a lesser extend of *An. funestus* [37]. However, as the species of the *An. gambiae* complex were not determined in these studies, a possible reason for this decrease would be a species shift from *An. gambiae* to *An. arabiensis*.

In other studies however, no evidence for a shift to outdoor biting of *An. gambiae* s.l. due to widespread IRS or ITNs use was found in Tanzania [42,50], Burkina Faso [53] and The Gambia [51]. Also widespread use of mostly untreated bed nets did not result in a higher outdoor biting rate of *An. gambiae* [5].

5.4. Shifts to zoophily

In Kenya, ITN-use caused a shift in host selection of *An. gambiae* s.l. and *An. funestus* [54] from humans towards cattle or other animals. Similar observations were made in Burkina Faso with *An. gambiae* [19]. In other studies in Kenya and The Gambia, the use of ITNs caused only small and insignificant decreases in human blood index (HBI) for *An. gambiae* s.l. [40,48,51] and *An. funestus* [40].

The use of ITNs, IRS, or insecticide treated curtains caused no shift in host selection (or decrease in HBI) for *An. arabiensis* in Zambia [56], for *An. gambiae* s.l. in Nigeria, Burkina Faso, The Gambia, Tanzania and Kenya [34,50,52,53,55], and for *An. funestus* in Tanzania and Kenya [34,50].

5.5. Shifts to exophily

As summarized in [57], different populations of *An. arabiensis*, e.g. in the Pare-Taveta malaria scheme, Mauritius, Madagascar, Zanzibar, Nigeria and other West African localities, became either completely exophilic or, at most, remained only partially endophilic after IRS campaigns. ITN distribution reduced the indoor resting fraction of *An. gambiae* s.l. in Niger and Kenya [37,48], and of *An. funestus* in Kenya [48]. No evidence for a resting place shift after introduction of ITNs or after IRS was observed in Tanzania [50].

6. Australasian, Oriental, and Neotropical Regions

6.1. Species shifts

In the Solomon Islands, IRS in the 1960s has nearly eliminated the major malaria vectors *An. koliensis* and *An. punctulatus*, which are mainly endophagic and late-biters. The density of *An. farauti*, a more exophagic and early-biting malaria vector, remained quite high, particularly in outdoor man-biting situations [58]. The latter species is now the primary vector in the Solomon Islands, with the former major malaria vectors being totally absent. *An. hinesorum*, which is not considered a vector, has now occupied the breeding sites commonly used by *An. koliensis* [59].

In the forested hilly areas of Thailand, IRS resulted in a higher proportional decrease of *An. dirus* s.l. as compared to *An. minimus* s.l. [60]. Widespread use of IRS resulted in a different behaviour of the *An. minimus* s.l. present [61], which probably reflects a species shift from *An. minimus* to *An. harrisoni*, as also observed in Vietnam as a result of widespread use of ITNs [62]. Residual spraying did effectively control indoor resting species in Nepal such as *An. annularis*, *An. culicifacies*, *An. splendidus* and *An. vagus*. The abundance of the partially outdoor resting species, *An. fluviatilis* s.l. and *An. maculatus* s.l. also decreased markedly after the spray application, but then rebounded rapidly within 1 or 2 months after treatment [63]. ITN use in China caused a higher decrease of the endophilic and anthropophilic *An. lesteri* (syn. *An. anthropophagus*) [64] and *An. minimus* s.l. [65] than of the exophagic and zoophilic *An. sinensis*.

In British Guiana, the primary malaria vector *An. darlingi* (both larvae and adults) was rapidly eliminated by IRS, whereas larvae and adults of a zoophilic species, *Anopheles aquasalis*, a possible malaria vector, were completely unaffected [66]. In Guatemala, *An. vestitipennis* decreased in abundance in communities with a wide distribution of ITNs, while *An. albimanus* did not change. Whether this change was an effect of the ITNs could not be concluded as the study was not designed for answering that question [67].

6.2. Shifts to early biting

In Papua New Guinea, ITN distribution immediately changed the biting cycles of both *An. farauti* and *An. koliensis* from a post-midnight peak towards a pre-midnight peak [68]. Also on the Solomon Islands, intervention and longitudinal studies have shown that IRS, ITNs, or a combination of both, changed the biting cycle of *An. farauti* to an earlier biting peak [58,69,70].

IRS changed the indoor biting peak of *An. dirus* s.l. in the forested hilly areas of Thailand to one hour earlier. Outdoors, the peak remained the same, but a higher proportion bite earlier. Also for *An. minimus* s.l., a shift to earlier biting was observed [60]. In the foothills on the other hand, where *An. minimus* s.l. was the main vector, no effect of DDT was seen on the already early biting *An. minimus* s.l. population [71]. Also recent studies in Vietnam have shown that in the prolonged presence of impregnated bed nets, 45% of the *Anopheles* bites are acquired before sleeping time in the forest, and 64% before sleeping time in the village [8]. In Cambodia, in a period when ITN coverage was still low, already 29% of the *Anopheles* bites were acquired before sleeping time [9].

Although we have not encountered studies in Latin-America with evidence for shifts to earlier biting, some studies indicated that also in this region, early biting vectors can maintain residual transmission. In an area in Brazil covered by IRS for example, blood-feeding of *An. darlingi* started at sunset, remained high during the first half of the night, and decreased gradually until early morning [72]. Also in the Bolivian Amazon, in an area with high ITN use, peak outdoor biting of *An. darlingi* occurred between 19:00 and 21:00 hours, when 48% of the total night's biting took place, and 83% of the night's biting had occurred by 22:00 hours when most local people go to bed [73].

6.3. Shifts to exophagy

On different islands of the Solomon, proportional shifts to outdoor biting (from 47% to 67%) were observed for *An. farauti* after IRS [58]. Moreover, compared to *An. koliensis* and *An. punctulatus*, the exophagic *An. farauti* population recovered completely within nine months after the spraying campaign. However, in other intervention and longitudinal studies on the Solomon Islands, the shift to outdoor biting of *An. farauti* due to ITNs and/or IRS was not so obvious [59,69].

IRS increased the outdoor biting rate of *An. dirus* s.l. [60,74], and of *An. minimus* s.l. in forested and foothill regions in Thailand [60,61]. In contrast, in another foothill region of Thailand, an initial effect of DDT was seen on the malaria transmission, but this was not sustained for this already outdoor biting *An. minimus* s.l. population [71]. Also wide scale use of ITNs caused a higher decrease in the indoor biting populations as compared to the outdoor biting populations of *An. sinensis*, *An. lesteri* (syn. *An. anthropophagus*) and *An. minimus* s.l. in China [64,65]. In Vietnam, after prolonged ITNs distribution, outdoor biting densities of the main vectors, *An. dirus*, *An. maculatus* s.l. and *An. minimus* s.l. were significantly higher than indoor biting density [8]. In Laos, in contrast, the use of ITNs did not stop *An. dirus* from entering the houses [75].

In an IRS area in Brazil, *An. darlingi* fed more frequently outdoors, whereas in earlier years before IRS this species mainly fed indoors [72]. In contrast, in Colombia, IRS did not stop malaria vectors to bite both indoors and outdoors [76]. The combined use of ITNs and IRS has preceded the collapse of a mainly exophagic *An. darlingi* population in Suriname. However, this collapse can also be attributed to an unusual, extensive flooding which coincided with the onset of the control interventions [77].

6.4. Shifts to zoophily

A significant decrease in HBI of *An. farauti* was observed immediately after the distribution of ITNs in Papua New Guinea, although this shift could be due to a slightly changed sampling method [68].

In Thailand, in the prolonged presence of DDT use in IRS, *An. minimus* s.l. exhibited a marked zoophily, whereas in villages with lower DDT pressure, no preference was observed [61], although this apparent 'change in behaviour' could have been due to a species shift within the *An. minimus* complex as observed in Vietnam [62]. In an intervention study in India, the HBI of *An. culicifacies* was lower in areas with ITNs as compared to areas with untreated bed nets or no nets [78].

In Mexico, a much lower HBI was observed in areas where IRS was implemented as compared to historical data [79]. Also in areas covered by IRS in Brazil, *An. darlingi* was mostly zoophilic [80].

6.5. Shifts to exophily

A very low endophily rate was observed for *An. farauti* after several DDT spraying campaigns in the Solomon Islands [58].

IRS also significantly reduced the indoor resting abundance of all anopheline species except for *An. fluviatilis* s.l. in Nepal [63], and of *An. dirus* s.l. in Thailand [74]. In India, *An. culicifacies* s.l. has been observed to be highly exophilic in areas where residual spraying with DDT was widely used [81]. Also in areas with wide scale use of ITNs in India fewer *An. culicifacies* s.l. were collected indoors (resting collections) as compared to control areas. However, in this area more *An. culicifacies* s.l. were found indoor-resting in individual houses with untreated bed nets as compared to houses with ITNs, both located in the ITN-area [78]. This suggests that this mosquito population did not shift entirely to exophily, but that this behaviour mainly reflects the excito-repellent effect of the permethrin.

IRS has brought the disappearance of *An. darlingi* from the interior of houses in Brazil and French Guiana [28,80]. However, outdoor-resting still persists, either in the vicinity of the houses [80] or outside the peridomestic environment [28]. ITNs as well caused less indoor-resting in an intervention trial in Guatemala [67]. In contrast, in Mexico, after prolonged use of DDT no deterrence was observed anymore for *An. pseudopunctipennis*, with as many mosquitoes seeking shelter in sprayed huts as in unsprayed huts [82].

Country	Vector control measure [a]	Insecticide [b]	Collection methods [c]	Species shift [d]	Shift to early-biting [d]	Shift to exophagy [d]	Shift to zoophily [d]	Reference
Australasian Region								
Papua New Guinea	ITN	Permethrin	Outdoor HLC	Not observed	Yes	ND	Yes?	[68]
Solomon Islands	IRS	DDT	HLC	Yes	Yes	Yes	ND	[58]
Solomon Islands	IRS, ITN	DDT, permethrin	Outdoor HLC, indoor CDC LT, outdoor pig baited traps	ND	Yes	Not clear	ND	[69]
Solomon Islands	IRS, ITN	DDT, lambda cyhalothrin Permethrin, unspecified LLIN	Indoor/ outdoor HLC, LD, animal baited trap	Yes	ND	ND	ND	[59]
Solomon Islands	ITN, IRS	Deltamethrin, lambda cyhalothrin	Indoor/ outdoor HLC, IRC, WET, LD	ND	yes	Yes, small	ND	[59]
Oriental region								

Country	Vector control measure [a]	Insecticide [b]	Collection methods [c]	Species shift [d]	Shift to early-biting [d]	Shift to exophagy [d]	Shift to zoophily [d]	Reference
China	ITN	Deltamethrin	Indoor/outdoor man-baited nets	Yes	ND	Yes	ND	[64]
China	ITN	Deltamethrin	?	Yes	ND	Yes	ND	In [65]
India	ITN	Lambdacyhalothrin	IRC, Indoor HLC, Outdoor Cattle collection	ND	ND	ND	Yes	[78]
Nepal	IRS	DDT, bendiocarb, malathion	Indoor/outdoor HLC, IRC, ORC, cattle collections, LD	Yes	ND	?	ND	[63]
Thailand	IRS	DDT	Indoor/outdoor HLC	Yes	Yes	Yes	ND	[60]
Thailand	IRS	DDT	Indoor/outdoor HLC	Not observed	Not observed	Not observed	ND	[71]
Thailand	IRS	DDT	Indoor/outdoor HLC, bovid-baited trap, IRC, ORC	Probably	ND	Yes	Yes	[61]
Thailand	IRS	DDT, fenitrothion	Indoor/outdoor HLC, IRC	ND	ND	Yes	ND	[74]
Vietnam	ITN	Permethrin	Indoor/outdoor HLC, IRC, CDC LT	Yes	ND	ND	ND	[62]
Neotropical Region								
Brazil	IRS	DDT	IRC, ORC, animal baited trap,	ND	ND	ND	Yes?	In [80]
Brazil	IRS	DDT	Indoor/outdoor HLC, outdoor animal baited trap	ND	ND	Yes	ND	[72]
British Guiana	IRS	DDT	IRC, LD	Yes	ND	ND	ND	[66]
Guatemala	ITN	Permethrin	Indoor/outdoor HLC, IRC, inspection of bed net surfaces, CMR	Yes?	ND	Not observed	ND	[67]
Mexico	IRS	DDT, bendiocarb	IRC, ORC	ND	ND	ND	Yes	[79]
Mexico	IRS	DDT (dieldrin before)	Entry traps, WET	ND	ND	ND	ND	[82]

[a] ITN: Insecticide treated nets; IRS: Indoor residual spraying; ITC: Insecticide treated curtains
[b] LLINs: Long lasting insecticidal nets
[c] IRC: Indoor resting collection; ORC: Outdoor resting collection; CDC LT: Center for Disease Control light trap; HLC: Human landing collection; WET: Window exit trap; LD: Larval dipping; CMR: Capture-Mark-Recapture
[d] ND: Not done

Table 2. Review of the effect of insecticide based indoor vector control measures on malaria vectors in the Australasian, Oriental and Neotropical regions

7. Discussion

7.1. The importance of residual transmission by outdoor and early biting malaria vectors

In this chapter we have shown that outdoor and early biting malaria vectors are widespread among malaria endemic countries and, as relative shifts to outdoor, early or animal-biting and outdoor resting vectors occur due to the use of IRS and ITNs, these vectors will increasingly contribute to malaria transmission in regions with a high coverage of ITNs and IRS. However the reported shifts are not always well documented: species identification of complexes are often missing, and confounding factors such as changes of the environment, habitat, human behaviour and occupation are not considered.

In Africa, most of the species shifts observed resulted in a large decrease of the important endophagic, endophilic and anthropophilic malaria vectors, *An. funestus* and *An. gambiae*, while the more exophagic, exophilic, and/or zoophilic species *An. arabiensis* persists. Reports on such species shift are recently increasing, with most of these shifts described in East-Africa. But also in the other geographical regions, shifts in species abundances have been observed. It is however important to note that the majority of shifts described are shifts in relative abundances, where the more endophagic, endophilic and/or anthropophilic species declines more (or is being eliminated) while the more exophagic, exophilic and/or zoophilic species maintains at the same density or declines less. Only in some cases, the density of the latter species actually increases (e.g. the non-vector species *An. rivulorum* [35] or *An. parensis* [36]), probably because they take over the breeding sites of the declining species. Moreover, as also mentioned in [83], the vectorial capacity of the species predominating after the intervention does not necessarily increase, but persisting species that are malaria vectors, such as *An. arabiensis*, will be responsible for the residual malaria transmission, while the role of e.g. *An. gambiae* or *An. funestus* decreases.

Therefore, one of the most plausible reasons for species shifts to occur in the presence of ITNs or IRS is the non-uniform exposure of the different species to the insecticides, as described above. This hypothesis is supported by a study in Kenya in which the persisting *An. arabiensis* in an area with high ITN coverage had little to no pyrethroid resistance compared to the declining *An. gambiae*, with moderate to high levels of pyrethroid resistance [41,43]. Moreover, in experimental hut trials on northeast Tanzania, the mortality of *An. arabiensis* measured in experimental huts was consistently lower than that of *An. gambiae* and *An. funestus* [83], which probably is a major contributing factor to the species shifts observed in East Africa following scale up of ITNs. The authors state that, as cone tests on the nets prior to the trials produced rather similar levels of mortality among *An. gambiae* and *An. arabiensis*, the most likely explanation for lower *An. arabiensis* mortality was behavioural avoidance of treated net surfaces. As feeding inhibition in this experiment was similar for *An. arabiensis* and *An. gambiae*, outdoor blood-feeding would be the major mechanism to which *An. arabiensis* avoids contact with the ITN, as opposed to abandoning host-searching when confronted with ITNs.

Besides the species shifts, shifts to earlier-, outdoor-, and animal-biting have been observed for primary vectors such as *An. gambiae*, *An. funestus*, *An. farauti*, *An. koliensis*, *An. dirus* s.l., *An.*

minimus s.l., *An. culicifacies*, and *An. darlingi*. These shifts might also be linked to the non-random exposure of subpopulations of vectors to insecticide treated surfaces (ITNs or IRS). Several studies have indeed shown that the feeding and resting behaviour of anophelines is consistent in certain subpopulations and/or linked to certain genetic markers. Most of the studies on genetic determination of biting and resting behaviour are based on chromosomal inversions. Alleles captured within chromosome rearrangements are protected from recombination and can as such favour local adaptation by capturing sets of locally adapted genes which might lead to reproductive isolated entities or subpopulations [84]. In the Garki District in Nigeria, chromosomal arrangements in *An. arabiensis* and *An. gambiae* have been associated with exophagy and exophily [85,86] and with zoophily [87]. Exophagy and exophily were associated with the standard chromosomal arrangements 2R+^{a} for *An. arabiensis* and 2R+^{b} for *An. gambiae*, and the inverted arrangement 2Rbc for *An. arabiensis*. Moreover, the chromosome arrangements associated with indoor biting or resting are the ones adapted to drier environments, while arrangements more frequent in outdoor collected specimens are those associated with more humid environments [85]. In the Zambesi valley, 2Rc *An. arabiensis* heterozygotes were associated with exophily and zoophily [57]. In Ethiopia *An. arabiensis* heterozygotes of the 2La and/or 2Rb chromosomal arrangements tended to bite later at night than the double homozygotes [88]. Also in laboratory experiments an association between chromosomal arrangements and circadian flight activity has been found [89]: female *An. stephensi* homozygotes for the 2Rb inversion showed more activity following light-on (corresponding to early morning) as compared to homozygous females for the standard 2R+^{b} arrangement. Other field-based evidence on the existence of subpopulations showing consistent behaviour was obtained by studying behaviour of *An. balabacensis* in a capture-mark-recapture experiment in Borneo (Malaysia) [90]. This study revealed significant trends of *An. balabacensis* to be recaptured on the same host or resting site of the original capture. In contrast, a similar capture-mark-recapture study on resting behaviour of *An. gambiae* s.l. in Tanzania showed no faithful tendencies of endo- or exophily [91]: the same individuals within the *An. gambiae* s.l. population mixed indoor and outdoor resting. More recent genetic studies are based on the frequencies of enzyme polymorphisms. In the Malaysian study [90], faithfully indoor and outdoor-resting populations showed significant differences in isozyme frequencies (loci *Est-3* and *Idh-3*). Also in Burundi, isozyme frequencies were significantly different between in- and out-door biting *An. arabiensis* (locus *Mdh-2*) and in- and out-door resting *An. gambiae* (*Mpi* and *Got-2* loci) [92]. Such differences were not observed for *An. gambiae* in Burkina Faso [93]. Moreover, mosquitoes carrying a specific genotype [93] or chromosome karyotypes [87] were found to be significantly more infected with sporozoites, suggesting the occurrence of subpopulations having different vector behaviours. These independent genetic studies, either based on karyotyping or on genotyping, provide evidence that active choice for the best place, time or host to bite, or the best place to rest can be associated with specific genotypes. This suggests the existence of subpopulations characterized by specific behavioural patterns which implies a non-uniform exposure to IRS or ITNs. Selection of specific behavioural patterns can then not be excluded.

However, other mechanisms can also explain these kinds of shifts. More early biting could occur as females that fail to obtain a blood meal during the previous night, might be more likely to commence host seeking in the early evening [44]. By disrupting the feeding behaviour, the ITNs would increase the length of the oviposition cycle of the overall population [68]. This mechanism could explain the immediate change in biting cycles of both *An. farauti* and *An. koliensis* after ITN distribution in Papua New Guinea. Both species shifted from a post-midnight biting peak towards a pre-midnight peak [68], with an extended oviposition cycle. Also in the Solomon Islands, the oviposition cycle was extended from 3 to 4 days due to ITN use, possibly explaining the higher tendency for early biting observed in the village with ITN use [69]. Shifts to outdoor biting by *An. farauti* also occurred immediately after DDT spraying [58]. This first effect would be caused by the deterrent effect of DDT, while only in second instance the endophilic fraction of *An. farauti* is being killed. Moreover, compared to *An. koliensis* and *An. punctulatus*, the *An. farauti* population recovered completely within nine months after the spraying campaign, indicating that this change of behaviour is due to a plastic response to the deterrent effect of DDT. Moreover, it has been shown that the occurrence of a shift in host selection does not necessarily reflect a selection of a more zoophilic vector subpopulation, but can also indicate plasticity in host selection. The *An. gambiae* population in Burkina Faso that showed a high proportion of cattle feeding (HBI of only 40%), had an innate preference for humans (88%) in a choice experiment using an odour-baited trap [19]. The weak accessibility of humans due to the use of ITNs, forces the mosquitoes to feed on cattle. According to the authors of the study, this suggests that in this area a plastic foraging strategy could provide greater benefits than a specialist strategy for this species.

Regardless of the mechanism that causes these behavioural shifts, the case studies show that in several areas the proportion of outdoor-, early- and/or animal biting primary vectors are relatively increasing, which will then be responsible for residual transmission. Moreover, in a similar way, transmission by 'secondary' vectors that have outdoor or early biting behaviour might become more important than transmission by primary vectors in contexts of high coverage of ITNs and IRS. In a malaria endemic region of Thailand, one specimen of the Barbirostris Subgroup (*An. barbirostris/campestris*) was found to contain *Plasmodium* oocysts, in the prolonged absence of the main malaria vectors, showing that *An. barbirostris* s.l., an outdoor biting mosquito [94], might be responsible for maintaining malaria transmission in the absence of the main vectors [95]. As secondary vectors are often less anthropophilic, and might be more exophagic and early biting, planning of vector control should also take into account their behaviour. Moreover, as pointed out in [8], secondary vectors might be better vectors of *P. vivax* as compared to *P. falciparum*, as the extrinsic incubation period of *P. vivax* is shorter. In British Guiana, for example, *An. aquasalis*, a mostly zoophilic and exophilic mosquito species breeding in brackish water, was vector of several Vivax malaria outbreaks after *An. darlingi* was eliminated by DDT spraying [96]. Also more recently in Vietnam, *An. sawadwongporni*, a very early biting secondary vector, was found positive for *P. vivax* [8].

7.2. ITNs and IRS are very effective, but additional measures are needed for reaching malaria elimination

ITNs and IRS have been shown to have a large impact on malaria infection and disease [97,98]. Moreover, several entomological studies have also shown that where the vectors are mostly endophagic, endophilic and anthropophilic, ITNs and IRS are very effective in reducing their population density. This was for example shown for *An. minimus* in India [99] and for *An. dirus* in Laos [100], both of them being anthropophilic, indoor- and late-biting in the respective study sites. A recent study in Zambia also showed that even at a high coverage of ITNs and IRS, the highest probability for malaria transmission based on human and vector behaviour, still occurs indoors [101], making ITNs and IRS valuable tools.

ITNs can also have an effect on malaria transmitted by more zoophilic and exophagic mosquitoes. In Sao Tomé for example, where *An. gambiae* is zoophilic and very exophagic, increased bed net use decreased the malaria prevalence in both bed net users and non-users [102]. The differences in prevalence between users and non-users were greatest in children under 5 years old, who are more likely to use the bed nets in the evening, showing that indeed the bed nets were the cause of the decrease. However, in older age groups, that are more likely to remain outside in the evening, no such difference was observed. Moreover, even at an almost 80% ITN coverage, still a 30% malaria prevalence was observed among bed net users. This means that, as expected, a part of transmission by these zoophilic and exophagic mosquitoes could not be prevented by ITNs [102]. Also in other parts of the world it has been shown that ITNs are less performing in areas with outdoor biting or resting vectors, for example in Peru and Nicaragua [11]. In the Garki District (Nigeria), the impact of the IRS campaign with propoxur was related to the prespraying ratio between the man-biting density and the indoor-resting density and to intraspecific cytogenetic variation [52]. Moreover, as reviewed in [103], even low levels of exophagy, exophily or zoophily may attenuate the impact of ITNs and IRS because this allows mosquitoes to obtain blood while avoiding fatal contact with insecticides.

As we have shown that outdoor-, animal- and early biting behaviour, as well as outdoor resting behaviour is widespread among malaria vectors all over the world and might be increasing as a result of widespread IRS or ITN use, there is an urgent need for additional control measures tackling malaria transmission by these vector populations [103–106]. In other words, there is a 'gap' in protection, not only before sleeping time, but also for people that remain outdoors during the night (Figure 2) and this gap needs to be tackled by additional vector control measures. There are many ways of additionally reducing host-vector contact, including the use of topical repellents, spatial repellents, insecticide treated clothing, long lasting insecticidal hammocks, etc. Recently much research is carried out on the effectiveness of these kind of tools. For example, in the Bolivian Amazon, where the primary vectors *An. darlingi* has a peak biting activity before sleeping time, a household based cluster randomized trial has shown that the combined use of a topical repellent (para-menthane-3,8-diol, PMD) and ITNs can reduce the incidence of malaria by 80%, which was only significant for *P. vivax* and not for *P. falciparum*, as compared to the use of ITNs alone [107]. DEET-based repellents also had an additional protective efficacy against malaria disease in a small scale community based trial in India [108], and DEET-based repellent soap against *P. falciparum* malaria in a household randomized trial in a refugee camp in Pakistan [109]. In an ongoing study in Cambodia, Picaridin based repellents are shown to provide a protection of more than 90% against the bites of the main malaria vectors *An. dirus* and *An. minimus* (MalaResT project led by ITM-Antwerp, preliminary results). Whether the mass use of this repellent will result in a decrease of malaria infection is currently under investigation using a cluster-randomized controlled trial in

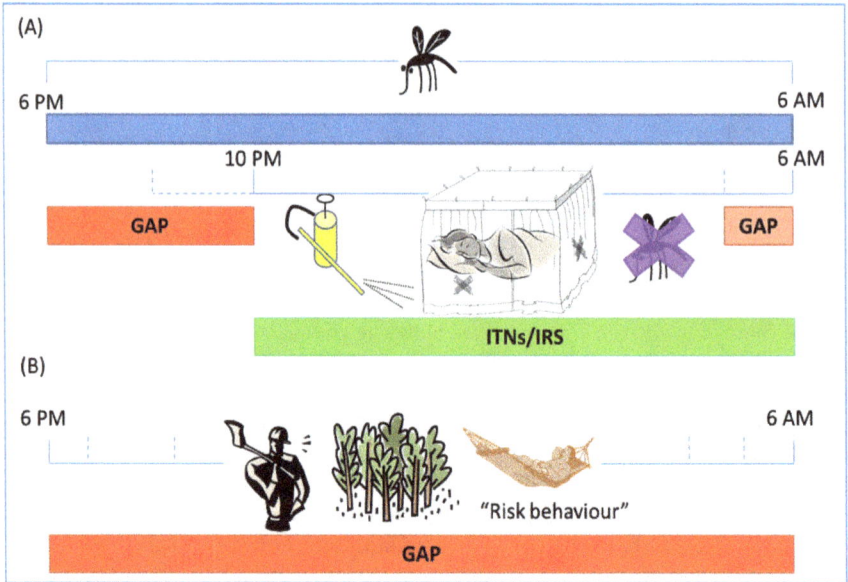

Figure 2. Protection 'gap' when only indoor insecticide-based vector control measures are applied. Anophelines generally bite between 6pm and 6am. ITNs will only protect from infective bites that are acquired indoors, and during sleeping time. IRS only target mosquitoes that rest indoors. Therefore, there is a gap in protection both indoors and outdoors before and after people go to bed (A), but also for people conducting outdoor activities during the night (i.e. 'risk behaviour') (B).

Ratanakkiri province in Cambodia. In a refugee camp in Kenya, permethrin treated clothing and blankets reduced malaria infection significantly [110]. In Southeast Asia, long lasting insecticidal hammocks have been shown to be effective against malaria disease [111] and against *An. minimus* bites, but not *An. dirus* bites [112]. For zoophilic mosquitoes, intervening in the host-vector contact could be more efficient by focusing on its preferred hosts, e.g. by insecticide treatment of cattle. However, killing partly zoophilic mosquitoes in sufficient numbers to suppress malaria transmission would require high protective coverage of both human and animal blood sources [104]. Moreover, it has been observed in Ethiopia that more than 90% of the blood meals taken by zoophilic vectors were taken from the legs of cattle [113], which are more difficult to treat.

Alternative personal protection measures are also of interest for people that work or reside in the forest, a risk area of malaria transmission in Southeast Asia [114]. For temporary shelters in the forest, insecticide treated plastic sheeting could be useful as this has proven to be effective in protecting against malaria disease in emergency camps [115]. Their effectiveness will rely both on their repelling effect and their killing effect, and whether mosquitoes will rest on this sheeting. Alternatively, other more accepted insecticide treated bed net-designs (V-shaped

Tool	Mosquito behaviour that is targeted				Personal (P) or community (C)[b] protection
	Time of biting (E/N)[a]	Host preference(I/O)[a] (A/Z)[a]	Place of biting	Place of resting (I/O)[a]	
Tools relying on host-vector contact					
ITNs	N	A	I	I	P & C
Long lasting insecticidal hammocks & other net designs adapted to outdoor conditions	(E &) N	A	O	O	P & C
Insecticide treated plastic sheeting for shelters in the forest	E & N	A & Z	I & O	O	P
Personal protection including Topical & spatial repellents, Insecticide treated clothing	E & N	A	I & O	I & O	P & C*
Insecticide treatment of cattle	E & N	Z	I & O	I & O	C*
Tools not relying on vector-host contact					
IRS	E & N	A & Z	I & O	I	C
Larval source management	E & N	A & Z	I & O	I & O	C*
Toxic sugar baits	E & N	A & Z	I & O	I & O	C*
Treatment of outdoor resting places, e.g. with fungal biopesticides	E & N	A & Z	I & O	O	C*

[a] E: Early evening & morning biting; N: Night biting; A: Antropophilic; Z: Zoophilic; I: Indoor; O: Outdoor
[b] Community protection can only be achieved if the coverage of the intervention is large enough.
* Community protection is assumed or shown in a limited number of studies, but more evidence is required for confirmation of community protection.

Table 3. Vector control tools and their targets.

nets, long lasting insecticidal hammocks, etc.), could provide protection for people staying in the forest during the night.

The more zoophilic, exophagic, or early biting a mosquito species or population, the more personal protection will act simply by blocking host-vector contact (through lethal or repellent effects). As shown by a mathematical model, malaria transmission involving zoophilic vectors (with 10% feeding on humans) can only be significantly decreased if the personal protection measures confer high levels of individual protection to users (80%) and be used by the majority of human population (80%) [116]. Therefore, the success of any intervention in this context will depend on its entomological efficacy, but also on the human behaviour, including acceptance and adherence to the preventive measures within the community. In São Tomé for example, many people watch communal television outdoors, posing them at risk for early-evening malaria transmission [117]. In Thailand, people do not take their ITN from the village to their farm plot [118]. Also in Vietnam, people often combine living in the village with a second home at their fields located in the forest [119], creating other malaria control needs, such as, for example, long lasting insecticidal hammocks. Taking into account human behaviour when adapting vector control strategies will then be crucial. In Bioko Island (Equatorial Guinea) for example, an increased trend of outdoor biting was observed for the main malaria vector *An. gambiae* [21]. However, the main malaria risk group, namely children under 15 years old, rarely stay outdoors when it is dark, and there is no evidence that children who report to stay outdoors during the night are at higher risk for malaria infection as compared to those who do not [120]. Implementing control measures that target outdoor biting mosquitoes in this age group would then provide no additional benefit and would be a waste of resources, as personal protection tools might be very expensive to implement.

Also other tools not relying on the host-vector contact can supplement ITNs and IRS as they are not specific for indoor biting and indoor resting mosquito populations [105,106]. Vector control tools could for example target key environmental resources such as the aquatic larval habitat, sugar sources, and resting behaviour. Very little is known about how to manipulate these environmental resources so that malaria transmission is interrupted [105]. Knowledge on vector ecology and behaviour therefore remains crucial. However, despite large knowledge gaps, several examples exist of malaria control by targeting non-blood meal related steps of the mosquito cycle. Larval source management has indeed shown to be effective where vectors breed in large water bodies [121]. However, when larval habitats are more dispersed and not permanent, this approach is considered less feasible. Renewed attention has been given to larval source management as complementary tool to ITNs as recent studies in Africa have shown that it provides substantial additional protection with a high cost-effectiveness in specific settings [122]. Moreover, other innovative ideas combined with knowledge on the vector behaviour can lead to successful vector control. Toxic sugar baits for example were successfully used in a targeted way for the control of the cistern dwelling malaria vector *An. claviger* in the desert oases of Israel [123]. Fungal biopesticides also have the potential to significantly reduce densities of malaria vectors [124] as well as associated malaria transmission [125]. These fungi could be delivered through outdoor odour-baited stations, and in this way slowly eliminate a high proportion of outdoor-resting vectors [126].

8. Conclusion

For malaria eradication to succeed, all elements in the transmission cycle must be sufficiently targeted. With the current vector control tools, only indoor- and late-biting, and indoor-resting vectors are tackled. In this paper, we have shown that there is a 'gap' in protection, not only before sleeping time, but also for people that remain outdoors during the night. Moreover, by describing different shifts in vector species, and vector behaviour within species or species complexes, we have shown that the importance of this gap can increase as a result of widespread ITN or IRS use. Therefore, to eliminate residual malaria transmission, additional vector control tools will be needed. These new vector control tools should be designed to target outdoor and early feeding mosquitoes. Moreover, they should be accessible and acceptable for the populations at risk. A specific mosquito behaviour assuring its vectorial status is only relevant in relation to a specific human behaviour and the relation people have with their surrounding environment. Interrupting malaria transmission may than require different combinations of mosquito control methods addressing each mosquito behaviour at risk for transmission, but also taking into account possible changes in soil occupation, housing conditions, sleeping habits, and outdoor occupation. In conclusion, there is no 'silver bullet' in vector control and malaria prevention. New paradigms for controlling and/or interrupting malaria transmission should then be explored for their protective efficacy and adapted to the local context for a good efficiency. Although implementation of such new approaches might be very expensive, they will be crucial if malaria elimination is the final aim.

Acknowledgements

This review was initiated under the impulse of the Roll Back Malaria - Vector Control Working Group – Work Stream Outdoor Malaria Transmission (http://www.rbm.who.int/mechanisms/vcwgWorkstream2.html), the MalaResT research Project (B&M Gates Foundation OPP1032354) and the Third ITM-DGCD Framework Agreement Programme. We would like to thank Vincent Sluydts and Sylvie Manguin for their critical review of this paper.

Author details

Lies Durnez[1] and Marc Coosemans[1,2*]

*Address all correspondence to: mcoosemans@itg.be; ldurnez@itg.be

1 Department of Biomedical Sciences, Institute of Tropical Medicine, Antwerp, Belgium

2 Department of Biomedical Sciences, Faculty of Pharmaceutical, Veterinary and Biomedical Sciences, University of Antwerp, Antwerpen (Wilrijk), Belgium

References

[1] Killeen, G F, Smith, T A, Ferguson, H M, Mshinda, H, Abdulla, S, Lengeler, C, & Kachur, S P. Preventing childhood malaria in Africa by protecting adults from mosquitoes with insecticide-treated nets. PLoS Medicine (2007). 4, e229.

[2] WHO. World Malaria Report 2011. World Health Organisation (2012).

[3] Alonso, P L, Brown, G, Arevalo-herrera, M, Binka, F, Chitnis, C, Collins, F, Doumbo, O K, Greenwood, B, Hall, B F, Levine, M M, Mendis, K, Newman, R D, Plowe, C V, Rodríguez, M H, Sinden, R, Slutsker, L, & Tanner, M. A research agenda to underpin malaria eradication. PLoS Medicine (2011). 8, e1000406.

[4] Shililu, J, Ghebremeskel, T, Seulu, F, Mengistu, S, Fekadu, H, Zerom, M, Asmelash,G, Sintasath, D, Mbogo, C, Githure, J, Brantly, E, Beier, J, & Novak, R. Seasonal abundance, vector behaviour, and malaria parasite transmission in Eritrea. Journal of the American Mosquito Control Association (2004). 20, 155-64.

[5] Killeen, G F, Kihonda, J, Lyimo, E, Oketch, F R, Kotas, M E, Mathenge, E, Schellenberg, J A, Lengeler, C, Smith, T A, & Drakeley, C J. Quantifying behavioural interactions between humans and mosquitoes: evaluating the protective efficacy of insecticidal nets against malaria transmission in rural Tanzania. BMC Infectious Diseases (2006). 6, 161.

[6] Maxwell, C A, Wakibara, J, Tho, S, & Curtis, C F. Malaria-infective biting at different hours of the night. Medical and Veterinary Entomology (1998). 12, 325-7.

[7] Okello, P E, Van Bortel, W, Byaruhanga, A M, Correwyn, A, Roelants, P, Talisuna, A, D'Alessandro, U, & Coosemans, M. Variation in malaria transmission intensity in seven sites throughout Uganda. The American Journal of Tropical Medicine and Hygiene (2006). 75, 219-25.

[8] Van Bortel, W, Trung, H D, Hoi, L X, Van Ham, N, Van Chut, N, Luu, N D, Roelants, P, Denis, L, Speybroeck, N, D'Alessandro, U, & Coosemans, M. Malaria transmission and vector behaviour in a forested malaria focus in central Vietnam and the implications for vector control. Malaria Journal (2010).9, 373.

[9] Durnez, L, Mao, S, Van Bortel, W, Denis, L, Roelants, P, Sochantha, T, & Coosemans, M. Outdoor malaria transmission in forested villages of Cambodia. Manuscript in preparation.

[10] Prakash, A, Bhattacharyya, D, Mohapatra, P, & Mahanta, J. Malaria transmission risk by the mosquito Anopheles baimaii (formerly known as An. dirus species D) at different hours of the night in North-east India. Medical and Veterinary Entomology (2005). 19, 423-7.

[11] Kroeger, A, González, M, & Ordóñez-González, J. Insecticide-treated materials for malaria control in Latin America: to use or not to use? Transactions of the Royal Society of Tropical Medicine and Hygiene (1999). 93, 565-70.

[12] Mouchet, J, & Hamon, J. Difficulties in malaria eradication campaigns due to the behavior of the vectors. Geneva: World Health Organisation (1963). WHO/Mal/394; WHO/Vector Control/35.

[13] Govella, N J, Okumu, F O, & Killeen, G F. Insecticide-treated nets can reduce malaria transmission by mosquitoes which feed outdoors. The American Journal of Tropical Medicine and Hygiene (2010). 82, 415-9.

[14] Molineaux, L, Shidrawi, G R, Clarke, J L, Boulzaguet, J R, & Ashkar, T S. Assessment of insecticidal impact on the malaria mosquito's vectorial capacity, from data on the man-biting rate and age-composition. Bulletin of the World Health Organization (1979). 57, 265-74.

[15] Molineaux, L, Shidrawi, G R, Clarke, J L, Boulzaguet, R, Ashkar, T, & Dietz, K. The impact of propoxur on Anopheles gambiae s.l. and some other anopheline populations,

and its relationship with some pre-spraying variables. Bulletin of the World Health Organization (1976). 54, 379-89.

[16] Smits, A, Coosemans, M, Van Bortel, W, Barutwanayo, M, & Delacollette, C. Readjustment of the malaria vector control strategy in the Rusizi Valley, Burundi. Bulletin of Entomological Research (1995). 85, 541-8.

[17] Griffin, J T, Hollingsworth, T D, Okell, L C, Churcher, T S, White, M, Hinsley, W, Bousema, T, Drakeley, C J, Ferguson, N M, Basáñez, M-G, & Ghani, A C. Reducing *Plasmodium falciparum* malaria transmission in Africa: a model-based evaluation of intervention strategies. PLoS Medicine (2010). 7, e1000324.

[18] Sinka, M E, Bangs, M J, Manguin, S, Coetzee, M, Mbogo, C M, Hemingway, J, Patil, A P, Temperley, W H, Gething, P W, Kabaria, C W, Okara, R M, Van Boeckel, T, Godfray, H C J, Harbach, R E, & Hay, S I. The dominant *Anopheles* vectors of human malaria in Africa, Europe and the Middle East: occurrence data, distribution maps and bionomic précis. Parasites & Vectors (2010). 3, 117.

[19] Lefèvre, T, Gouagna, L-C, Dabiré, K R, Elguero, E, Fontenille, D, Renaud, F, Costantini, C, & Thomas, F. Beyond nature and nurture: phenotypic plasticity in blood-feeding behaviour of *Anopheles gambiae* s.s. when humans are not readily accessible. The American Journal of Tropical Medicine and Hygiene (2009). 81, 1023-9.

[20] Sousa, C A, Pinto, J, Almeida, A P, Ferreira, C, Do Rosário, V E, & Charlwood, JD. Dogs as a favored host choice of *Anopheles gambiae* sensu stricto (Diptera: Culicidae) of São Tomé West Africa. Journal of Medical Entomology (2001). 38, 122-5.

[21] Reddy, M R, Overgaard, H J, Abaga, S, Reddy, V P, Caccone, A, Kiszewski, A E, & Slotman, M A. Outdoor host seeking behaviour of *Anopheles gambiae* mosquitoes following initiation of malaria vector control on Bioko Island, Equatorial Guinea. Malaria Journal (2011). 10, 184.

[22] Trung, H D, Van Bortel, W, Sochantha, T, Keokenchanh, K, Briët, O J T, & Coosemans, M. Behavioural heterogeneity of *Anopheles* species in ecologically different localities in Southeast Asia: a challenge for vector control. Tropical Medicine & International Health (2005). 10, 251-62.

[23] Vythilingam, I, Sidavong, B, Chan, S T, Phonemixay, T, Vanisaveth, V, Sisoulad, P, Phetsouvanh, R, Hakim, S L, & Phompida, S. Epidemiology of malaria in Attapeu-Province, Lao PDR in relation to entomological parameters. Transactions of the Royal Society of Tropical Medicine and Hygiene (2005). 99, 833-9.

[24] Obsomer, V, Defourny, P, & Coosemans, M. The *Anopheles dirus* complex: spatial distribution and environmental drivers. Malaria Journal (2007). 6, 26.

[25] Sinka, M E, Rubio-Palis, Y, Manguin, S, Patil, A P, Temperley, W H, Gething, P W, Van Boeckel, T, Kabaria, C W, Harbach, R E, & Hay, S I. The dominant *Anopheles*

vectors of human malaria in the Americas: occurrence data, distribution maps and bionomic précis. Parasites & Vectors (2010). 3, 72.

[26] Hiwat, H, Issaly, J, Gaborit, P, Somai, A, Samjhawan, A, Sardjoe, P, Soekhoe, T, & Girod, R. Behavioural heterogeneity of *Anopheles darlingi* (Diptera: Culicidae) and malaria transmission dynamics along the Maroni River, Suriname, French Guiana. Transactions of the Royal Society of Tropical Medicine and Hygiene (2010). 104, 207-13.

[27] Moutinho, P R, Gil, LHS, Cruz, R B, & Ribolla, P E M. Population dynamics, structure and behaviour of *Anopheles darlingi* in a rural settlement in the Amazon rainforest of Acre, Brazil. Malaria Journal (2011). 10, 174.

[28] Girod, R, Gaborit, P, Carinci, R, Issaly, J, & Fouque, F. *Anopheles darlingi* bionomics and transmission of *Plasmodium falciparum*, *Plasmodium vivax* and *Plasmodium malariae* in Amerindian villages of the Upper-Maroni Amazonian forest, French Guiana. Memórias Do Instituto Oswaldo Cruz (2008). 103, 702-10.

[29] Muirhead-Thomson, R C. The significance of irritability, behaviouristic avoidance and allied phenomena in malaria eradication. Bulletin of the World Health Organization (1960). 22, 721-34.

[30] Grieco, J P, Achee, N L, Chareonviriyaphap, T, Suwonkerd, W, Chauhan, K, Sardelis, M R, & Roberts, D R. A new classification system for the actions of IRS chemicals traditionally used for malaria control. PloS One (2007). 2, e716.

[31] Siegert, P Y, Walker, E, & Miller, J R. Differential behavioural responses of *Anopheles gambiae* (Diptera: Culicidae) modulate mortality caused by pyrethroid-treated bednets. Journal of Economic Entomology (2009). 102, 2061-71.

[32] Badyaev, A V. Stress-induced variation in evolution: from behavioural plasticity to genetic assimilation. Proceedings. Biological Sciences / The Royal Society (2005). 272, 877-86.

[33] Pothikasikorn, J, Chareonviriyaphap, T, Bangs, M J, & Prabaripai, A. Behavioural responses to DDT and pyrethroids between *Anopheles minimus* species A and C, malaria vectors in Thailand. The American Journal of Tropical Medicine and Hygiene (2005). 73, 343-9.

[34] White, G. Blood feeding habits of malaria vector mosquitos in the South Pare district of Tanzania 10 years after cessation of a dieldrin residual spraying campaign. Geneva: World Health Organisation (1969). WHO/MAL/69.684 – WHO/VBC/69.144.

[35] Gillies, M, & Smith, A. The effect of a residual house-spraying campaign in East Africa on species balance in the *Anopheles funestus* group. The replacement of *A. funestus* Giles by *A. rivulorum* Leeson. Bulletin of Entomological Research (1960). 51, 243-52.

[36] Gillies, M, & Furlong, M. An investigation into the behaviour of *Anopheles parensis* Gillies at Malindi on the Kenya coast. Bulletin of Entomological Research (1963). 55,1-16.

[37] Labbo, R, Czeher, C, Djibrila, A, Arzika, I, Jeanne, I, & Duchemin, J-B. Longitudinal follow-up of malaria transmission dynamics in two villages in a Sahelian area of Niger during a nationwide insecticide-treated bednet distribution programme. Medical and Veterinary Entomology (2012). 26, 386-95.

[38] Iyengar, R. The bionomics of salt-water *Anopheles gambiae* in East Africa. Bulletin of the World Health Organization (1962). 27, 223-9.

[39] Lindblade, K, Gimnig, J, Kamau, L, Hawley, W, Odhiambo, F, Olang, G, TerKuile, F O, Vulule, J, & Slutsker L. Impact of sustained use of insecticide-treated bednets on malaria vector species distribution and culicine mosquitoes. Journal of Medical Entomology (2006). 43, 428-32.

[40] Mutuku, F M, King, C H, Mungai, P, Mbogo, C, Mwangangi, J, Muchiri, E M, Walker, E D, & Kitron, U. Impact of insecticide-treated bed nets on malaria transmission indices on the south coast of Kenya. Malaria Journal (2011). 10, 356.

[41] Bayoh, M N, Mathias, D K, Odiere, M R, Mutuku, F M, Kamau, L, Gimnig, J E,Vulule, J M, Hawley, W A, Hamel, M J, & Walker, E D. *Anopheles gambiae*: historical population decline associated with regional distribution of insecticide-treated bednets in western Nyanza Province, Kenya. Malaria Journal (2010). 9, 62.

[42] Russell, T L, Govella, N J, Azizi, S, Drakeley, C J, Kachur, S P, & Killeen, G F. Increased proportions of outdoor feeding among residual malaria vector populations following increased use of insecticide-treated nets in rural Tanzania. Malaria Journal (2011). 10, 80.

[43] Mathias, D K, Ochomo, E, Atieli, F, Ombok, M, Bayoh, M N, Olang, G, Muhia, D,Kamau, L, Vulule, J M, Hamel, M J, Hawley, W A, Walker, E D, & Gimnig, J E. Spatial and temporal variation in the kdr allele L1014S in *Anopheles gambiae* s.s. and phenotypic variability in susceptibility to insecticides in Western Kenya. Malaria Journal (2011). 10, 10.

[44] Mathenge, E M, Gimnig, J E, Kolczak, M, Ombok, M, Irungu, L W, & Hawley, W A. Effect of permethrin-impregnated nets on exiting behaviour, blood feeding success, and time of feeding of malaria mosquitoes (Diptera: Culicidae) in western Kenya. Journal of Medical Entomology (2001). 38, 531-6.

[45] Derua, Y A, Alifrangis, M, Hosea, K M, Meyrowitsch, D W, Magesa, S M, Pedersen, E M, & Simonsen, P E. Change in composition of the *Anopheles gambiae* complex and its possible implications for the transmission of malaria and lymphatic filariasis in northeastern Tanzania. Malaria Journal (2012). 11, 188.

[46] Braimah, N, Drakeley, C, Kweka, E, Mosha, F, Helinski, M, Pates, H, Maxwell, C, Massawe, T, Kenward, M G, & Curtis, C. Tests of bednet traps (Mbita traps) for mon-

itoring mosquito populations and time of biting in Tanzania and possible impact of prolonged insecticide treated net use. International Journal of Tropical Insect Science (2005). 25, 208-13.

[47] Moiroux, N, Gomez, M B, Pennetier, C, Elanga, E, Djènontin, A, Chandre, F, Djègbé, I, Guis, H, & Corbel, V. Changes in *Anopheles funestus* biting behaviour following universal coverage of Long-Lasting Insecticidal Nets in Benin. The Journal of Infectious Diseases (2012). 206, 1622-9.

[48] Mbogo, C N, Baya, N M, Ofulla, A V, Githure, J I, & Snow, R W. The impact of permethrin-impregnated bednets on malaria vectors of the Kenyan coast. Medical and Veterinary Entomology (1996). 10, 251-9.

[49] Njau, R, Mosha, F, & Nguma, J. Field trials of pyrethroid impregnated bednets in northern Tanzania 1. Effect on malaria transmission. International Journal of Tropical Insect Science (1993). 14, 575-84.

[50] Magesa, S M, Wilkes, T J, Mnzava, A E, Njunwa, K J, Myamba, J, Kivuyo, M D, Hill, N, Lines, J D, & Curtis, C F. Trial of pyrethroid impregnated bednets in an area of Tanzania holoendemic for malaria. Part 2. Effects on the malaria vector population. Acta Tropica (1991). 49, 97-108.

[51] Quiñones, M L, Lines, J D, Thomson, M C, Jawara, M, Morris, J, & Greenwood, B M. *Anopheles gambiae* gonotrophic cycle duration, biting and exiting behaviour unaffected by permethrin-impregnated bednets in The Gambia. Medical and Veterinary Entomology (1997). 11, 71-8.

[52] Molineaux, L, & Gramiccia, G. The Garki Project: Research on the Epidemiology and Control of Malaria in the Sudan Savanna of West Africa. World Health Organisation (1980), 331pp.

[53] Ilboudo-Sanogo, E, Cuzin-Ouattara, N, Diallo, D A, Cousens, S N, Esposito, F, Habluetzel, A, Sanon, S, & Ouédraogo, A P. Insecticide-treated materials, mosquito adaptation and mass effect: entomological observations after five years of vector control in Burkina Faso. Transactions of the Royal Society of Tropical Medicine and Hygiene (2001). 95, 353-60.

[54] Bøgh, C, Pedersen, E M, Mukoko, D A, & Ouma, J H. Permethrin-impregnated bednet effects on resting and feeding behaviour of lymphatic filariasis vector mosquitoes in Kenya. Medical and Veterinary Entomology (1998). 12, 52-9.

[55] Lindsay, S W, Alonso, P L, Armstrong Schellenberg, JR, Hemingway, J, Adiamah, J H, Shenton, FC, Jawara, M, & Greenwood, B M. A malaria control trial using insecticide treated bed nets and targeted chemoprophylaxis in a rural area of The Gambia, west-Africa. 7. Impact of permethrin-impregnated bed nets on malaria vectors. Transactions of the Royal Society of Tropical Medicine and Hygiene (1993). Suppl , 2, 45-51.

[56] Fornadel, C M, Norris, L C, Glass, G E, & Norris, D E. Analysis of *Anopheles arabiensis* blood feeding behaviour in southern Zambia during the two years after introduction of insecticide-treated bed nets. The American Journal of Tropical Medicine and Hygiene (2010). 83, 848-53.

[57] White, G. *Anopheles gambiae* complex and disease transmission in Africa. Transactions of the Royal Society of Tropical Medicine and Hygiene (1974). 68, 278-301.

[58] Taylor, B. Changes in the feeding behaviour of a malaria vector, *Anopheles farauti* Lav., following use of DDT as a residual spray in houses in the British Solomon Islands Protectorate. Transactions of the Royal Entomological Society of London (1975). 127, 277-92.

[59] Bugoro, H, Iro'ofa C, Mackenzie, D O, Apairamo, A, Hevalao, W, Corcoran, S, Bobogare, A, Beebe, N W, Russell, T L, Chen, C-C, & Cooper, R D. Changes in vector species composition and current vector biology and behaviour will favour malaria elimination in Santa Isabel Province, Solomon Islands. Malaria Journal (2011). 10, 287.

[60] Ismail, I A, Notananda, V, & Schepens, J. Studies on malaria and responses of *Anopheles balabacensis balabacensis* and *Anopheles minimus* to DDT residual spraying in Thailand. Acta Tropica (1975). 32, 206-31.

[61] Nustsathapana, S, Sawasdiwongphorn, P, Chitprarop, U, & Cullen, J R. The behavior of *Anopheles minimus* Theobald (Diptera: Culicidae) subjected to differing levels of DDT selection pressure in northern Thailand. Bulletin of Entomological Research (1986). 76, 303-12.

[62] Garros, C, Marchand, R P, Quang, N T, Hai, N S, & Manguin, S. First record of *Anopheles minimus* C and significant decrease of *An. minimus* A in central Vietnam. Journal of the American Mosquito Control Association (2005). 21, 139-43.

[63] Reisen, W K, Pradhan, S P, Shrestha, J P, Shrestha, S L, Vaidya, R G, & Shrestha, J D. Anopheline mosquito (Diptera: Culicidae) ecology in relation to malaria transmission in the inner and outer terai of Nepal, 1987-1989. Journal of Medical Entomology (1993). 30, 664-82.

[64] Li, Z Z, Zhang, M C, Wus, Y G, Zhong, B L, Lin, G Y, & Huang, H. Trial of deltamethrin impregnated bed nets for the control of malaria transmitted by *Anopheles sinensis* and *Anopheles anthropophagus*. The American Journal of Tropical Medicine and Hygiene (1989). 40, 356-9.

[65] Zhang, Z, & Yang, C. Application of deltamethrin-impregnated bednets for mosquito and malaria control in Yunnan, China. The Southeast Asian Journal of Tropical Medicine and Public Health (1996). 27, 367-71.

[66] Giglioli, G. Nation-wide malaria eradication projects in the Americas III. Eradication of *Anopheles darlingi* from the inhabited areas of British Guiana by DDT residual spraying. Journal of the National Malaria Society (1951). 10, 142-61.

[67] Richards, F, Flores, R Z, Sexton, J D, Beach, R F, Mount, D L, Cordon-Rosales, C, Gatica, M, & Klein, R E. Effects of permethrin-impregnated bed nets on malaria vectors of Northern Guatemala. Bulletin of PAHO (1994). 28, 112-21.

[68] Charlwood, J D, & Graves, P M. The effect of permethrin-impregnated bednets on a population of *Anopheles farauti* in coastal Papua New Guinea. Medical and Veterinary Entomology (1987). 1, 319-27.

[69] Hii, J L, Birley, M H, Kanai, L, Foligeli, A, & Wagner, J. Comparative effects of permethrin-impregnated bednets and DDT house spraying on survival rates and oviposition interval of *Anopheles farauti* (Diptera: Culicidae) in Solomon Islands. Annals of Tropical Medicine and Parasitology (1995). 89(1), 521-9.

[70] Bugoro, H, Cooper, R D, Butafa, C,Iro'ofa, C, Mackenzie, DO, Chen, C-C, & Russell, T L. Bionomics of the malaria vector *Anopheles farauti* in Temotu Province, Solomon Islands: issues for malaria elimination. Malaria Journal (2011). 10, 133.

[71] Ismail, I A, Phinichpongse, S, & Boonrasri, P. Responses of *Anopheles minimus* to DDT residual spraying in a cleared forested foothill area in central Thailand. Acta Tropica (1978). 35, 69-82.

[72] Lourenço-de-Oliveira, R, Guimarães, A E, Arlé, M, Da Silva, T F, Castro, M G, Motta, M A, & Deane, L M. Anopheline species, some of their habits and relation to malaria in endemic areas of Rondônia State, Amazon region of Brazil. Memórias Do Instituto Oswaldo Cruz (1989). 84, 501-14.

[73] Harris, A F, Matias-Arnéz, A, & Hill, N. Biting time of *Anopheles darlingi* in the Bolivian Amazon and implications for control of malaria. Transactions of the Royal Society of Tropical Medicine and Hygiene (2006). 100, 45-7.

[74] Suwonkerd, W, Amg-Ung, B, Rimwangtrakul, K, Wongkattiyakul, S, Kattiyamongkool, B, Chitprarop, U, & Takagi, M. A Field Study on the Response of *Anopheles dirus* to DDT and Fenitrothion Sprayed to Huts in Phetchabun Province, Thailand. Tropical Medicine (Nagasaki) (1990). 32, 1-5.

[75] Pongvongsa, T, Ha, H, Thanh, L, Marchand, R P, Nonaka, D, Tojo, B, Phongmany, P, Moji, K, & Kobayashi, J. Joint malaria surveys lead towards improved cross-border cooperation between Savannakhet province, Laos and Quang Tri province, Vietnam. Malaria Journal (2012). 11, 262.

[76] Elliott, R. Studies on man vector contact in some malarious areas in Colombia. Bulletin of the World Health Organization (1968). 38, 239-53.

[77] Hiwat, H, Mitro, S, Samjhawan, A, Sardjoe, P, Soekhoe, T, & Takken, W. Collapse of *Anopheles darlingi* populations in Suriname after introduction of insecticide-treated

nets (ITNs); malaria down to near elimination level. The American Journal of Tropical Medicine and Hygiene (2012). 86, 649-55.

[78] Sampath, T R, Yadav, R S, Sharma, V P, & Adak, T. Evaluation of lambdacyhalothrin impregnated bednets in a malaria endemic area of India. Part 2. Impact on malaria vectors. Journal of the American Mosquito Control Association (1998). 14, 437-43.

[79] Loyola, E G, Rodríguez, M H, González, L, Arredondo-Jimenez, J I, Bown, D N, & Vaca, M A. Effect of indoor residual spraying of DDT and bendiocarb on the feeding patterns of *Anopheles pseudopunctipennis* in Mexico. Journal of the American Mosquito Control Association (1990). 6, 635-40.

[80] Giglioli, G. Biological variations in *Anopheles darlingi* and *Anopheles gambiae*; their effect on practical malaria control in the neotropical region. Bulletin of the World Health Organization (1956). 15, 461-71.

[81] Barai, D, Hyma, B, & Ramesh, A. The scope and limitations of insecticide spraying in rural vector control programmes in the states of Karnataka and Tamil Nadu in India. Ecology of Disease (1982). 1, 243-55.

[82] Martinez-Palacios, A, & De Zulueta, J. Ethological changes in *Anopheles pseudopunctipennis* in Mexico after prolonged use of DDT. Nature (1964). 203, 940-1.

[83] Kitau, J, Oxborough, R M, Tungu, P K, Matowo, J, Malima, R C, Magesa, S M, Bruce, J, Mosha, F W, & Rowland, M W. Species shifts in the *Anopheles gambiae* complex: do LLINs successfully control *Anopheles arabiensis*? PloS One (2012). 7, e31481.

[84] Ayala, D, Fontaine, M C, Cohuet, A, Fontenille, D, Vitalis, R, & Simard, F. Chromosomal inversions, natural selection and adaptation in the malaria vector *Anopheles funestus*. Molecular Biology and Evolution (2011). 28, 745-58.

[85] Coluzzi, M, Sabatini, A, Petrarca, V, & Di Deco, M A. Behavioural divergences between mosquitoes with different inversion karyotypes in polymorphic populations of the *Anopheles gambiae* complex. Nature (1977). 266, 832-3.

[86] Coluzzi, M, Sabatini, A, Petrarca, V, & Di Deco MA. Chromosomal differentiation and adaptation to human environments in the *Anopheles gambiae* complex. Transactions of the Royal Society of Tropical Medicine and Hygiene (1979). 73, 483-97.

[87] Coluzzi, M. Malaria vector analysis and control. Parasitology Today (1992). 8, 113-8.

[88] White, G B. Biological effects of intraspecific chromosomal polymorphism in malaria vector populations. Bulletin of the World Health Organization (1974). 50, 299-306.

[89] Jones, M. Inversion polymorphism and circadian flight activity in the mosquito *Anopheles stephensi* List. (Diptera, Culicidae). Bulletin of Entomological Research (1974). 64, 305-11.

[90] Hii, J L, Chew, M, Sang, V Y, Munstermann, L E, Tan, S G, Panyim, S, & Yasothornsrikul, S. Population genetic analysis of host seeking and resting behaviours in the

malaria vector, *Anopheles balabacensis* (Diptera: Culicidae). Journal of Medical Entomology (1991). 28, 675-84.

[91] Lines, J D, Lyimo, E O, & Curtis, C F. Mixing of indoor- and outdoor-resting adults of *Anopheles gambiae* Giles s.l. and *A. funestus* Giles (Diptera: Culicidae) in coastal Tanzania. Bulletin of Entomological Research (2009). 76, 171.

[92] Smits, A, Roelants, P, Van Bortel, W, & Coosemans, M. Enzyme polymorphisms in the *Anopheles gambiae* (Diptera: Culicidae) complex related to feeding and resting behaviour in the Imbo Valley, Burundi. Journal of Medical Entomology (1996). 33,545-53.

[93] Coosemans, M, Smits, A, & Roelants, P. Intraspecific isozyme polymorphism of *Anopheles gambiae* in relation to environment, behaviour, and malaria transmission in southwestern Burkina Faso. The American Journal of Tropical Medicine and Hygiene (1998). 58, 70-4.

[94] Sinka, M E, Bangs, M J, Manguin, S, Chareonviriyaphap, T, Patil, A P, Temperley, W H, Gething, P W, Elyazar, I R F, Kabaria, C W, Harbach, R E, & Hay, S I. The dominant *Anopheles* vectors of human malaria in the Asia-Pacific region: occurrence data, distribution maps and bionomic précis. Parasites & Vectors (2011). 4, 89.

[95] Limrat, D, Rojruthai, B, Apiwathnasorn, C, Samung, Y, & Prommongkol, S. *Anopheles barbirostris* /*campestris* as a probable vector of malaria in Aranyaprathet, Sa Kaeo Province. The Southeast Asian Journal of Tropical Medicine and Public Health (2001). 32,739-44.

[96] Giglioli, G. Ecological change as a factor in renewed malaria transmission in an eradicated area. A localized outbreak of *A. aquasalis*-transmitted malaria on the Demerara river estuary, British Guiana, in the fifteenth year of *A. darlingi* and malaria eradication. Bulletin of the World Health Organization (1963). 29, 131-45.

[97] Lengeler, C. Insecticide-treated bed nets and curtains for preventing malaria. Cochrane Database of Systematic Reviews (2004). 2, CD0003632009.

[98] Pluess, B, Tanscer, F C, Lengeler, C, & Sharp, B L. Indoor residual spraying for preventing malaria. Cochrane Database of Systematic Reviews (2010). 4, CD006657.

[99] Jana-Kara, B R, Jihullah, W A, Shahi, B, Dev, V, Curtis, C F, & Sharma, V P. Deltamethrin impregnated bednets against *Anopheles minimus* transmitted malaria in Assam, India. The Journal of Tropical Medicine and Hygiene (1995). 98, 73-83.

[100] Kobayashi, J, Phompida, S, Toma, T, Looareensuwan, S, Toma, H, & Miyagi, I. The effectiveness of impregnated bed net in malaria control in Laos. Acta Tropica (2004). 89, 299-308.

[101] Seyoum, A, Sikaala, C H, Chanda, J, Chinula, D, Ntamatungiro, A J, Hawela, M, Miller, J M, Russell, T L, Briët, O J, & Killeen, G F. Human exposure to anopheline mos-

quitoes occurs primarily indoors, even for users of insecticide-treated nets in Luangwa Valley, South-east Zambia. Parasites & Vectors (2012). 5, 101.

[102] Charlwood, J D, Alcântara, J, Pinto, J, Sousa, C A, Rompão, H, Gil, V, & Rosário, V E. Do bednets reduce malaria transmission by exophagic mosquitoes? Transactions of the Royal Society of Tropical Medicine and Hygiene (2005). 99, 901-4.

[103] Govella, N J, & Ferguson, H. Why use of interventions targeting outdoor biting mosquitoes will be necessary to achieve malaria elimination? Frontiers in Physiology (2012).3, 199.

[104] Kiware, S S, Chitnis, N, Devine, G J, Moore, S J, Majambere, S, & Killeen, G F. Biologically meaningful coverage indicators for eliminating malaria transmission. Biology Letters (2012). 8, 874-877.

[105] Ferguson, H M, Dornhaus, A, Beeche, A, Borgemeister, C, Gottlieb, M, Mulla, M S, Gimnig, J E, Fish, D, & Killeen, G F. Ecology: a prerequisite for malaria elimination and eradication. PLoS Medicine (2010). 7, e1000303.

[106] The malERA Consultative Group on Vector Control. A research agenda for malaria eradication: vector control. PLoS Medicine (2011). 8, e1000401.

[107] Hill, N, Lenglet, A, Arnéz, A M, & Carneiro, I. Plant based insect repellent and insecticide treated bed nets to protect against malaria in areas of early evening biting vectors: double blind randomised placebo controlled clinical trial in the Bolivian Amazon. BMJ (Clinical Research Ed.) (2007).335, 1023.

[108] Dutta, P, Khan, A M, Khan, S A, Borah, J, Sharma, C K, & Mahanta, J. Malaria control in a forest fringe area of Assam, India: a pilot study. Transactions of the Royal Society of Tropical Medicine and Hygiene (2011). 105, 327-32.

[109] Rowland, M, Downey, G, Rab, A, Freeman, T, Mohammad, N, Rehman, H, Durrani, N, Reyburn, H, Curtis, C, Lines, J, & Fayaz, M. DEET mosquito repellent provides personal protection against malaria: a household randomized trial in an Afghan refugee camp in Pakistan. Tropical Medicine & International Health (2004). 9, 335-42.

[110] Kimani, E W, Vulule, J M, Kuria, I W, & Mugisha, F. Use of insecticide-treated clothes for personal protection against malaria: a community trial. Malaria Journal (2006). 5, 63.

[111] Thang, N D, Erhart, A, Speybroeck, N, Xa, N X, Thanh, N N, Van Ky, P, Hung, L X, Thuan, L K, Coosemans, M, & D' Alessandro, U. Long-lasting Insecticidal Hammocks for controlling forest malaria: a community-based trial in a rural area of central Vietnam. PloS One (2009). 4, e7369.

[112] Sochantha, T, Van Bortel, W, Savonnaroth, S, Marcotty, T, Speybroeck, N, & Coosemans, M. Personal protection by long-lasting insecticidal hammocks against the bites of forest malaria vectors. Tropical Medicine & International Health (2010). 15,336-41.

[113] Habtewold, T, Prior, A, Torr, S J, & Gibson, G. Could insecticide-treated cattle reduce Afrotropical malaria transmission? Effects of deltamethrin-treated Zebu on *Anopheles arabiensis* behaviour and survival in Ethiopia. Medical and Veterinary Entomology (2004). 18, 408-17.

[114] Coosemans, M, & Van Bortel, W. Malaria Vectors in the Mekong Countries: a Complex Interaction between Vectors, Environment and Human Behaviour. In: International Conference Hubs, Harbours and Deltas in Southeast Asia. Royal Academy of Overseas Sciences (2006). 551-569.

[115] Burns, M, Rowland, M, Guessan, R, Carneiro, I, Beeche, A, Ruiz, S S, Kamara, S, Takken, W, Carnevale, P, & Allan, R. Insecticide-treated plastic sheeting for emergency malaria prevention and shelter among displaced populations: an observational cohort study in a refugee setting in Sierra Leone. The American Journal of Tropical Medicine and Hygiene (2012). 87, 242-50.

[116] Kiware, S S, Chitnis, N, Moore, S J, Devine, G J, Majambere, S, Merrill, S, & Killeen, G F. Simplified models of vector control impact upon malaria transmission by zoophagic mosquitoes. PloS One (2012). 7, e37661.

[117] Charlwood, J D, Pinto, J, Ferrara, P R, Sousa, C A, Ferreira, C, Gil, V, & Do Rosário V E. Raised houses reduce mosquito bites. Malaria Journal (2003). 2, 45.

[118] Somboon, P, Lines, J, Aramrattana, A, Chitprarop, U, & Prajakwong, S. Entomological impregnated evaluation of community-wide use of lambdacyhalothrin-bed nets against malaria in a border area of north-west Thailand. Transactions of the Royal Society of Tropical Medicine and Hygiene (1995). 89, 248-54.

[119] Grietens, K P, Xuan, X N, Ribera, J M,Duc, T N, Van Bortel, W, Ba, N T, Van, K P, Xuan, H L, D'Alessandro, U, & Erhart, A. Social Determinants of Long Lasting Insecticidal Hammock-Use Among the Ra-Glai Ethnic Minority in Vietnam: Implications for Forest Malaria Control. PLoS One (2012). 7, e29991.

[120] Bradley, J, Matias, A, Schwabe, C, Vargas, D, Monti, F, Nseng, G, & Kleinschmidt, I. Increased risks of malaria due to limited residual life of insecticide and outdoor biting versus protection by combined use of nets and indoor residual spraying on Bioko Island, Equatorial Guinea. Malaria Journal (2012). 11, 242.

[121] Fillinger, U, & Lindsay, S W. Larval source management for malaria control in Africa: myths and reality. Malaria Journal (2011). 10, 353.

[122] Worrall, E, & Fillinger, U. Large-scale use of mosquito larval source management for malaria control in Africa: a cost analysis. Malaria Journal (2011). 10, 338.

[123] Müller, G C, & Schlein, Y. Efficacy of toxic sugar baits against adult cistern-dwelling *Anopheles claviger*. Transactions of the Royal Society of Tropical Medicine and Hygiene (2008). 102, 480-4.

[124] Scholte, E-J, Ng'habi, K, Kihonda, J, Takken, W, Paaijmans, K, Abdulla, S, Killeen, GF, & Knols, BGJ. An entomopathogenic fungus for control of adult African malaria mosquitoes. Science (2005). 308, 1641-2.

[125] Blanford, S, Chan, BHK, Jenkins, N, Sim, D, Turner, RJ, Read, AF, &Thomas, MB. Fungal pathogen reduces potential for malaria transmission. Science (2005). 308, 1638-41.

[126] Lwetoijera, D W, Sumaye, R D, Madumla, E P, Kavishe, D R, Mnyone, L L, Russell, T L, & Okumu, F O. An extra-domiciliary method of delivering entomopathogenic fungus, *Metharizium isopliae* IP 46 for controlling adult populations of the malaria vector, *Anopheles arabiensis*. Parasites & Vectors (2010). 3, 18.

Chapter 7

Vector Control: Some New Paradigms and Approaches

Claire Duchet, Richard Allan and Pierre Carnevale

Additional information is available at the end of the chapter

1. Introduction

1.1. Context

The World Malaria Report 2012 [1] summarizes data received from 104 malaria-endemic countries and territories for 2011. Ninety-nine of these countries had on-going malaria transmission. According to the latest World Health Organization (WHO) estimates, there were about 219 million cases of malaria in 2010 and an estimated 660,000 deaths. Africa is the most affected continent: about 90% of all malaria deaths occur there.

Malaria surveillance systems detect now only around 10% of the estimated global number of cases. In 41 countries around the world, it is not possible to make a reliable assessment of malaria trends due to incompleteness or inconsistency of reporting over time.

Actually another estimation of mortality [2] gave the following figures of 1,238,000 (929,000-1,685,000) deaths in 2010. This "one to two" ratio for the same year is matter of concern when considering that the main target of RBM is to reduce by 50% the burden of malaria.

The Lives Saved Tool (LiST) was developed to provide national and regional estimates of cause-specific mortality based on the extent of intervention coverage scale-up in sub-Saharan Africa and it appeared that it "performed reasonably well at estimating the effect of vector control scale-up on child mortality when compared against measured data from studies across a range of malaria transmission settings and is a useful tool in estimating the potential mortality reduction achieved from scaling-up malaria control interventions" [3].

Three major issues deserve special attention: tools for vector control, resistance of mosquito to insecticides, of *Plasmodium* to drugs, of human population to change their behavior, and costs. To tackle these issues new paradigms must be developed with the objectives of efficacy, acceptability and cost-efficiency.

Vector control remains the most generally effective measure to prevent malaria parasite transmission and therefore was one of the four basic technical elements of the Global Malaria Control Strategy [4]. Through the 1980s', vector control was mainly based upon Indoor Residual Spraying (IRS) and, in some circumstances, larval control, but an important break-through occurred with Insecticide Treated Nets (ITNs) then Long Lasting Insecticide treated Nets (LNs) (Figure 1) were introduced. The large scale implementation of ITN has, in several epidemiological settings, produced striking reductions in malaria transmission (-90%), incidence rate of malaria morbidity (-50%) and overall infant mortality (-17%) [5].

For WHO to achieve universal access to long-lasting insecticidal nets (LLINs), 780 million people at risk would need to have access to LLINs in sub-Saharan Africa, and approximately 150 million bed nets would need to be delivered each year. The number of LLINs delivered to endemic countries in sub-Saharan Africa dropped from a peak of 145 million in 2010 to an estimated 66 million in 2012 [1]. This will not be enough to fully replace the LLINs delivered 3 years earlier, indicating that total bed net coverage will decrease unless there is a massive scale-up in 2013. A decrease in LLIN coverage is likely to lead to major resurgences in the disease. In 2011, 153 million people were protected by indoor residual spraying (IRS) around the world, or 5% of the total global population at risk. In the WHO African Region, 77 million people, or 11% of the population at risk were protected through IRS in 2011.

Recent field observations have shown that LLINs may not be as durable as previously estimated and the majority of the most commonly distributed LLINs may have a shorter effective material life, which induce a higher than scheduled cost of global malaria control when LLIN have to be changed more frequently than expected. The problem of cost is a burning issue. International disbursements for malaria control rose steeply during the past eight years and were estimated to be US$ 1.66 billion in 2011 and US$ 1.84 billion in 2012. National government funding for malaria programmes has also been increasing in recent years, and stood at an estimated US$ 625 million in 2011. However, the currently available funding for malaria prevention and control is far below the resources required to reach global malaria targets. An estimated US$ 5.1 billion is needed every year between 2011 and 2020 to achieve universal access to malaria interventions. In 2011, only US$ 2.3 billion was available, less than half of what is needed ([1] fact sheet).

In its 23rd meeting in Senegal, the RBM Partnership Board concluded with an urgent call to governments of malaria endemic countries and development partners to secure the US$2.4 billion needed over the next two years to maintain high levels of coverage with life-saving malaria prevention and treatment interventions in eight African countries. This call follows a decade of success where *malaria deaths have fallen by over one-third in sub-Saharan Africa.*

Overall, out of a total of US$6.8 billion required, US$3.2 billion has been mobilized leaving a US$3.6 billion gap to make sure all affected countries in Africa have enough insecticide treated nets, effective treatments and rapid diagnostic tests for all populations at risk of malaria to achieve the target of near-zero deaths by 2015.

In term of vector control several issues deserve special attention. The change in vector behavior from indoor to outdoor feeding under insecticide pressure may limit the impact of classical control interventions such as LNs and IRS which target indoor feeding and resting mosquitoes and new tools are obviously needed. On the other hand, species that naturally bite and spend most of their time outdoors such as *Anopheles dirus* in S.E. Asia are poorly controlled by these classical tools and new approaches are urgently needed.

Vector control is also threatened by *the development of insecticide resistance* [4-9]. The frequency of resistance, has risen sharply over the last decade and the relationship between current indicators of resistance and the impact of vector control interventions is still unclear according to the different mechanisms of resistance, though most scientists believe that at some point in the near future resistance will begin to compromise control efforts, and new active ingredients to replace the current ones are urgently needed. Mosquito resistance to at least one insecticide used for malaria control has been identified in 64 countries around the world. In May 2012, WHO and the Roll Back Malaria Partnership released the Global Plan for Insecticide Resistance Management in malaria vectors, a five-pillar strategy for managing the threat of insecticide resistance.

Overcoming insecticide resistance will require novel chemical modes of action or combined interventions, with multiple active agreements, used as part of an integrated vector management strategy or completely new tools to delay the emergence of resistance by reducing selection pressure (e.g. rotations), or kill resistant vectors by exposing them to multiple insecticides (e.g. mixtures, when they become available).

Thus, new paradigms and approaches to vector control will expand the range of species that can be controlled and the chemical modes of action that can be employed, as well as potentially reducing the costs and complications of delivering them.

1.2. Definitions (from Innovative Vector Control Consortium IVCC)

A paradigm can be defined as a mean to deliver an active ingredient to the vector by targeting certain behaviors or ecologies. Paradigms can be associated with general chemical modes of action. Tools that target mosquito resting employ contact toxins. Those based on sugar feeding employ the so-called stomach poisons, etc. New paradigms open the door for exploitation of new chemical modes of action. An intervention paradigm (current examples: Insecticidal Nets or Indoor Residual Spray) is characterized by a primary mode of action (e.g. kills insect that land on the walls) and key characteristics such as the way it applied, its distribution process, economics, user, acceptability etc.

A paradigm may be served by several categories of products, each of which is described by a Target Product Profile (TPP) (e.g. ITNs *vs.* LLINs). The TPP will describe the primary functionality and characteristics that are required of a product to achieve a particular epidemiological outcome. Individual products within the category are defined by specifications.

Figure 1 illustrates the relationship among behaviors, paradigms and chemical mode of action. Where new paradigms do not exist in public health an example from agriculture or home and garden products is listed instead.

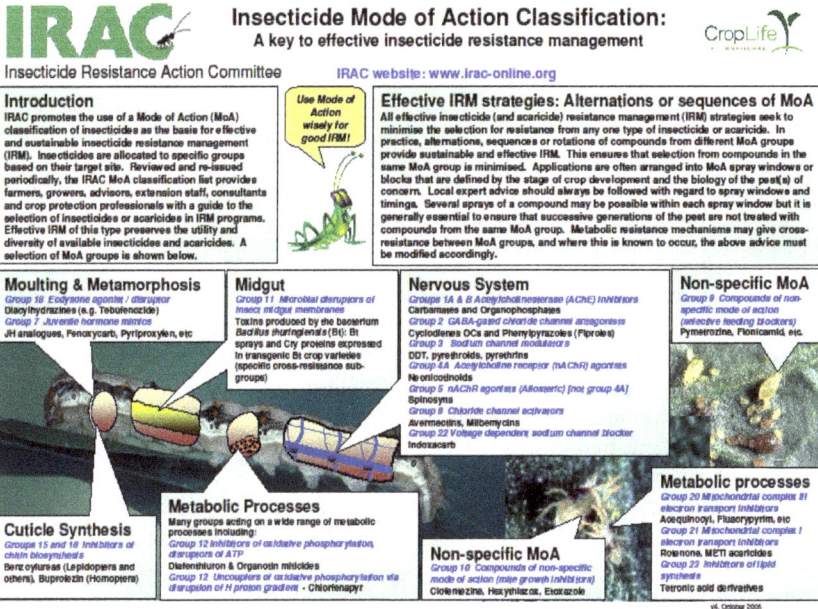

Figure 1. Relationship among behaviors, paradigms and chemical mode of action of insecticides.

2. New approaches to existing paradigms

2.1. New long lasting insecticide formulation for IRS

A microencapsulated formulation (CS) of the organophosphate chlorpyrifos methyl has recently been developed as long lasting i.e., alternative to DDT. In experimental huts in South Benin, against pyrethroid resistant (*kdr* + metabolic resistance) *An. gambiae* M form (and *Cx. quinquefasciatus*), chlorpyrifos methyl (Figure 2) was used to treat mosquito nets, and for IRS, and was compared to other commonly used insecticides: DDT and lambdacyhalothrin [10].

On nets, for N'Guessan et al [10] "the percentage of mortality among *An. gambiae* was 45.2% with the chlorpyrifos methyl-treated net and only 29.8% with the lambacyhalothrin-treated net. Mortality rates among *Cx. quinquefasciatus* were lower than among *An. gambiae* and did not exceed 15% with either type of treated net". While "Mortality of pyrethroid resistant *An. gambiae* was 95.5% with chlorpyrifos methyl-IRS compared to 50.4% in the hut sprayed with DDT and 30.8% in the hut sprayed with lambdacyhalothrin. The mortality of *Cx. quinquefas-*

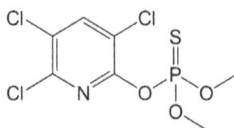

Figure 2. Chemical formula of chlorpyrifos methyl

ciatus in the chlorpyrifos methyl-IRS huts was 66.1% whereas in the DDT and lambdacyhalo-thrin-IRS huts it was only 14%". Therefore "chlorpyrifos methyl-IRS showed greater potential than DDT of lambdacyhalothrin-IRS for control of pyrethroid resistant *An. gambiae* M form and *Cx. quinquefasciatus* in areas of high *kdr* frequency" [11].

In terms of mortality the short residual activity of chlorpyrifos methyl on ITN is of great concern with a mortality rate decreasing from 100% to 9.7% within just one month while as IRS on cement it was observed "no loss of activity during the nine months of follow-up" compared to the fast decay of DDT and lambdacyhalothrin observed within the first month of spraying. A 9-month efficacy could be very valuable in many West and East African endemic countries with malaria transmission seasons lasting less than 8 months, and where IRS application of chlorpyrifos methyl each year could be adequate. In areas with developing pyrethroid resistance one might envisaged continued use of pyrethroid LLIN in combination with IRS, rotating the use of chlorfenapyr and CS long lasting chlorpyrifos methyl formulation.

2.2. New insecticides paints combining several insecticides and an insect growing regulator for IRS

Insecticide paints are new interesting paradigm for vector control with several advantages regarding classical IRS. It may provide future possibilities to combine several active ingredients in one product and therefore be used to help manage insecticide resistance. Paints can be produced in different colors to fit with people's choice. They may also be potentially implementable by households without the need for a specialized team to deliver the intervention, as is the case with IRS. This could improve community and household acceptance and uptake. Paints may also have the potential of being longer lasting than IRS. Insect growth regulator (IGR), a product usually used as larvicides, is also now being evaluated in Inesfly® 5A IGR™, a paint designed to target adult mosquitoes. Inesfly® 5A IGR™ is composed of two organophosphates (OPs), chlorpyriphos (1.5%), and diazinon (1.5%) and pyriproxyfen (0.063%) an IGR which was successfully used against *Triatoma infestans* [12]. The product is white vinyl paint with an aqueous base. Active ingredients reside within Ca CO3 + resin microcapsules. The formulation allows a gradual release of active ingredients, increasing its persistence.

In Benin the Inesfly® insecticide paint has been tested in laboratory [13] and in field [14] studies. In the laboratory study, the paint was tested against laboratory strains of the urban pest *Cx. quinquefasciatus* the susceptible (S-Lab) strain and the SR homozygote for the ace-1R resistant gene involved in the resistance to OPs and carbamates, with classical bioassay cones (tests on 30 min). Efficacy was measured not only in terms of induced mortality but also in terms of fecundity (number of eggs laid), fertility (% hatching) and larval development (%

pupation and % emergence). Insecticidal paints were tested at different time points: T0, 6 (= 6 months), 9 (= 9 months) and 12 months after application on four different surfaces: softwood, hard plastic (non-porous materials), ready-mixed cement and ready-mixed stucco (porous materials) at two doses, 1kg/6 m² (manufacturer's recommended dose to obtain surfaces completely white) and 1 kg/12 m². Female mosquitoes were given a blood meal 36 hours after standardized exposure to the painted surfaces. The study showed that the highest rates of mortality were obtained by both doses on susceptible as well as resistant strains even 12 months after treatment, on non-porous surfaces (softwood, plastic), whereas, on porous surfaces (cement, stucco) efficacy was much lower on resistant than on susceptible strain and it dropped to almost 0 at 6 and 12 months in both strains.

Thus long-term efficacy was an issue of porosity of materials rather than the pH of materials or the dose applied. It should be noted that 100% mortality was achieved on non-porous surface even against the OP resistant strain.

In terms of fecundity, fertility, and larval development, "a significant reduction in the number of eggs laid was shown at 0 and 9 months after treatment at either dose. A reduction in egg hatching was observed at T0, but not at T9. An increased mortality from the nymph to the adult stage was shown 9 months after treatment at the higher dose. No differences were found on the duration of the larval development. No IGR effect was observed 12 months after treatment". The percentage of emergence (i.e. adult emerging from pupa) dropped from 80% in control to #53% in samples from exposed females. Hence an adulticide could have impact not only on longevity of females exposed but also on their offspring which is a great advantage for mosquito population control.

Field trials were conducted in area where the local population of *An. gambiae* is composed of the M molecular form with resistance to pyrethroids and DDT, *kdr* is present at a high frequency, but is susceptible to OPs and carbamates, the ace-1R mutation was absent. *Cx. quinquefasciatus* shows high resistance to DDT, pyrethroids and carbosulfan with high *kdr* frequency and elevated levels of esterases and GST activity but the ace-1R mutation was absent [9]. In these trials, experimental huts were treated with either 1 or 2 layers of insecticide paint at one dose (6 kg/m²). Treatments were applied to either just walls, or to walls plus the ceiling. Unfed females of the lab-reared *An. gambiae* Kisumu strain (sensitive to all insecticides), were tested against local resistant wild strain *An. gambiae* and *Cx. quinquefasciatus*. The *An. gambiae* Kisumu strain mosquitoes were placed inside the huts at a distance of 1 m from two perpendicular walls, and left from 19:00 to 7:00 h [14]. The wild strains were tested using the standard WHO bioassay method.

Mortality of wild resistant *An. gambiae* was high with 83% even 9 months after treatment (2 paint layers on walls). Mortality of wild resistant *Cx. quinquefasciatus* was >50% even 9 months after treatment (2 paint layers on walls). No deterrent or excito-repellent effect was observed against *An. gambiae* nor *Cx. quinquefasciatus*. Mortality rates of exposed *An. gambiae* Kisumu strain in distance experiments in huts (1 m from two perpendicular walls; see above) with 2 layers were most striking, because even one year after treatment 100% of these sensitive mosquitoes were killed (Figure 3C).

Classical cone bioassay showed that in huts with 2 layers "twelve months after treatment mortality rates were of 70-80% against *An. gambiae* and *Cx. quinquefasciatus*". Release of insecticide susceptible unfed *An. gambiae* specimens in huts treated but without net (untreated) showed that 2-13% of females took their blood meal while 72% were well blood fed in control huts. Mortality rates observed in distance experiments were most striking, (Figures 3A & 3B) and even one year after treatment 100% of exposed *An. gambiae* Kisumu strain specimens were killed in huts with 2 layers (Figure 3C).

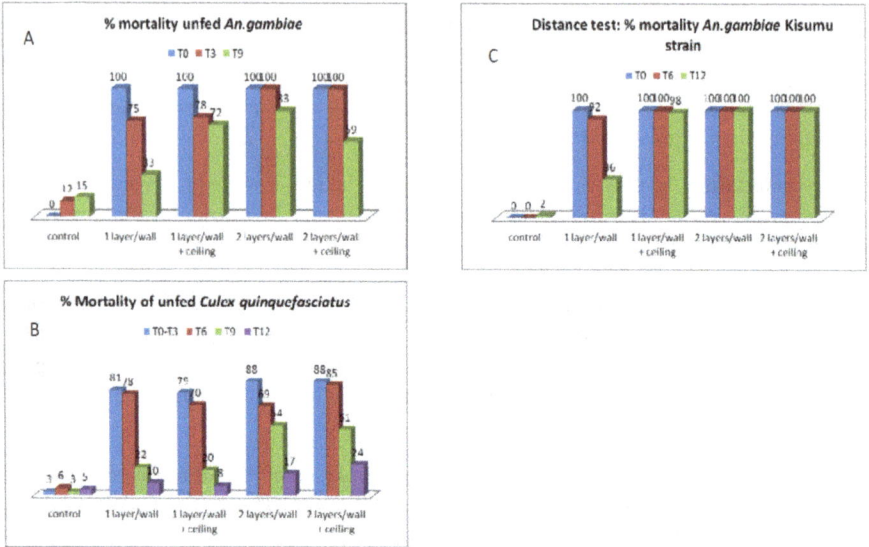

Figure 3. Mortality rates observed in distance experiments of exposed unfed *Anopheles gambiae* (A), unfed *Culex quinquefasciatus* (B), and *Anopheles gambiae* Kisumu strain (C) observed after 3 or 6 or 9 or 12 months after treatment (T3, T6, T9, T12 respectively).

These observations of "volume effect", "layer effect", "substrate effect", residual efficacy duration, and its efficacy against susceptible and resistant strains of the malaria vector *An. gambiae* and the nuisance insect *Culex quinquefasciatus*, are very encouraging. The paints ability to reduce mosquito fecundity and egg hatching opens up interesting new perspectives on malaria and mosquito control for urban settings where walls are commonly constructed with brick, concrete and plaster and provide suitable surfaces for paints, unlike classical mud made wall houses that characterize most rural communities. The paints ability to also reduce *Culex* mosquitoes is likely to increase community acceptance and maintenance of paint.

2.3. New mode of action families for IRS usage: Neonicotinoids

Neonicotinoid insecticides act on the central nervous system of insects by binding of agonist on postsynaptic nicotinic receptors [15]. Discovered in 1998, dinotefuran is a novel neonicotinoid insecticide which belongs to the third-generation neonicotinoids (sub-class: furanicotinyl compounds) [16]. It is a neonicotinoid agonist of the nicotinoid acetylcholine receptor with no cross-resistance to other insecticides such as organochlorine (OC), organophosphate (OP), carbamates or pyrethroids. Its efficiency is not greatly diminished by the presence of resistance mechanisms such as *kdr* or ace-1^R in mosquitoes.

In studies comparing the impact of dinotefuran, permethrin and propoxur on resistant strains of *Cx. quinquefasciatus*, dinotefuran was about 10 times more effective than permethrin on the BKPER strain, and 1000 times more effective than propoxur on resistant R-LAB strain [17]. If this product can be incorporated into material (e.g. LNs) or IRS applications then it should be useful in areas where resistance to pyrethroids and carbamates has developed.

The option of associating insecticides with different modes of action is one of the possible strategies for resistance management (as developed in another Chapter by Corbel & N'Guessan). An interesting approach that has recently been studied, combined Piperonyl butoxide (PBO), organic compound used as pesticide synergist, and dinotefuran in an attempt to restore the efficacy of deltamethrin treated mosquito net against resistant *An. gambiae* [18]. Darriet and Chandre [18] have also conducted classical laboratory cone tests of nets treated with deltamethrin, PBO (the classical synergist, inhibitor of oxidases) and dinotefuran alone or in combination against susceptible ("KIS") and resistant '("VKPR") strains of laboratory reared *An. gambiae*. Results of these tests are summarized in Table 1.

Product/ strain	KIS			VKPR		
	mortality	KDt50	KDt95	mortality	KDT50	KDT95
Deltamethrin	100%	8'	18'	7.5%	31'	194'
Dinotefuran				39%	No	No
PBO				4%	No	No
Deltamethrin +PBO				58%	13'	36'
Dinotefuran + PBO				28%	No	No
Deltamethrin+ Dinotefuran + PBO				99%	10'	23'

Table 1. Effects of mosquito nets treated with deltamethrin, PBO and dinotefuran on susceptible ("KIS"), and resistant '("VKPR") strains of *Anopheles gambiae*.

WHO's minimum mortality level for insecticides is 80% and this provides a reasonable operational guideline for effectiveness. In this study PBO combined with deltamethrin increased significantly its efficacy (synergistic effect), but not to a level adequate for control against pyrethroid-resistant mosquitoes, "suggesting that the acetylcholine concentration within the synaptic gap probably also increased". Interestingly, PBO had an antagonistic effect when combined with dinotefuran, decreasing this insecticide's efficacy. However, when PBO and Dinotefuran were combined with deltamethrin, the combination resulted in 99% mortality against the pyrethroid resistant mosquito strain, comparable with deltamethrin treated nets (in terms of mortality and KD effect) on the fully susceptible mosquito strain. For Darriet and Chandre [18] "the concomitant action of enhanced acetylcholine concentration in the synaptic gap and inactivation of nicotinic receptors by dinotefuran probably explains the strong synergy observed after exposure to the three-compound mixture, which caused nearly 100% mortality in a pyrethroid-resistant strain of *An. gambiae*".

2.4. New Insecticide Treated Plastic Sheeting (ITPS) and Durable Wall Linings (DL or WL)

Insecticide Treated Plastic Sheeting (ITPS) was developed in 2001 to provide a dual purpose tool capable of providing effective shelter and malaria control to displaced families in human-itarian crises. Durable wall linings (DL), developed in 2005, follow similar principles to ITPS, but are designed to be applied to the surface of existing rural house walls. In both cases these tools were developed to overcome the operational complexities and short comings of IRS, increase user acceptance (as the materials are available in different colors), and to increase residual insecticide activity (from classical 3-6 months with IRS to multiple years with ITPS or DL), and to increase community participation with a tool that households can implement themselves, and finally to provide new tools and new insecticide delivery mechanisms within the framework of insecticide resistance management. To date all factories produced ITPS based on solid format of polyethylene treated with pyrethroid insecticide, either permethrin or deltamethrin. The first generation of DL is also a polyethylene, but in 50% shading material format (woven polyethylene threads, with equal sized spaces between the threads).

One study group [19] has used "plastic sheeting impregnated with carbamates combined with long-lasting insecticidal mosquito nets for the control of pyrethroid-resistant malaria vectors" but this version of ITPS is unlikely to be tested at Phase III level or commercialized due to significant toxicity and fire risk problems associated with carbamates in this format. Different commercial products have been developed with different deltamethrin surface concentrations such as "ZeroVector (DL)" (170 mg a.i./m^2) or "Zero Fly" (360 mg a.i./m^2). Zerofly ITPS have been studied (Phase II) in refugee's camps in Afghanistan [20], in Sierra Leone (Phase III) [21], as well as in India (in endemic area with *An. culicifacies* and *An. fluviatilis* vectors or laborer settlements with *An. culicifacies* and *An. stephensi* as vectors) [22-23].

In Angola, a Phase III field trial was implemented in rural area, 8 villages around Balombo which were paired and received LLIN PermaNet 2.0 (55 mg a.i./m^2; Figures 3) or DL/WL ZeroVector or LLIN + ITPS "Zero Fly" or IRS with lambdacyhalothrin (25 mg a.i./m^2) with comprehensive evaluation: entomology, parasitology and immunology; focus group and KAP surveys were also implemented to follow the household acceptability of the vector control methods introduced.

The main vector in these villages was *An. funestus*. Entomological and parasitological first studies results showed that deltamethrin treated DL ZeroVector alone gave same results as IRS (lambdacyhalothrin) or LLIN (PermaNet®) alone or both PermaNet + ITPS Zero Fly in reducing by 55% the *P. falciparum* prevalence and parasitic load in children 2-9 years old (Figure 5) [24].

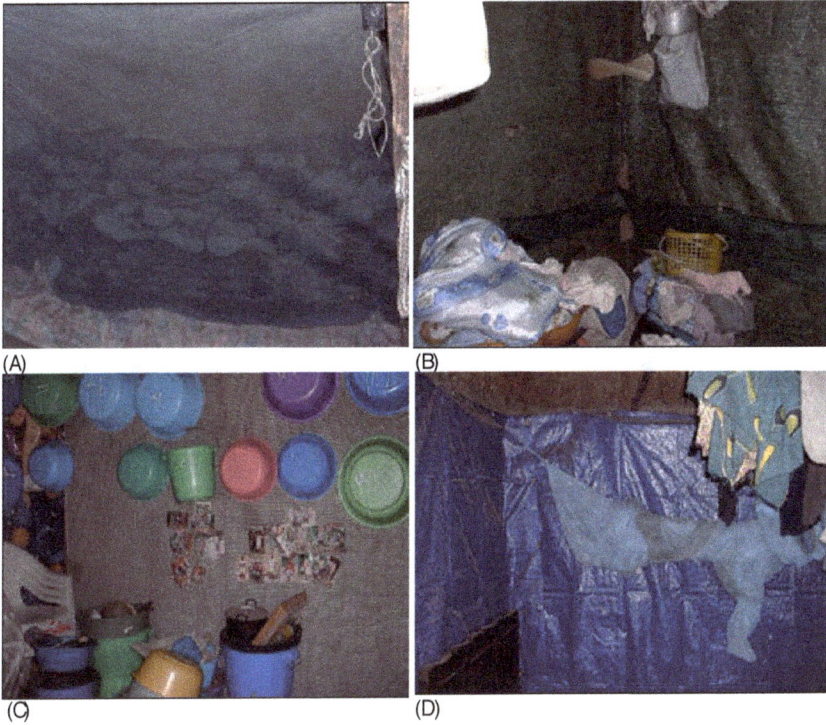

Figure 4. LLIN PermaNet 2.0 inside a house in Caala village (A); Green DL/WL ZeroVector inside a house in Chisséquélé village (B); Silver DL/WL ZeroVector inside a house in Barragem village (C); LLIN PermaNet 2.0 + ITPS Zero Fly in a house of Capango village (D) (Photos by P. Carnevale).

Entomological data obtained by classical CDC light traps inside houses before/after implementation of vector control measures were in line with the clinical results i.e. similar level of reduction of number of *Anopheles* in each village (Figure 6) such as 79.1% reduction all villages combined [24].

Immunological analysis of antibodies directed against saliva proteins of *Anopheles* [23] (Figure 7) confirmed the actual reduction of man/*Anopheles* contact with ITPS as well as IRS while association LLIN + ZF gave the best result.

A series of smaller Phase II DL/WL feasibility and acceptability studies, with entomological monitoring have also been conducted in Angola and Nigeria [25], Equatorial Guinea, Ghana, Mali, South Africa and Vietnam [26], and Papua New Guinea [27]. In each of these Phase II village studies, DL/WL acceptability data were collected using a standardized household survey used by each of the different study groups, with the conclusive result that DL/WL had an extremely high acceptance level amongst all cultures and communities in which it was

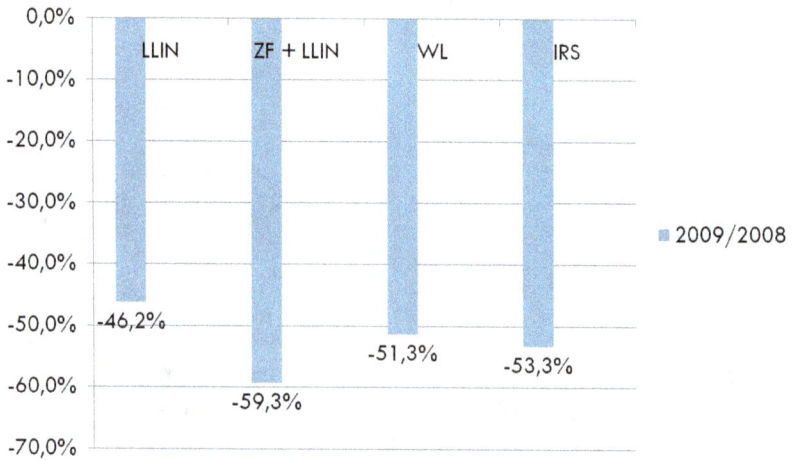

Figure 5. Regressive evolution of endemicity indice (plasmodic indices of 2 – 9 years old children) before/after implementation of each one of the four vector control methods.

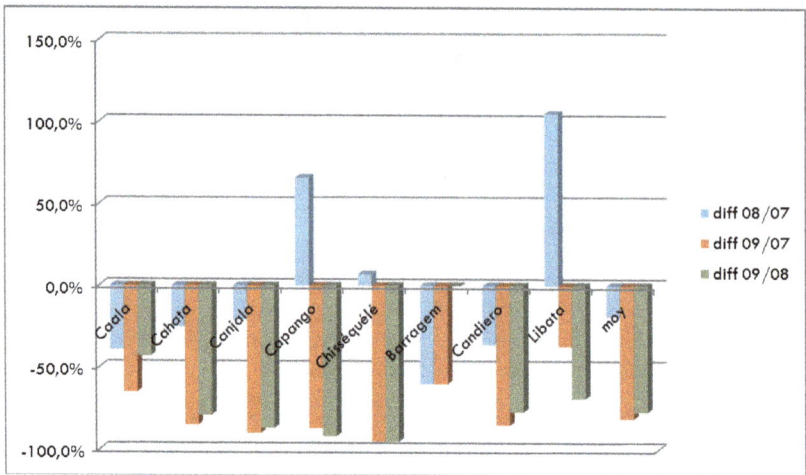

Figure 6. Reduction of number of *Anopheles* in CDC light trap sampling inside houses in villages before (2007-2008) and after (2009) vector control implementation [Caala and Cahata = LLIN alone; Canjala and Capango = LLIN + ZF; Barragem and Chisséquélé = WL alone; Candiero and Libata = IRS.

tested, and that when compared to IRS it was the preferred malaria prevention tool in every study. DL/WL proved feasible in every country study and in all house construction types tested, including brick, mud, wooden, and concrete walled rural houses. In each of these

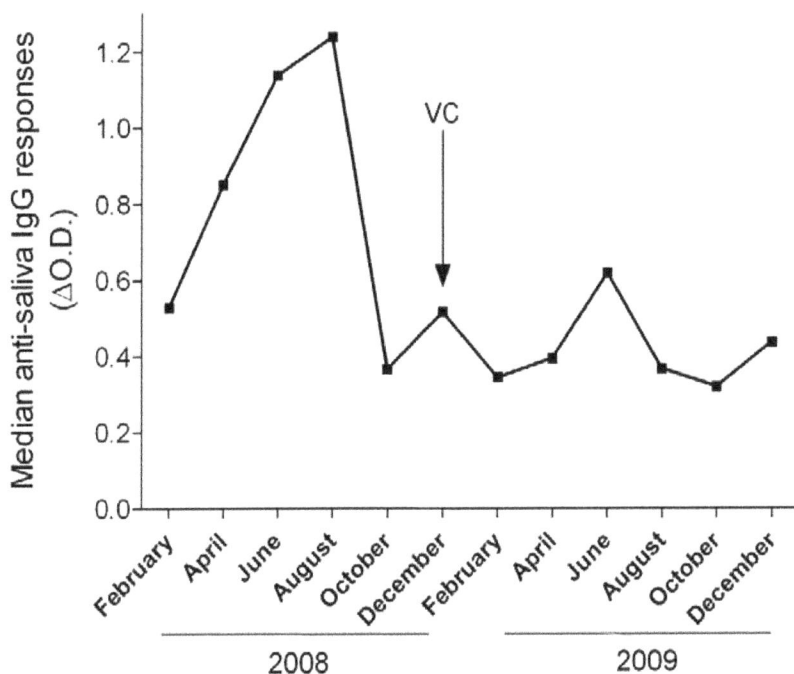

Figure 7. Evolution of the median values of the IgG antibody response to *Anopheles* saliva for all 6 villages combined according to the survey period in 2008 and 2009 (VC: vector control methods implemented in December 2008) [24].

studies, samples of DL/WL were collected at 4 monthly time intervals and were examined for deltamethrin residual content and bioassay impact on vector mosquitoes. The different studies produced very similar results regardless of house construction type, and in all cases DL/WL retained full activity and achieved >90% mortality of vector mosquitoes for the full monitoring periods of each study. The minimum study monitoring period was 6 months and the maximum was 4 years.

In Sierra Leone, Burns et al [21] conducted a Phase III study of ITPS. They constructed two refugee camps, Largo and Tobanda, using ITPS in 50% of each camp for shelter construction. The remaining 50% of each camp had shelter constructed out of untreated plastic sheeting (UPS). In Largo Camp, ITPS/UPS was applied onto walls and the ceiling of each shelter. In Tobanda Camp, ITPS/UPS was used only on ceilings. In Largo, the *Plasmodium falciparum* incidence rate in children up to 3 years of age who were cleared of parasites and then monitored for 8 months, was 163/100 person-years under UPS and 63 under ITPS. In Tobanda, incidence rate was 157/100 person-years under UPS and 134 under ITPS. Protective efficacy was 61% under fully lined ITPS shelters, and 15% under roof lined ITPS alone. Anemia rates improved under ITPS in both camps. Burns et al [21] concluded that "this novel tool proved to be a convenient, safe, and long-lasting method of malaria control when used as a full shelter lining in an emergency setting". Of note Burns et al [21] observed great difference of ITPS on walls + ceiling *versus* ceiling only at *P. falciparum* incidence rate level. Diabate et al [28] found similarly significant entomological difference in experimental huts of Burkina Faso lined with permethrin treated plastic sheeting on walls only or walls + ceiling reporting that "ITPS had a major effect on the mortality of mosquitoes, the proportion killed being dependent upon the surface area covered" and "deterred entry of mosquitoes and inhibition of blood feeding were also correlated with surface area covered."

2.5. New tools for LNs

2.5.1. Combined LN with PBO or two different class of insecticide

Pyrethroid treated LNs are the principle tool upon which malaria control has relied for the last decade, however, the rapid ongoing spread of pyrethroid resistance in Africa, is likely to increasingly compromise their protective efficacy. This concern has highlighted the urgent need to develop alternative active ingredients for LNs. While a study on bitreated (OP or C + pyr) [29] nets showed positive results they have not been commercially developed or operationalised due to safety concerns. To tackle the issue of pyrethroid resistance a new model of LLIN call "Permanet 3" (P3) was recently developed by Vestergaard Frandsen SA, Aarhus, Denmark [30] with *a top panel* made of monofilament polyethylene fabric incorporating deltamethrin ($121mg/m^2$) and PBO ($759mg/m^2$) plus side panels made of multifilament polyester fabric coated with a wash-resistant formulation of deltamethrin ($85mg/m^2$) (while the usual concentration was 55 mg a.i./m^2 in classical Permanet 2 and 25 mg a.i./m^2 in former hand treated nets "ITN"). PBO is the synergist of pyrethrins and pyrethroids without intrinsic insecticidal activity. The action of the synergist PBO is due to inhibition of oxidative enzymes in the insect which can detoxify the insecticide (metabolic resistance). The inhibition or blocking of the detoxification enzyme significantly increases mortality of resistant insects. PBO is used in a ratio ranging generally from 3 to 8 with the active ingredient used, depending on the type of formulation and target insects. LLIN "Permanet 3" (P3) was recently tested in several countries of West, Central [31] and East Africa such as Tanzania [32] and Ethiopia [33].

In southern Benin, N'Guessan et al [11] tested LLIN Permanet 3 against *An. gambiae* M molecular form (highly resistant owing to knockdown resistance (*kdr*) site insensitivity and elevated oxidase and esterase metabolic mechanisms) and *Cx. quinquesfasciatus,* and showed that in experimental huts "the level of personal protection against *An. gambiae* biting from PermaNet 3.0 (50%) was similar to that from PermaNet 2.0 (47%)" and "protection fell significantly after 20 washes to 30% for PermaNet 3.0 and 33% for PermaNet 2.0".

In Côte d'Ivoire, in experimental huts of Yaokoffikro where *An. gambiae* population is mainly composed of S form (90%) *versus* M form (10%) and is strongly resistant with high *kdr* frequency (94%) and Cyt P 450 metabolic resistance, Permanet 3 (unwashed and washed 20x) were compared against the standard Permanet 2 (unwashed and washed 20x), and hand treated ITNs ("CTN") with K Otab® (washed 5x), with untreated nets as control [34]. It appeared that both unwashed and washed P3 reduced entry rate (- 60%) and increased exit rate as well as other treated nets. On the other hand "a significantly higher mortality rate of *An. gambiae* s.s was recorded for unwashed PermaNet® 3.0 (55%) than for unwashed PermaNet® 2.0. However, for washed nets, there was no statistical difference between the mortality rates of *An. gambiae* s.s for washed PermaNet® 2.0, washed PermaNet® 3.0 and the CTN. Classical cone bioassays were conducted with the same nets (testing side panels and roofs) using either susceptible Kisumu strain of *An. gambiae* or local wild resistant population. Against Kisumu strain, all treatments including the washed CTN showed a mean KD rate over the threshold of 95% and a mean mortality rate >80%, (the official cut off).

Against pyrethroid-resistant wild caught *An. gambiae* s.s cone bioassays showed a mean KD rate < 95% and a mean mortality rate < 80% for all treatment arms, except with a mean KD of 94.3% and 98.6% and a mean mortality rate of 93.5% and 99.5%, respectively on side and roof showing a great efficacy even against polyresistant populations. The unwashed PermaNet® 3.0 gave the best results (KD 95.8% and mortality 97.0%)

In Tanzania, laboratory and experimental huts trial compared PermaNet 3.0 (P3), PermaNet 2.0 (P2) and a conventional deltamethrin treated net [32] against pyrethroid susceptible *An. gambiae* and pyrethroid resistant *Cx. quinquefasciatus*, (elevated oxidase and *kdr* mechanisms), Bioassays tests showed that against the susceptible *An. gambiae* P3 and P2 were still efficient after 20 washes while conventionally treated nets lost its efficacy. Against the pyrethroid resistant strain of *Cx. quinquefasciatus* Masimbani strain, it clearly appeared that the treated roof (with PBO) was much more efficient than sides (without PBO) of the LLIN. In experimental huts, general results of P3 and P2 (washed and unwashed) were comparable against pyrethroid susceptible *An. gambiae* and pyrethroid resistant *Cx. quinquefasciatus* and gave high similar personal protection. Mortality induced by unwashed P3 on resistant *Cx. quinquefasciatus* was higher than P2 (both washed and unwashed) and 20x washed P3, showing the increased efficacy achieved by PBO against pyrethroid resistant mosquitoes but this efficacy disappeared after 20 washes. Chemical concentration of the P3 roof decreased from 136 mg a.i./m^2 to 132 mg a.i./m^2 after 20 washes; whereas deltamethrin concentration of the P3 sides decreased from 103-109 mg a.i./m^2 before washing to 53 mg a.i./m^2 after 20 washes. The concentration of PBO decreased from 1142 mg/m^2 before wash to 684 mg/m^2 after 20 washes. Finally, chemical concentration of deltamethrin in P2 decreased from 61-77 mg a.i./m^2 to 25 77 mg a.i./m^2 after the classical 20 washes.

Tungu et al [32] observed that "the tunnel tests demonstrated a synergistic interaction of PBO and deltamethrin on roof netting against susceptible *An. gambiae* and both susceptible and resistant *Cx. quinquefasciatus* relative to netting from side panels treated with deltamethrin alone. This synergy was manifested in higher mortality, reduced passage through the holes and reduced feeding rates with netting treated with PBO-deltamethrin. The synergy in tunnels against pyrethroid resistant *Cx. quinquefasciatus* was progressively lost over 10 washes and fully lost after 20 washes. Cone bioassays on resistant *Cx. quinquefasciatus* confirmed the loss of synergy over 20 wash".

Sumitomo have also recently released a new LLIN (Olyset Plus®) treated with a combination of permethrin and PBO, and they claim similar increased efficacy against resistant strains of mosquitoes. However, questions do remain about the efficacy of adding PBO and its impact on the development of resistance amongst mosquitoes [35].

2.5.2. New kit: New formulation and binder for long lasting treating net

The efficacy of the long-lasting treatment kits ICON® Maxx (Syngenta) (slow release 10% capsule suspension formulation of lambdacyhalothrin + a polymer binding agent) was evaluated under laboratory conditions and in an experimental hut trial in various situations [36].

Laboratory and field trials were recently implemented in central Côte d'Ivoire, where *Anopheles gambiae* s.s. are resistant to pyrethroid insecticides [37]. In laboratory studies, classical bioassays were conducted on Kisumu SS susceptible *An. gambiae* strain, with polyester and polyethylene nets with up to 20 classical washes. Unwashed the treated polyester net resulted in 89% KD and 52% mortality while the polyethylene treated net achieved 98% KD and 46% mortality. Washing these nets had a serious negative impact on efficacy, in terms of both KD at 1 hour and mortality at 24 hours. After 20 washes, KD rates dropped to 59% with polyethylene and 55% for polyester net i.e. below the mean KD defined for LLINs by WHO Pesticide Evaluation Scheme (WHOPES) guideline (i.e. 95% after 20 washings). After 20 washes the mean mortality also decreased for both netting materials to around 20%, falling well below the WHOPES criteria for long-lasting nets (KD ≥ 95% and/ or mortality ≥ 80% for at least 20 standards WHO washes under laboratory conditions using an *An. gambiae* Kisumu-susceptible strain). Field evaluation of 2 ICON Maxx polyester treated nets and 2 untreated ones (= control) was carried out over one year in the experimental huts of M'bé. The wild *An. gambiae* population (mainly S form, 92%) used in these studies showed a high frequency of *kdr* (# 97% pyrethroid resistant heterozygotes) with 2 ICON Maxx polyester treated nets and 2 untreated one (= control). Blood feeding rate was reduced and mortality was significantly increased (70% for 8 months) in huts with treated nets even against the resistant wild *An. gambiae* population. It is worth noting this impact on insecticide resistant *An. gambiae* population and further epidemiological studies should be carried out.

2.6. New non chemical approaches of larviciding

2.6.1. New formulations of entomopathogen fungus

Laboratory and field bioassays have been implemented "to develop formulations that facilitate the application of *Metarhizium anisopliae* and *Beauveria bassiana* spores (to improve spreading) for the control of anopheline larvae [*An. gambiae* and *An. stephensi*], and also to improve their persistence under field conditions" [36]. These studies showed that the pathogenicity of dry *M. anisopliae* and *B. bassiana* spores against *An. stephensi* larvae is however too short (# 5 days) to have any application in control settings; with ShellSol T fungal spores only somewhat more persistent. In field bioassays (Western Kenya), the percentage of pupation observed in *An. gambiae* larvae treated with ShellSol T formulated spores was much lower than with unformulated treatment: 43 to 49% with *M. anisopliae* and 39 to 50% with *B. bassiana* (at 10 mg and

20 mg respectively). Bukhari et al [38] suggest that "these formulated fungi can be utilized in the field, providing additional tools for biological control of malaria vectors".

2.6.2. Another new class of product: Spinosad

Spinosad has been considered as "a new larvicide against insecticide-resistant mosquito larvae" [39] representing a new class of insect control products [40] and it has been tested in several trials [41].

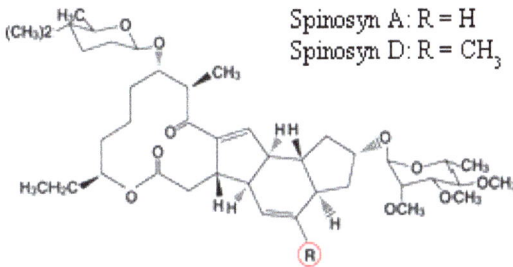

Figure 8. Two toxins of spinosad (Spinosyn A and Spinosyn D).

Spinosad is a fermented product derived from the mixture of two toxins (A and D spinosyns; Figure 8) secreted by soil based bacteria, *Saccharopolyspora spinosa*. It is traditionally used for crop protection [36] against pest insects. In the European Union, the active substance is included in Annex I to Directive 91/414/EEC by Directive 2007/6/EC and the rate of the pesticide residues in food is regulated in Europe. In France, the active substance is authorized for use in approved market products.

Spinosad acts on the nervous system of insects, by external contact or ingestion. It induces involuntary muscle contractions, prostration with tremors and paralysis. An insect stops feeding and paralysis may occur within minutes after ingestion of the product, death ensuing within one to three days. Spinosad has low toxicity to mammals, birds, fish and crustaceans but it is highly toxic to bees and aquatic invertebrates [42]. Spinosad (Group 5 insecticide) when used as a larvicide could be considered in rotation with another insecticide from a different class of pesticides.

Laboratory larval bioassays of spinosad on *Aedes aegypti*, *Cx. quinquefasciatus*, and *An. gambiae* (specimens that were either susceptible or resistant to pyrethroids, carbamates, and organophosphates) have shown that this product has a lethal action (mortality after 24 h of exposure) regardless of the original status, susceptible or resistant, of the mosquito larvae and was significantly more effective against *An. gambiae* than against the two other species and more effective against *Cx. quinquefasciatus* than *Ae. aegypti* [39] (Table2).

species	status	LC$_{50}$	LC$_{100}$
An. gambiae	SS	0.01	0.032
	RR (Kdr)	0.011	0.073
Cx. quinquefasciatus	SS	0.093	0.49
	RR (Ace-1^R)	0.12	0.59
Ae. aegypti	SS	0.35	0.92
	RR (Kdr)	0.32	0.72

Table 2. LC50 and LC100 of spinosad for *An. gambiae*, *Cx. quinquefasciatus*, and *Ae. aegypti* (SS, homozygote susceptible, RR: homozygote resistant).

Several other studies showed the potential of this bioinsecticide against different genera and species of mosquitoes [41, 43-44]. Different concentrations of spinosad were tested against larval instar and pupa of *An. stephensi* [45]. It was observed that "the reduction percentage of *Anopheles* larvae was 82.7%, 91.4% and 96.0% after 24, 48, 72 hours, respectively, while more than 80% reduction was observed after 3 weeks". A CS Spinosad formulation was tested in classical laboratory bioassays and successfully used for the control of *Ae. aegypti* and *An. albimanus* larvae in Mexico [46]. A spinosad shows an absence of cross resistance with insecticides commonly used in Public Health and it may be an interesting product to integrate into vector borne diseases control strategies where vectors are resistant to current insecticides.

3. Other new paradigms

3.1. Slow Acting Product (SAP) — Entomopathogens fungus

A completely new paradigm in vector control would be *slow acting products* called «Late Life Acting products » [47]. As malaria parasite sporogonic development last at least 10 days, any product which kills mosquito vectors within that time frame will automatically reduce the number of infected vectors and therefore almost certainly also reduce *Plasmodium* inoculation rates.

Formulated as biopesticides, fungal entomopathogens may have a great potential for application in indoor residual spraying of house wall surfaces or other resting places in human or animal dwellings. Once infected the fungus physically proliferates within the insect and results in the production of various secondary metabolites that have negative impacts on insect physiology [48-49] and performance and eventual death [50]. Histopathological studies of tissues infected by fungus suggest that the insect dies due to the combination of nutrient depletion, mechanical damage, and toxicosis. These biopesticides, if they can be successfully applied, could be useful for malaria control [51-52] especially if they prove effective against insecticide-resistant mosquitoes [53-55].

3.1.1. Entomopathogen fungus on clay

In recent trials [56] adult females of *An. stephensi* mosquitoes were exposed with cone tests to clay tiles sprayed with an oil formulation of spores of the entomopathogenic fungus *Beauveria bassiana* using different concentrations or time of exposure. A mortality rate of 100% was observed in less than one week, even when no KD effect was observed.

In addition to reducing longevity, it was noticed that fungal infection also reduces feeding propensity and fecundity [56-57] which added to the reduction of longevity could have a significant impact on vectorial capacity and therefore also on malaria transmission. Blanford et al [56] showed that "fungal exposed mosquitoes showed a declining response to the feeding stimulus over time, with 77, 60 and 50% of mosquitoes initiating feeding behaviors on days 1, 2 and 3, respectively and no mosquitoes responding on day 4. Combining the proportion of mosquitoes alive with the proportion attempting to feed gives a measure of overall transmission blocking (biting risk) on any given day. For treated mosquitoes, this combination of pre-lethal and lethal effects revealed reductions in biting risk of 36, 52, 72 and 100% on days 1–4, respectively. This represents complete transmission blocking within a feeding cycle".

Fungal infection was also observed to have a negative impact on flight performance which may be an important consideration for malaria control at focal level. Another very important character of entomopathogen fungus is its ability to control insecticide resistant mosquito strains. Exposure to the fungal biopesticide on clay tiles using the standard dose and a 30 minute-exposure period before classical bioassay (WHO cone test) of colonies of 3 species, *An. gambiae s.s.*, *An. arabiensis* and *An. funestus*, (ranging from fully susceptible to resistant to DDT, and/or Bendiocarb, and/or Malathion, and/or Deltamethrin) showed 100% mortality by day 6 irrespective of mosquito species or the level of resistance to insecticides. Blanford et al. [56] who reported that "the *An. gambiae* colony "TONGS", which was fully resistant to all chemical classes, had an Median Lethal Time (MLT) of 4 (3.93–4.07) days and all individuals were dead by day 5 (± 0.0) which was not dissimilar to the fully susceptible *An. gambiae* colony "SUA" which had an MLT of 4 (3.82–4.18) days and were all dead by day 6 "(±0.25)". It clearly appeared that "insecticide resistance confers no cross resistance to fungal pathogens in the key African malaria vectors" and this point must be taken into account in the management of insecticide resistance. For Blanford et al [56] "what is striking here is that when the effects of blood feeding are added in, risk of malaria transmission is essentially reduced to zero within a day of fungal exposure and never recovers".

3.1.2. Entomopathogen fungus on nets

Howard et al [58] implemented several classical tube bioassays to compare the fungal-susceptibility of an insecticide-resistant (VKPER) and insecticide-susceptible strain (SKK) of *An. gambiae* and test the activity (and longevity) of *M. anisopliae* and *B. bassiana* conidia on white polyester netting (Table 3). It appeared that *M. anisopliae* and *B. bassiana* significantly increased mortality of both resistant and susceptible strains of *An. gambiae* exposed to 2 or 7 days after treatment of nets (Table 3). *B. bassiana* was significantly more pathogenic than *M. anisopliae* both for SKK and VKPER (Table 3). The insecticide-resistant mosquito strain VKPER was significantly more susceptible to fungal infection than the SKK strain after exposure to 2 or 7 days after treatment of nets (table) while other studies did not find any difference in efficacy of dry conidia of B. bassiana on resistant or susceptible strain. It is possible that the discrepancies in data could be due to the mode of formulation of conidia (dry or ShellSol T suspensions in this study). The mosquito pathogenicity was maintained seven days after net application, but the viability of the two fungal species after seven days at 27°C was low, 62% and 2% respectively, for B. bassiana and M. anisopliae, hampering their practical application in LLINs.

Fungus	An. gambiae strain	Days after treatment	
		2	7
M. anisopliae	SKK	3.2	2.6
	VKPER	17.1	29.9
B. bassiana	SKK	11.0	7.4
	VKPER	32.2	43.5

Table 3. Comparison of mortality rates of fungal-susceptibility (M. anisopliae and B. bassiana) between an insecticide-resistant (VKPER) and insecticide-susceptible strain (SKK) of Anopheles gambiae.

Trials of entomopathogen fungus on mosquitoes have generated various results according to the protocol followed: formulation of fungus (dry/suspension); substrata (mud wall, cloth etc); field/lab trials; doses, exposure times; species of fungus; species/strain of mosquitoes, etc. Of note, Howard et al [58] successfully demonstrated the efficacy of nets treated with B. bassiana and tested against a resistant strain of An. gambiae. Even though the residual efficacy duration was short, the authors logically concluded that "Field trials over a longer trial period need to be carried out to see if wild insecticide-resistant mosquitoes are as susceptible as the colony strain used in this trial". Further studies, against resistant An. gambiae VKPER strain showed that "B. bassiana infection caused significantly increased mortality with the daily risk of dying being increased by 2.5 × for fungus-exposed mosquitoes compared to control mosquitoes. However, the virulence of the B. bassiana conidia decreased with increasing time spent exposed to the tropical field conditions, the older the treatment on the net, the lower the fungus-induced mortality rate. This is likely to be due to the tropical climate because laboratory trials found no such decline within the same trial time period. Conidial viability also decreased with increasing exposure to the net and natural abiotic environmental conditions. After 20 days field exposure the conidial viability was 30%, but the viability of control conidia not exposed to the net or field conditions was 79%" [59].

3.1.3. Influence of temperature

Kikankie et al [55] did several trials "to assess the susceptibility of insecticide-susceptible ("MBN") and resistant ("SENN") laboratory strains and wild-collected An. arabiensis to infection with the fungus B. bassiana under two different laboratory temperature regimes (21 ± 1°C or 25 ± 2°C)".

It appeared that exposure to dry *B. bassiana* spores resulted in significant reductions in longevity of the wild *An. arabiensis* mosquitoes and virulence was significantly higher at 25°C than 21°C, and exposure to *B. bassiana* spores resulted in significant reductions in longevity in all mosquito colonies regardless of their insecticide susceptibility levels and temperature regimes. Fungal susceptibility was not affected by resistance to insecticides.

It was also noted that "fungus-induced mortality rates were relatively rapid at 25°C, with 100% mortality taking 10-12 days post-fungus exposure in the baseline colonies (MBN and SENN) and field-collected mosquitoes" i.e. a lapse of time shorter than the duration of the sporogonic cycle of *P. falciparum* at this temperature, an important element for actual reduction of malaria transmission through vector control.

3.1.4. Influence of physiological stage and age

Mnyone et al [60] conducted bioassays using fed and unfed adult females of *An. gambiae* maintained in colony for several years with two fungal isolates: *M. anisopliae* and *B. bassiana* I93-825. Mosquitoes were exposed to conidia for 6 hours, with a follow up of 28 days. To study the effect of age, "three different age groups of female mosquitoes were exposed to both fungal isolates (2–4 days, 5–8 days, and 9–12 days post emergence), whereas to study the effect of physiological stage, five groups with differing blood-feeding status were exposed to both fungal isolates (non-fed, 3, 12, 36, or 72 h post-blood feeding). Results showed that, with both fungus, "older mosquitoes died relatively earlier than younger ones" and "blood-fed mosquitoes had a lower risk of dying relative to unfed ones". Increased risk of death in older than younger individuals has also been reported elsewhere [61-62]. Mnyone et al [60] considered that "the fact that blood-fed mosquitoes are less susceptible to fungal infection could be beneficial in terms of evolution proofing against resistance development. Although fungal infection reduces the fecundity of female mosquitoes [57], they are still able to pass their genes to the subsequent generation reducing selection pressure on resistance against fungi [55]. Furthermore, fungal infections suppress the successful development of *Plasmodium* parasites in the vectors [51], and hence both effects (i.e., fungus-induced mortality and parasite resistance) lead to a significantly reduced parasite transmission risk".

3.2. Attractive Toxic Sugar Bait (ATSB) methods

Recent studies on sugar feeding behavior of *Anopheles* [63-73] have been conducted in order "to optimize strategies for malaria vector control in Africa using attractive toxic sugar bait methods" [74] and to develop a new approach for mosquito control [75-78]. Stone et al [79] developed "an effective indoor mesocosm for studying populations of *An. gambiae* in temperate climates" and used the mesocosm concept to "determine whether the sugar-or-blood meal choice of *An. gambiae* females one day after emergence is influenced by blood-host presence and accessibility, nectariferous plant abundance, and female size" [80].

Stone et al. [80] noted that with a sleeping human present in the mesocosm, the majority of one day-old females obtained a blood meal. This was the case even with treated mosquito net use. But when a blood host was not present, or access was restricted through the use of a net, sugar meals became more frequent. The feeding choices of female *An. gambiae* were determined to a great degree by the presence and accessibility of the blood host, and not by the abundance of potential nectar sources in the mesocosm. Concerning the use of sugar baits as a malaria vector control, the strong tendency to feed on blood, even at one day post-emergence, suggests that in areas where larval development sites are close to human habitations, the method may be useful mainly as a complement to mosquito nets. If larval development sites are located at considerable distance from humans, the dominance of blood feeding is a smaller issue. Though females are willing to feed on humans as early as 24 h after emergence, in nature they may not come into contact with humans that early, and attraction to sugar sources would be paramount. Males and small females are particularly likely to seek a sugar meal when access to blood hosts is restricted by mosquito nets, suggesting that a plant-based method may be an effective control tool for such endgame scenarios. The combination of sugar baits (for instance, placed indoors or near a house) and treated mosquito nets, is one of these options. Its feasibility will require bait substantially more attractive than the plant species used in this experiment, such as the one used in Mali [78].

Based on highly successful demonstrations in Israel [75-77, 81] that attractive toxic sugar bait (ATSB) methods can decimate local populations of mosquitoes, Muller et al [78] implemented a study "to determine the effectiveness of ATSB methods for malaria vector control in the semi-arid Bandiagara District of Mali, West Africa". The *Anopheles* vector population was mainly composed of *An. gambiae* s.l. (mainly *An. gambiae* s.s. 86% and *An. arabiensis* 14%) and *An. funestus* [82]. The *Attractive Sugar Bait* (ASB) was composed, among other, by Guava (30%) (*Psidium guajava*) and honey melons (30%) (*Cucumis melo*) highly present in the area of the trial and known to be attractive for *An. gambiae s.l.* [83] while "ATSB was made by adding the boric acid [84-85] 1% (W/V) to ASB liquid". The ASB (in "control areas") and ATSB (in "treated areas") solutions were sprayed on the vegetation around the ponds and rice paddies and mosquitoes collected by CDC Light Traps at fixed positions between the ponds, during the 38 days of the trial, implemented at the end of the peak of malaria transmission period. It was observed that "ATSB treatment reduced densities of female and male *An. gambiae* s.l. by about 90%. After spraying ATSB in the treatment site, population densities of female and male *An. gambiae* s.l. declined rapidly over a week and then stabilized at low levels"; this impact on males is worth underlining as it could have an impact on decreased fertilized females and therefore on progeny. Furthermore, "ATSB treatment correspondingly affected the longevity of female *An. gambiae* s.l."

According to their data, Müller et al [78] considered that "ATSB methods differ from, and potentially complement, LLIN and IRS methods. In terms of malaria vector control in Africa, the ATSB methods when used operationally will likely reduce both total numbers of recently emerged female anophelines before they enter houses to feed on humans, and the proportion of females exiting houses to oviposit and then returning to houses to re-feed on humans. It is likely that ATSB approaches could soon be added as a major component of Integrated Vector Management (IVM) based malaria vector control programs" [86-88].

Along with their studies in Mali on the attractiveness of various local plants, fruits, flowers to mosquitoes *versus* human scents, Müller et al [83] noticed a very interesting "different rhythm of attractivity as plants showed peaks of *An. gambiae* s.l. attraction between 19:30-22:00 and 04:00-05:00, which differed considerably from the response to human odors, which peaked at around midnight". The well-known local *Acacia macrostachya* and *Acacia albida* (Fabaceae) appeared very attractive, and *Hyptis suaveolens* (Lamiaceae) appeared highly repellent.

It is clear that a great lot of questions still remain to be solved about ATSB such as, among others: What is the side effect of spraying vegetation on non-target fauna? What is the actual epidemiological efficacy in various epidemiological settings? Which attractant is the best in different ecological and entomological conditions? Which "toxin" is the most effective in various entomological conditions? And should it be used inside as well as outside and following which method and what about the acceptability and actual community participation, etc?

Nevertheless ATSB is another interesting approach worth further study for potential use, in complement to other classical methods such as IRS and LLIN, to reduce the number and the longevity of vectors i.e. malaria transmission and hence incidence of parasite infection and malaria morbidity.

3.3. New mathematical modeling of impacts of vector control

Since Roos and Macdonald, many mathematical models have been developed [89-90] for example (Figure 9):

- to evaluate the influence of environmental variables (climate, rain, relative humidity etc) [91];

- to facilitate the mathematicians to further develop suitable models and help the biologists and public health personnel to adopt better understanding of the modeling strategies to control the disease [92];

- to evaluate the potential mortality impact achievable by different long lasting, insecticide-treated net delivery strategies [93];

- to develop "a novel, convenient and versatile method to model *Plasmodium falciparum* infection that accounts for the essential in-host processes: parasite replication and its regulation by innate and adaptive immunity" [94];

- to improve malaria elimination strategies in areas where data are still scarce or not fully reliable [95];

- to develop a flexible and user-friendly *website* with an online mathematical model of malaria elimination that is being developed interactively with end users [96]; the website can be accessed at http://www.tropmedres. ac/elimination (see Malaria Elimination Model. http:// elimination.tropmedres.ac and Internet Model of Malaria Elimination User Guide http:// www.tropmedres.ac/images/modelling/userguide.pdf;

- to inform resistance management practices [97] determining the impact of different mosquito control intervention strategies including the protection conferred by mosquito nets [98];

• to develop new approaches such as the idea of evolution-proof insecticide [99-100].

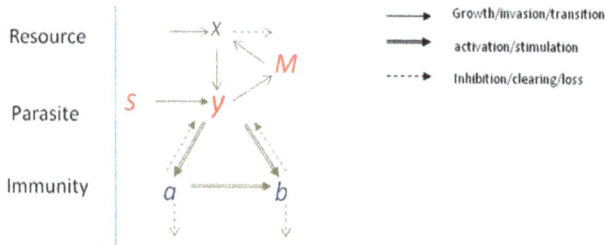

Figure 9. Schematic representation of model. The population of uninfected red blood cells (x) provides the source for the infected population (y). Level I immune effector (a) is stimulated by y. Level II immune effector (b) is stimulated by y interacting with a+b. M represents the number of merozoites, S represents an external source of inoculation

Mathematical models are useful in exposing what may otherwise be non-intuitive results, for example indoor residual spray (IRS) of insecticides in conjunction with mosquito nets can show antagonism, arising via interference of their modes of action while it is generally assumed that the two tools have synergistic benefits in reducing malaria transmission [101]. However, few have considered the spread of resistance in a variable selection pressure context [102]. A mathematical model [35] was recently developed to explore the effects on mosquito populations of spatial heterogeneous deployment of insecticides, to predict changes in mosquito fitness and resistance allele frequency, to identify important parameters in the evolution of insecticide resistance, to examine the contribution of new generation long-lasting insecticidal mosquito nets, that incorporate a chemical synergist on the roof panel, in delaying insecticide resistance.

Four niches were considered:

• Insecticide free (n): it can be an area either inside or outside a household;

• Non public-health related insecticide deployment: typically insecticide use in agriculture and households. These are deployed outwith of public health mosquito control campaigns, and generally out of the control of public health officials; mosquito coils, would also be included in this class;

• Insecticide-treated mosquito nets (ITN);

• Insecticide-treated mosquito nets with synergist on the top of the net (ITN + Synergist).

It appeared that resistance spreads slower in the presence of a synergist. The effect of synergist in males and females was not strictly comparable but was overall similar. The delay in the spread of resistance caused by the synergist was not very large; however, in approximately 10% of cases the rate of allele spread was higher when the synergist was fully effective. The predicted frequency of the resistance allele under different values of k at generation 70, the predicted frequency when the synergist is inefficient ($k = 1$), is 0.11 and when is fully effective ($k = 0$) is 0.26. The synergist has only a small impact in controlling the population, but even small values of k will help to recover the effect of the insecticide, and this is may be the main contribution of the synergist. Nevertheless adding synergists to mosquito nets does decrease the rate at which resistance spreads in about 90% of scenarios. If a fully effective synergist ($k = 0$) is present, the fitness of all genotypes inside the house will be zero (k affects the 3 genotypes equally, so all mosquitoes die irrespective of their genotype) and the next generation will be mostly composed by progeny of survivors from the niche outside the household where selection for resistance was high. One hypothesis is that in this particular case the synergist removes the refugia of weak selection in the house thereby magnifying the effects of selection for resistance outside the house.

According to Barbosa and Hastings [35], "The finding that a situation can arise in which having a fully effective synergist in place contributes to intensify the spread of resistance is the most interesting result of this work, a very important fact often overlooked in modeling resistance: that it is highly dangerous to consider selection in only a single niche, isolated from other selection pressures, and to then extrapolate the results from the single niche to the whole population. In this case it seems reasonable to conclude that adding effective synergists will reduce selection for resistance in the household niche because all three genotypes are killed. The level of impact that a fully effective synergist could have on disease transmission is a question that cannot be directly answered by the results presented here, because it is not clear how the genetic concept of fitness translates into the demographic factors, such as mosquito population size and longevity that determine the intensity of disease transmission. On the other hand, as noted above, if synergist throws most of the selection pressure onto another niche then overall the rate of selection for resistance may increase. Consequently the impact of the use of insecticide within the home (predominantly as wall sprays and/or mosquito nets) on mosquitoes cannot easily be isolated from other insecticide applications that mosquitoes may encounter during their lifetime. This suggests that the malaria community is correct in being alarmed at the often uncontrolled use of insecticides in applications such as agriculture".

Ghani et al [103] developed a very interesting model to consider the possibility that a large reduction in malaria transmission may result in a loss of immunity, and how useful integrated malaria control measures could be to counterbalance such an eventuality. They prepared "a mathematical model for malaria transmission which incorporates the acquisition and loss of both clinical and parasite immunity", to "explore the impact of the trade-off between reduction in exposure and decreased development of immunity on the dynamics of disease following a transmission-reducing intervention such as insecticide treated nets". It is worth noticing how their model "predicts that initially rapid reductions in clinical disease incidence will be observed as transmission is reduced in a highly immune population. However, these benefits in the first 5–10 years after the intervention may be offset by a greater burden of disease decades later as immunity at the population level is gradually lost. The negative impact of having fewer immune individuals in the population can be counterbalanced either by the implementation of highly-effective transmission-reducing interventions (such as the combined use of insecticide-treated nets and insecticide residual sprays) for an indefinite period, or the concurrent use of a pre-erythrocytic stage vaccine or prophylactic therapy in children to protect those at risk from disease as immunity is lost in the population".

One of the key issues is the still current lack of sound knowledge about "malaria immunity" called "premunition" which involves immunity against the parasite, and therefore against the disease. For Ghani et al [103] "Clinical immunity develops over time dependent on the force of infection in the population and reduces the probability that an individual will develop clinical disease. Parasite immunity develops as individuals' age, and reduces the amount of time spent in the asymptomatic patent infection state (mimicking a reduction in parasite density and hence onward infectiousness)". Their previous model "suggests that the loss of both clinical and parasite immunity occurs over a period of years rather than weeks or months" [104] and according to a study in Madagascar, it seems that "immunity" could be of long duration [105]. In their model, Ghani et al [103] "assume that clinical immunity is developed at a rate proportional to the EIR in each setting and has a half-life of approximately 7 years and that parasite-clearance immunity has a half-life of approximately 14 years". They consider that 3 phrases are crucial: sustain intervention/integrated measures/sustain financial support and "Sustaining both control interventions and effective case management for many years, possibly decades, should remain the primary goal of all intervention programmes and it is essential that these long-term goals are matched with financial commitments".

3.4. New ecological care

Special attention is now devoted to the environment, especially environmental modifications that may result because of the impact of insecticides on the environment and its biodiversity.

3.4.1. Environmental Risk Assessment (ERA) and Insect Pest Management IPM

No pesticide is completely safe. Only through their careful use are we able to gain an understanding of the risks and control them. The environmental impact of biocides is generally studied in the context of scientific investigations conducted beyond the regulatory requirements for approval. This helps to generate better understanding of the biocides and provides opportunity to assess their potential impact and overall effectiveness when used in various control strategies. Although vector control methods are generally confined to urban and suburban areas, these areas may have a significant vegetation cover that provides both refuge and food for wildlife (insects, reptiles, birds, bats etc)...). This shows the need of environmental risk assessments prior to large scale vector control interventions. It also highlights the need for further studies to determine direct, indirect short and long-term potential effects. Risk assessment of control methods must be addressed in an integrated strategy taking into account the relationships between species in regards of the local biodiversity. In fact, environmental risk assessment of these treatments cannot be limited only to consider information on hazards, such as acute toxicity of the biocides used. Every effort needs to be made to minimize the use of chemical pesticides. A great deal of improvement can be made in vector control programs if the existing, methods and materials are more effectively used. The idea of integrated vector control which effectively combines a package of appropriate control methods i.e. insecticidal, environmental, biological and physical, in an orderly and coordinated manner can impact upon insect vectors and diseases with positive results of economic, ecological and sociological consequences [106].

Programs based on Insect Pest Management (IPM) must be designed to reduce vector bites and disease transmission, but also mitigate any potentially negative effects, i.e., such as environmental damage, harm of non-target organisms exposed to insecticides, or increase of insecticide resistant in target organisms [107]. Such programs do already exist notably in the USA (for example in Santa Barbara County) and in Australia [108]. In these programs, process are very well defined step by step: 1) vector surveillance and identification of target vector species to develop species-specific pest management strategies based on developmental and behavioral considerations for each species; 2) threshold measures to determine when action is necessary; 3) public education, control, prevention; 4) monitoring of efficacy and environmental impacts to identify the occurrence of unexpected/unwanted effects of treatments.

3.4.2. Impact of insecticides used for vector control

The impact of insecticides on the environment depends not only on the active substance, but also the formulation and the method of applying: indoor residual spraying, space spraying or treated nets will have different impacts.

3.4.2.1. Indoor Residual Spraying (IRS)

Domestic livestock (particularly chickens) and organisms in the environment may be harmed if operations, cleanup, and disposal are not conducted according to best practices.

Table 4 describes the potential ecological effects of each recommended IRS chemical. There is a lack of data concerning toxicity of IRS insecticides on non-target fauna. However, most insecticides are highly toxic for aquatic and terrestrial arthropods like bees (in particular pyrethroid), and some of them can also be toxic for mammals (some pyrethroids and organophosphates).

3.4.2.2. Space spraying and larviciding

Space spraying has only occasionally been used in malaria epidemic control program and as a complementary measure against exophilic vectors. Nevertheless, pyrethroids, which have a short remanence, have been the predominant insecticides [123], and then care must be taken to avoid applications near fish-bearing water bodies. It is also recommended that such applications should not be carried out directly over water bodies and that a no-treated barrier of 100 m should be maintained to prevent fish mortality. Home owners should be advised to cover domestic fish tanks and bird cages during the applications [123].

Blom [124] examined the effects of aerial, barrier, and ground based ultra-low volume (ULV) sprays with sumithrin and deltamethrin, in Massachusetts on non-target insects. Malaise traps, targeting the flying insect population, were collected in regular intervals before and after sprays, then the captured insects were sorted by order and counted. The results have shown little effect on non-target insects from the ground based sprays, and a temporary knockdown from the aerial spray. However, Coleoptera were affected in the short term by the ULV sprays and, suffered long term effects from aerial spraying.

IRS insecticides	Mammal	Bird	Fish	Aquatic invertebrate	Bee	References
α-cypermethrin	0	0	++	++	++	[109]
Bendiocarb	0	0	+	+	++	[110]
Bifenthrin	+	+	++	++	++	[111], [112]
Cyfluthrin	+	0	++	++	++	[113]
DDT	+	+	++	++	+	[114]
Deltamethrin	+	0	++	++	++	[115]
Etofenprox	0	0	+	+	++	[116], [112]
Fenitrothion	0	+	0	++	++	[117]
λ-cyhalothrin	+	0	++	++	++	[118]
Malathion	+	+	0	++	++	[119], [120], [112]
Pirimiphos-methyl	++	0	++	++	++	[121], [112]
Propoxur	++	++	++	++	++	[122]

Key: 0: non-toxic; +: potentially toxic; ++: highly toxic

Table 4. Toxicity of chemicals used for IRS on non-target organisms

Davis and Peterson [125] assessed long-term impacts of permethrin on non-target terrestrial arthropods after repeat ULV applications in the context of West Nile Virus Management in the USA. The authors concluded that although small flying insects that were active at the same time as mosquitoes were slightly impacted, effects on non-target arthropods exposed to adulticides applied via ULV sprayer would be small in the ecosystem studied.

Several classes of recommended larvicides are used in vector control management such as: the bio-insecticides (*Bacillus thuringiensis* var. *israelensis* (*Bti*), *Bacillus sphaericus* (*Bs*) and spinosad), the organophosphates (chlorpyrifos, fenthion, pirimiphos-methyl, and temephos), and the insect growth regulators (diflubenzuron, methoprene, pyriproxyfen). The results of some studies concerning the environmental risk assessment of these larvicides are summarized in the Table 5.

3.4.2.3. Treated net

Long-Lasting Insecticide-Treated Nets (LLINs) have many important advantages as there is no need for re-treatment, the insecticide consumption is reduced, and release of insecticide in natural water bodies during washing is also reduced [142]. However, there is considerable misuse of mosquito nets for drying fish and fishing, in particular along Lake Victoria [143]. In their study, Minakawa et al. [143] surveyed 7 fishing villages along the lake and estimated that 239 LLIN were used for fishing and drying fish from the 1040 LLINs distributed by NGO in these villages. This could have an impact on aquatic organisms while the net are immersed into the lake water. On the other hand, LLIN can also moderately impact non-target household

Larvicides	Mammal	Bird	Fish	Aquatic invertebrate	Bee	References
Bti and *Bs*	0	0	0	0ᵃ	0	[126]
Spinosad	0	0	0	++	++	[127-129]
Chlorpyrifos	+	++	++	++	++	[130]
Fenthion	++	++	++	++	++	[131-132]
Pirimiphos-methyl	++	0	++	++	++	[133-134]
Temephos	+	0	+	+	++	[135-136]
Diflubenzuron	0	0	+	+	+	[137-139]
Methoprene	0	0	0	++	+	[134]
Pyriproxyfen	+	0	+	++	+	[140-141]

Key: 0: non-toxic; +: potentially toxic; ++: highly toxic

ᵃ In some cases non-target Nematocera such as Chironomidae can be impacted by *Bti*, depending on the dose and the formulations applied (Boisvert and Lacoursière, 2004)[126].

Table 5. Toxicity of larvicides chemicals on non-target organisms

pests such as house fly, American cockroach, head louse, and mosquito bug after 30-min exposure [144].

3.4.3. Environmental management

Mosquitoes breed in shallow-water habitats, so it is not surprising that most environmental management interventions for malaria control are associated with the manipulation of wetland environments. If applied correctly, these strategies can have very good results by modifying vector-breeding habitats [145]. But these habitats can include freshwater wetlands (swamps, flood plains, riverine forest, and swamp forest), mangroves, and coastal wetlands (lagoons, estuaries, and tidal mudflats) [146]. In some geographical regions, there are also semi-arid grasslands, which maintain areas of temporary flooding. Wetlands provide a wide range of ecological services including soil erosion and flood control, water purification and pollutant and nutrient retention, groundwater discharge and recharge, and provision of habitat and breeding grounds for wildlife. Disturbing wetlands through environmental management may alter the quantity and quality of the services that wetlands provide. Increasing water runoff (or, alternatively, a change in the composition or clearing of wetland vegetation by drainage or clearing vegetation) may also decrease the ability of the wetland to take up pollutants, potentially diminishing the quality of water resources. It may also cause higher peak water flows in streams and rivers during rain events, resulting in flood damage. Vegetation clearance may also decrease spawning ground for aquatic species and decrease breeding habitats for migratory birds and animals [147].

Larvivorous fish (such as *Gambusia*) are often introduced for biological control. However, the introduction of exotic fish species into the natural environment (e.g., wetlands and marshes) could disrupt existing predator–prey relationships and alter ecosystem composition. In some cases, the introduction of *Gambusia* has led to the destruction of native fish [145].

3.4.4. Methodological approach for ERA in the context of vector control

Measurements of toxicity based on the impact of a chemical on a species of interest, such as the LC_{50} (concentration that kills 50% of a population), and the no observable effect concentration for reproduction, are used extensively in determining ecological risk. But these methods are too simplistic to establish relationship between the results obtained and the response observed [148] and are not always representative of real life settings. As a consequence, new assessment methodologies to predict and anticipate the risks associated with new chemicals, and improve knowledge about existing chemicals are needed. The last decade has seen some development in this area, but there have been very few studies on the effects of large scale vector control published [149]. Recently, indirect effects of *Bti* treatments on birds such as house martins *Delichon urbicum* have been shown via measuring impact on their insect food sources [150]. In this study, the authors have measured foraging rates and chick diet and have shown that clutch size and fledgling survival were significantly lower at treated sites relative to control. Their hypothesis is that intake of Nematocera (Diptera) and their predators (spiders and dragonflies) decreased significantly in the sites treated with *Bti*, hindering the breeding success of the house martins. Another study on *Bti* monitored Chironomidae populations [151] in three wetlands treated with *Bti*-treatment to control mosquitoes, and three untreated wetlands. Results showed no reduced production of chironomids in *Bti*-treated as compared to untreated wetlands. However, the same authors [152] identified possible indirect effects of *Bti*-treatments in a further study that showed a higher specific richness of chironomids in treated wetlands, compared to control wetlands. They hypothesized that this was the result of reduced competition from mosquito larvae.

These studies demonstrate the need for more suitable methodologies and protocols to be developed for long-term monitoring of ecosystems. Several studies in Europe have monitored long term mosquito control effects, including programmes efforts in western France [153-154], and another in Ramsar area of southern France [155] where the Life-Environment European Program has been studying methods for the sustainable management of mosquito control. The French Ministry for Ecology, Sustainable Development and Spatial Planning via the National Programme for Ecotoxicology (PNETOX; APR2003) are studying the harmonisation of mosquito control methods in terms of their impact on non-target invertebrates in Mediterranean and Atlantic coastal wetlands [156].

A Life-Environment project, sustained by the European Commission, called "Control of noxious or vector mosquitoes: implementation of integrated management consistent with sustainable development (IMCM/n° n°LIFE08 ENV/F/000488)" is also under way in France. Its objective is to validate integrated methodologies and techniques allowing (1) a precise and up to date knowledge of target species' presence, biology, colonized habitats, using GIS/GPS tools, (2) the development of control methods fully appropriate to the health and environmental risks faced, (3) an evaluation of nuisance thresholds based on knowledge of social demands through sociological surveys, in order to optimise the communication strategies, (4) traceability of operations by means of retrospective and prospective analyses, and (5) the adoption of valid procedures and methodologies for the monitoring of the non-intentional effects on Man and the environment that can result from these control methods. This project will implement these decision-making tools with five public bodies that are involved in mosquito control efforts in Metropolitan France (Entente InterDepartementale pour la Démoustication du Littoral méditerranéen, EID Méditerranée, Entente InterDépartementale Rhône-Alpes pour la démoustication, EID Rhône-Alpes, General Council of Southern Corsica) and overseas (General Councils of Martinique and Guyana). The project prioritises environmental care and uses complementary methods for environmental risk assessment (in aquatic and terrestrial compartments) for mosquito control methods in temperate or tropical zones. All these projects have focused on consideration of the indirect possible effects of mosquito control on the invertebrates' communities in order to preserve the local biodiversity and endangered species. These projects have highlighted the importance of using methodologies adapted to the habitats and specific organisms, with relevant bio-indicators, implemented infield settings that represent the context in which the vector control management is to be undertaken. The studies also underlined the necessity of post-approval monitoring of the insecticides used in vector control management.

4. Conclusion — Discussion

The history of vector control for malaria control can roughly be divided in 3 main periods: before DDT: from general control to "eradication"; the DDT era and the "Malaria Eradication Programme" (MEP); after DDT: insecticide treated nets (ITN-LLIN), Integrated Vector Management (IVM) and new paradigms.

4.1. Before DDT

Since his discovery of the role of mosquito as vector of malaria parasite, Ross advocated the vector control for malaria control and in 1899, in Sierra-Leone; he "carried out the first project based on his discovery. His principal weapon was "illuminating oil" (kerosene)". It "was a transient success" not sustained due to lack of funds [157]. "In 1907 Ross was invited to Mauritius to organize antimalaria operations there. His recommendations were sound and the results were good if the government had given them more support" (Bruce-Chwatt, loc.cit.). It is interesting to underline some of the main issues observed at that time: the lack of financial and political support and the financial support is still matter of concerns when referring to the recent RBM statement. The greatest and most successful programme was malaria control in the Panama Canal zone by Gorgas [158] who, helped by Joseph Le Prince, successfully planned and implemented "*sanitation measures*" based on the principle to deal with the situation by all available means based on the role of mosquitoes. He could be therefore considered as the actual precursor of IVM.

Still underlined by Bruce-Chwatt (loc. Cit) "among the early projects one carried out by Malcolm Watson in Malaya deserves special mention, because of the ingenious combination of open and subsoil-drainage with naturalistic methods of control of *Anopheles* [159]. These measures were adapted to the behavioral characteristics of malaria in a given area and formed the basis for the concept of *"species sanitation"* [160].

After the success of Watson, several other "naturalistic methods" were developed such as altering the salinity of breeding site of *An. ludlowae* control in Indonesia, introduction of natural enemies of mosquitoes, use of *Gambusia* in California, Florida, then in Cyprus, Spain, Italy, Russia, Chile, etc [161].

Some of the best example of environmental modifications based upon drainage for successful malaria control were observed in Italy with reclamation of marshy areas (with resettlement of population in new land) for *"bonifica integrale"* of Pontine Marshes of the Roman Campagna [162-164] or Algeria in the marshy area of Mitidja Plaine [165-166].

Such programs could also be considered as precursor in the field of biological control which currently received great attention with the ecological issues of insecticide and insecticide resistance of main vectors.

In term of chemical control, 2 schools of thought were opposed: larva control, based upon Paris Green dust successfully used in Sardinia and Calabria and in several other places such as Brazil to get rid of invaders *An. gambiae* which caused severe epidemics of malaria in 1930s'; and adult control, with the use of the well known oriental daisy *Chrysanthemum cinerariaefolium*, (used for long time as fumigants in China against biting insects) the powder made of it contains powerful insecticide compounds such as pyrethrins and cinerins and as soon as 1932 Park-Ross and De Meillon instituted systematic house to house weekly sprayings of pyrethrum solution in kerosene for the control of adults *Anopheles* in Natal and Zululand and this program is somehow still ongoing with the regular inside resting spraying (with DDT) operations added to case management to control malaria in KwaZulu Natal [167]. Instead of pyrethrins, National Malaria control programme uses now pyrethroid but they are chemically developed from natural pyrethrins used formerly. Somehow history of approaches for malaria control repeats itself.

It is interesting to notice the variety of approaches and techniques involved (species sanitation, sanitation measures, bonifica integrale (reclamation of marshy area and resettlement of populations on the new land), pursued by Italian governments for many years, larval control through different measures from source reduction to Paris Greendust spraying, adult control with spray of pyrethrin, …) based on some knowledge of entomological, ecological and socio-economical situation for improvement of Public Health, control of outbreak or achievement of large constructions (dams, Panama Canal, etc). In a way these measures paved the way for new approaches developed after the failure of the Global Malaria Eradication Programme and the development of IVM with new paradigms for vector control.

4.2. The DDT era 1957 – 1969: Global malaria eradication programme

"In 1874 a Viennese student of chemistry, Othmar Zeidler, published in the Berichtungen (Proceedings) of the German Chemical Society a paper under the title "Verdindungen von

Chlral mit Brom und Chlorbenzol"; the compound described in it was DDT (Bruce-Chwatt, loc cit) but its insecticidal properties remained unknown until 1939 [168].

The first Expert Malaria Committee (Ciuca, Gabaldon, Hamilton, Fairley, Pampana, Russell) met in Geneva in 1947 to deal with "the enormous social and economic damage that malaria was causing to the developing tropical countries", Russell [169] estimating that throughout the world there were some 300 million cases of malaria every year with at least a million deaths, it is interesting to underline that such evaluation of the burden of malaria was regularly reported during the following decades. And as Bruce-Chwatt [157] rightly underlined: "this was also the time when the new concept of malaria control by imagocidal measures was stimulated by the reports of the extraordinary properties of an obscure compound synthesized 65 years before the outbreak of the Second World War. They were observed by a Swiss chemist, Müller who was looking for a substance active against clothes moths, and with the biologist Wiesmann they realized in 1939 the insecticidal properties of this product, named Gesarol or Neocid and first used in agriculture [170] then sent to USA and Britain (where it received the acronym DDT). This product presented 3 important operational properties: long persistence of residues on sprayed surfaces; high toxicity for insects and low for man; killing insects by simple contact. The advent of DDT revolutionized malaria control as the residual indoor spraying as this product appeared simple, and could be successfully and economically used even in rural areas where malaria was the worse. Actually a lot of successful campaigns were done in Sardinia (Italy) (for eradication of *An. labranchiae*), Cyprus, Greece, Venezuela, British Guiana, Bombay State, etc [171]. In 1955, Pampana and Russell [172] underlined the needs of "plans to eradicate malaria from a territory within a few years, so that eventually the recurring item of malaria control could be struck from the annual budget". And the Eighth World Health Assembly in 1955 decided "that the World Health Organization should take the initiative, provide technical advice, and encourage research and co-ordination of resources in the implementation of a programme having as its ultimate objective the world-wide eradication of malaria".

DDT appeared as a "magic bullet" but the great mistake was that the original policy relied only on the use of residual insecticide, DDT then other organochlorines (BHC, dieldrin,...) along with drug use for reducing human reservoir, with the same strategy to be implemented everywhere without taking care of biodiversity, epidemiological diversity, social, economical, entomological diversity. The basic concept was one malaria and therefore one strategy to be implemented faster than insecticide resistance spreading, already noticed in the main vectors such as *An. gambiae*. In 1956, the Ninth World Health Assembly recommended the policy of eradication and stimulation of inter-countries cooperation. The strategy was defined as "operation aimed at cessation of transmission of malaria and elimination of the reservoir of infected cases in a campaign limited in time and carried to such a degree of perfection that, when it comes to an end, there is no resumption of transmission". It was based upon 3 successive steps: "attack phase" with total coverage with inside residual spraying, then "consolidation phase" to eradicate any remaining foci after the IRS rounds, then the "maintenance phase" where the malaria eradication programme doesn't exist as such and comes under the responsibility of general health services involves in "vigilance" to check any imported cases.

During the following decades malaria was actually eradicated from Europe, part of Russia, Middle East, North America, Australia, Japan, Singapore, Korea, Taiwan, almost all West Indies Islands and about 53% of the population of the originally malarious areas became free of malaria. But "the magnitude of the malaria problem in Tropical Africa has been daunting" (Bruce-Chwatt, loc cit). A re-examination of the global strategy of malaria eradication was carried in the 60' and the results presented at the 22nd World Health Assembly in 1969. One of the conclusion was that "in countries where eradication does not appear to be feasible because of the inadequacy of financial resources, manpower requirements or shortcomings of basic health services, malaria control operations should move to a transitional control programme stage, with the aim of launching of an eradication programme in the future". This is political wording that recognizes the failure of the rigid Global Eradication Programme and the reality that this may translate to "malaria control" involving the use of every available effective method to tackle first malaria mortality and morbidity, rather than malaria transmission specifically, as it was targeted by the MEP.

After the illusion of the Malaria eradication came the time of pragmatism, and the recognition of the biodiversity concept with IVM which takes into account all biological but also economical, socio-cultural components of the vector-borne parasitic disease and tools available (or to be developed) to tailor vector control measures to each epidemiological settings, to reach its full efficacy in the aim of sharply reduce, then eliminating malaria steps by steps. In this concept of biodiversity, a flexible and multifaceted approach is requested and paradigms were developed accordingly. For example, it is generally considered that tools for vector control must have a quick action to kill vectors before they transmit the parasites to any other human being, but slow acting products are now envisaged considering that if life is shortening to become less than the duration of the sporogonic cycle there couldn't be any transmission of the pathogenic agent even if this takes slightly more time than the "killing" product. Another approach is to mix different products for LLIN or IRS to deal with insecticide resistance and even to join IGR usually used against larvae in product targeting adults such as insecticide paints and even LLIN. The main impact should therefore be observed in term of reducing fecundity and fertility which would impact new generations of adults and more generally *Anopheles* populations.

Nevertheless for the time being the only new tools operational for vector control at large is insecticide treated nets (ITN) currently industrialized treated to become Long Lasting nets and which clearly showed their efficacy if well used and maintained. But the field is largely open for new tools mainly dealing with insecticide, and sometimes social resistance.

A great attention is now devoted to the cultural and social aspects of vector control methods implemented from outside, the "non usage" or "mis-usage" of mosquito nets are good example of the misfit between International agencies which gave large number of LLIN free of charge and the local social acceptability or local financial constraints.

A great care is also given to ecological impact and Malaria control programme must take lessons from the large multicountries Onchocerciasis Control Programme for managing insecticide resistance and care of non targeted fauna.

We must keep in mind the sentences of late Prof Bruce-Chwatt [173]: "the present approach to the control of this disease envisages a progressive incorporation of all general and specific antimalarial activities into the primary health care structures. This opens up many possibilities for research on the use of different technical resources together with the involvement of indigenous communities. But this is a different story!".

List of abbreviations

ATSB - Attractive toxic sugar bait

ASB - Attractive Sugar Bait

C - Carbamate

CS - Microencapsulated formulation

CTN - hand treated ITN

DL - Durable wall linings

EID - Entente InterDepartementale pour la Démoustication

ERA - Environmental Risk Assessment

IGR - Insect Growth Regulator

IPM - Insect Pest Management

IRS - Indoor Residual Spraying

ITN - Insecticide Treated Nets

ITPS - Insecticide-Treated Plastic Sheeting

IVCC - Innovative Vector Control Consortium

IVM - Integrated Vector Management

KD - KnockDown

KDR - KnockDown Resistance

LC50 - median Lethal Concentration of a substance

LC100 - absolute Lethal Concentration

LiST - Lives Saved Tool

LLIN - Long-Lasting Insecticidal Net

LN - Long lasting insecticide treated Net

MEP - Malaria Eradication Programme

MLT - Median Lethal Time

OC - Organochlorine

OP - Organophosphate

P3 - Permanet 3

PBO - Piperonyl Butoxide

Pyr - Pyrethroid

RBM - Roll Back Malaria

SAP - Slow Acting Product

TPP - Target Product Profile

ULV - Ultra-Low Volume

UPS - Untreated Plastic Sheeting

WHO - World Health Organization

WHOPES - WHO Pesticide Evaluation Scheme

WL - Durable Wall Linings

Acknowledgements

We are grateful to Dr Kate Aultman for her helful suggestions and comments all along the writing of this document.

Author details

Claire Duchet[1,2], Richard Allan[3] and Pierre Carnevale[4]

*Address all correspondence to: pjcarnevale2001@yahoo.fr; cduchet.eid@gmail.com

1 Entente InterDépartementale de Démoustication du Littoral Méditerranéen, Montpellier, France

2 Community Ecology Laboratory, Institute of Evolution and Department of Evolutionary & Environmental Biology, University of Haifa, Israel

3 The MENTOR Initiative, Crawley, UK

4 Portiragnes, France

References

[1] WHO. Global Malaria Report –World Malaria Report. World Health Organization: Geneva; 2012.

[2] Murray CJ, Rosenfeld LC, Lim SS, Andrews KG, Foreman KJ, Haring D, Fullman N, Naghavi M, Lozano R, Lopez AD. Global malaria mortality between 1980 and 2010: a systematic analysis. Lancet Infect Dis 2012; 379: 413–31.

[3] Larsen D, Friberg I, Eisele T. Comparison of Lives Saved Tool model child mortality estimates against measured data from vector control studies in sub-Saharan Africa. BMC Public Health 2011; 11 (3): S34.

[4] WHO. Global malaria control and elimination: report of a technical review. World Health Organization: Geneva; 2009.

[5] Lengeler C, Cattani J, De Savigny D. Net gain - A new method for preventing malaria deaths. IDRC Books; 1996. 189pp.

[6] Ranson H, N'Guessan R. Lines J, Moiroux N, Nkuni Z, Corbel V. Pyrethroid resistance in African anopheline mosquitoes: what are the implications for malaria control? Trends in Parasitology 2011; 27: 91–98.

[7] Nauen R. Insecticide resistance in disease vectors of public health importance. Pest Management Science 2007; 63: 628–633.

[8] Labbé P, Alout H, Djogbénou L, Pasteur N, Weill M. Evolution of Resistance to Insecticide in Disease Vectors. Massachusetts, USA: Elsevier; 2011.

[9] Corbel V, N'Guessan R, Brengues C, Chandre F, Djogbénou L, Martin T, Akogbéto M, Hougard J, Rowland M. Multiple insecticide resistance mechanisms in *Anopheles gambiae* and *Culex quinquefasciatus* from Benin, West Africa. Acta Tropica 2007; 101: 207-16.

[10] N'Guessan R, Boko P, Odjo A, Chabi J, Akogbeto M, Rowland M. Control of pyrethroid and DDT-resistant *Anopheles gambiae* by application of indoor residual spraying or mosquito nets treated with a long-lasting organophosphate insecticide, chlorpyrifos-methyl. Malaria Journal 2010; 9: 44.

[11] N'Guessan R, Asidi A, Boko P, Odjo A, Akogbeto M, Pigeon O, Rowland M. An experimental hut evaluation of PermaNet® 3.0, a deltamethrin–piperonyl butoxide combination net, against pyrethroid-resistant *Anopheles gambiae* and *Culex quinquefasciatus* mosquitoes in southern Benin. Transactions of the Royal Society of Tropical Medicine and Hygiene 2010; 104: 758–765.

[12] Amelotti I, Catalá S, Gorla D. Experimental evaluation of insecticidal paints against *Triatoma infestans* (Hemiptera: Reduviidae), under natural climatic conditions. Parasites & Vectors 2009; 2: 30-6.

[13] Mosqueira B, Duchon S, Chandre F, Hougard J, Carnevale P, Mas-Coma S. Efficacy of an insecticide paint against insecticide-susceptible and resistant mosquitoes - part 1: laboratory evaluation. Malaria Journal 2010; 9: 340.

[14] Mosqueira B, Chabi J, Chandre F, Akogbeto M, Hougard J, Carnevale P, Mas-Coma S. Efficacy of an insecticide paint against malaria vectors and nuisance in West Africa - part 2: field evaluation. Malaria Journal 2010; 9: 341.

[15] Jones A, Sattelle D. Diversity of insect nicotinic acetylcholine receptor subunits. Advances in Experimental Medicine and Biology 2010; 683: 25-43.

[16] Wakita T, Kinoshita K, Yamada E, Yasui N, Kawahara N, Naoi A, Nakaya M, Ebihara K, Matsuno H, Kodaka K. The discovery of dinotefuran: a novel neonicotinoid. Pest Management Science 2003; 59: 1016-22.

[17] Corbel V, Duchon S, Zaim M, Hougard J. Dinotefuran: a potential neonicotinoid insecticide against resistant mosquitoes. Journal of Medical Entomology 2004; 41: 12-7.

[18] Darriet F, Chandre F. Combining piperonyl butoxide and dinotefuran restores the efficacy of deltamethrin mosquito nets against resistant *Anopheles gambiae* (Diptera: Culicidae). Journal of Medical Entomology 2011; 48: 952-5.

[19] Djènontin A, Chandre F, Dabiré K, Chabi J, N'Guessan R, Baldet T, Akogbéto M, Corbel V. Indoor use of plastic sheeting impregnated with carbamate combined with long-lasting insecticidal mosquito nets for the control of pyrethroid-resistant malaria vectors. The American Journal of Tropical Medicine and Hygiene 2010; 83: 266-70.

[20] Graham K, Mohammad N, Rehman H, Nazari A, Ahmad M, Kamal M, Skovmand O, Guillet P, Allan R, Zaim M, Yates A, Lines J, Rowland M. Insecticide-treated plastic tarpaulins for control of malaria vectors in refugee camps. Medical and Veterinary Entomology 2002; 16: 404-8.

[21] Burns M, Rowland M, N'Guessan R, Carneiro I, Beeche A, Ruiz S, Kamara S, Takken W, Carnevale P, Allan R. Insecticide-Treated Plastic Sheeting for Emergency Malaria Prevention and Shelter among Displaced Populations: An Observational Cohort Study in a Refugee Setting in Sierra Leone. The American Journal of Tropical Medicine and Hygiene 2012; 87: 242-50.

[22] Sharma S, Upadhyay A, Haque M, Tyagi P, Mohanty S, Mittal P, Dash A. Field evaluation of ZeroFly--an insecticide incorporated plastic sheeting against malaria vectors & its impact on malaria transmission in tribal area of northern Orissa. Indian Journal of Medical Research 2009; 130: 458-66.

[23] Mittal P, Sreehari U, Razdan R, Dash A. Evaluation of the impact of ZeroFly®, an insecticide incorporated plastic sheeting on malaria incidence in two temporary labour shelters in India. Journal of Vector Borne Disease 2011; 48: 138-43.

[24] Brosseau L, Drame PM, Besnard P, Toto JC, Foumane V, Le Mire J, Mouchet F, Remoue F, Allan R, Fortes F, Carnevale P, Manguin S. Human antibody response to

Anopheles saliva for comparing the efficacy of three malaria vector control methods in Balombo, Angola. PLoS One 2012; 7(9):e44189.

[25] Messenger LA, Miller NP, Adeogun AO, Awolola TS, Rowland M. The development of insecticide-treated durable wall lining for malaria control: insights from rural and urban populations in Angola and Nigeria. Malaria Journal 2012; 11:332.

[26] Messenger LA, Matias A, Manana AN, Stiles-Ocran JB, Knowles S, Boakye DA, Coulibaly MB, Larsen ML, Traoré AS, Diallo B, Konaté M, Guindo A, Traoré SF, Mulder CE, Le H, Kleinschmidt I, Rowland M. Multicentre studies of insecticide-treated durable wall lining in Africa and South-East Asia: entomological efficacy and household acceptability during one year of field use. Malaria Journal 2012; 11(1):358.

[27] Pulford J, Tandrapah A, Atkinson JA, Kaupa B, Russell T, Hetzel MW. Feasibility and acceptability of insecticide-treated plastic sheeting (ITPS) for vector control in Papua New Guinea. Malaria Journal 2012; 11:342 doi:10.1186/1475-2875-11-342.

[28] Diabate A, Chandre F, Rowland M, N'Guessan R, Duchon S, Dabire K, Hougard J. The indoor use of plastic sheeting pre-impregnated with insecticide for control of malaria vectors. Tropical Medicine & International Health 2006; 11: 597-603.

[29] Chandre F, Dabire R, Hougard J, Djogbenou L, Irish S, Rowland M, N'Guessan R. Field efficacy of pyrethroid treated plastic sheeting (durable lining) in combination with long lasting insecticidal nets against malaria vectors. Parasites & Vectors 2010; 3: 65.

[30] WHOPES. Report of the Twelfth WHOPES Working Group Meeting, Review of: Bioflash® GR, Permanet® 2.0, Permanet® 3.0, Permanet® 2.5, Lambda-cyhalothrin® LN. WHO/HTM/NTD/WHOPES/2009.

[31] Corbel V, Chabi J, Dabiré Roch K, Etang J, Nwane P, Pigeon O, Akogbeto M, Hougard J. Field efficacy of a new mosaic long-lasting mosquito net (PermaNet® 3.0) against pyrethroid resistant malaria vectors: a multi centre study in Western and Central Africa. Malaria Journal 2010; 9: 113.

[32] Tungu P, Magesa S, Maxwell C, Malima R, Masue D, Sudi W, Myamba J, Pigeon O, Rowland M. Evaluation of PermaNet 3.0 a deltamethrin-PBO combination net against *Anopheles gambiae* and pyrethroid resistant *Culex quinquefasciatus* mosquitoes: an experimental hut trial in Tanzania. Malaria Journal 2010; 9: 21.

[33] Yewhalaw D, Asale A, Tushune K, Getachew Y, Duchateau L, Speybroeck N. Bio-efficacy of selected long-lasting insecticidal nets against pyrethroid resistant *Anopheles arabiensis* from south-western Ethiopia. Parasites & Vectors 2012; 5: 159.

[34] Koudou B, Koffi A, Malone D, Hemingway J. Efficacy of PermaNet® 2.0 and PermaNet® 3.0 against insecticide-resistant *Anopheles gambiae* in experimental huts in Côte d'Ivoire. Malaria Journal 2011; 10: 172.

[35] Barbosa S, Hastings I. The importance of modeling the spread of insecticide resist-ance in a heterogeneous environment: the example of adding synergists to bed nets. Malaria Journal 2012; 11: 258.

[36] WHO: Report of the 11th WHOPES Working Group Meeting. Review of Spinosad 7.48% DT, Netprotect®, Duranet®, Dawaplus®, Icon® maxx. World Health Organi-zation, Geneva, WHO/HTM/NTD/WHOPES/2008.1. 2007.

[37] Winkler M, Tchicaya E, Koudou B, Donzé J, Nsanzabana C, Müller P, Adja A, Ut-zinger J. Efficacy of ICON® Maxx in the laboratory and against insecticide-resistant *Anopheles gambiae* in central Côte d'Ivoire. Malaria Journal 2012; 11: 167.

[38] Bukhari T, Takken W, Koenraadt C. Development of *Metarhizium anisopliae* and *Beau-veria bassiana* formulations for control of malaria mosquito larvae. Parasites & Vectors 2011; 4: 23.

[39] Darriet F, Duchon S, Hougard JM. Spinosad: a new larvicide against insecticide-re-sistant mosquito larvae. Journal of the American Mosquito Control Association 2005; 21: 495-496.

[40] Thompson G, Michel K, Yao R, Myderse J, Mosburg C, Worden T, Chio E, Sparks T, Hutchins S. The discovery of *Saccharopolyspora spinosa* and a new class of insect con-trol products. Down Earth 1997; 52: 1-5.

[41] Bret B, Larson L, Shoonoever J, Sparks T, Thompson G. Biological properties of spi-nosad. Down Earth 1997; 2: 6-13.

[42] Duchet C, Caquet T, Franquet E, Lagneau C, Lagadic L. Influence of environmental factors on the response of a natural population of *Daphnia magna* (Crustacea: Clado-cera) to spinosad and *Bacillus thuringiensis israelensis* in Mediterranean coastal wet-lands. Environmental Pollution 2010; 158: 1825-1833.

[43] Romi R, Proietti S, Di Luca M, Cristofaro M. Laboratory evaluation of the bioinsecti-cide Spinosad for mosquito control. Journal of the American Mosquito Control Asso-ciation 2006; 22: 93-6.

[44] Kumar A, Murugan K, Madhiyazhagan P, Prabhu K. Spinosad and neem seed kernel extract as bio-controlling agents for malarial vector, *Anopheles stephensi* and non-bit-ing midge, *Chironomus circumdatus*. Asian Pacific Journal of Tropical Medicine 2011; 4: 614-8.

[45] Prabhu K, Murugan K, Nareshkumar A, Bragadeeswaran S. Larvicidal and pupicidal activity of spinosad against the malarial vector *Anopheles stephensi*. Asian Pacific Jour-nal of Tropical Medicine 2011; 4: 610-3.

[46] Bond J, Marina C, Williams T. The naturally derived insecticide spinosad is highly toxic to *Aedes* and *Anopheles* mosquito larvae. Medical and Veterinary Entomology 2004; 18: 50-56.

[47] Read A, Lynch P, Thomas M. How to make evolution-proof insecticides for malaria control. PLoS Biol 2009; 7: e1000058.

[48] Kershaw M, Moorehouse E, Bateman R, Reynolds S, Charnley AK. The role of des-truxins in the pathogenicity of *Metarhizium anisopliae* for three species of insect. Journal of Invertebrate Pathology 1999;74: 213–223.

[49] Hajek A, St Leger R. Interactions between fungal pathogens and insect hosts. Annual Review of Entomology 1994; 39: 293–322.

[50] Bell A, Blanford S, Jenkins N, Thomas M, Read A. Real-time quantitative PCR analy-sis of candidate fungal biopesticides against malaria: Technique validation and first applications. Journal of Invertebrate Pathology 2009; 100: 160–168.

[51] Blanford S, Chan B, Jenkins N, Sim D, Turner R. Fungal pathogen reduces potential for malaria transmission. Science 2005; 308: 1638–1641.

[52] Thomas M, Read A. Can fungal biopesticides control malaria? Nature Reviews Mi-crobiology 2007; 5: 377–383.

[53] Farenhorst M, Mouatcho J, Kikankie C, Brooke B, Hunt R. Fungal infection counters insecticide resistance in African malaria mosquitoes. Proceedings of the National Academy of Sciences 2009; 106: 17443–17447.

[54] Farenhorst M, Knols B, Thomas M, Howard A, Takken W. Synergy of fungal ento-mopathogens and permethrin against West African insecticide-resistant *Anopheles gambiae* mosquitoes. PLoS One 2010; e12801.

[55] Kikankie C, Brooke B, Knols B, Koekemoer L, Farenhorst M. The infectivity of the en-tomopathogenic fungus *Beauveria bassiana* to insecticide-resistant and susceptible *Anopheles arabiensis* at two different temperatures. Malaria Journal 2010; 9: 71.

[56] Blanford S, Shi W, Christian R, Marden J, Koekemoer L. Lethal and Pre-Lethal Effects of a Fungal Biopesticide Contribute to Substantial and Rapid Control of Malaria Vec-tors. PLoS ONE 2011; 6.

[57] Scholte E, Knols B, Takken W. Infection of the malaria mosquito *Anopheles gambiae* with the entomopathogenic fungus *Metarhizium anisopliae* reduces blood feeding and fecundity. Journal of Invertebrate Pathology 2006; 91: 43–49.

[58] Howard A, Koenraadt C, Farenhorst M, Knols B, Takken W. Pyrethroid resistance in *Anopheles gambiae* leads to increased susceptibility to the entomopathogenic fungi *Metarhizium anisopliae* and *Beauveria bassiana*. Malaria Journal 2010; 9: 168.

[59] Howard A, N'Guessan R, Koenraadt C, Asidi A, Farenhorst M, Akogbéto M, Knols B, Takken W. First report of the infection of insecticide-resistant malaria vector mosqui-toes with an entomopathogenic fungus under field conditions. Malaria Journal 2011; 10: 24.

[60] Mnyone L, Kirby M, Mpingwa M, Lwetoijera D, Knols B, Takken W, Koenraadt C, Russell T. Infection of *Anopheles gambiae* mosquitoes with entomopathogenic fungi:

effect of host age and blood-feeding status. Parasitological Research 2011; 108: 317–322.

[61] Harrington L, Buonaccorsi J, Edman J, Costero A, Kittayapong P, Clark G, Scott T. Analysis of survival of young and old *Aedes aegypti* (Diptera: Culicidae) from Puerto Rico and Thailand. Journal of Medical Entomology 2001; 38: 537–547.

[62] Styer L, Carey J, Wang J, Scott T. Mosquitoes do senesce: departure from the paradigm of constant mortality. The American Journal of Tropical Medicine and Hygiene 2007; 76: 111–117.

[63] Yuval B: The other habit: sugar feeding by mosquitoes. Bull. Soc. Vector Ecol 1992; 17:150-156.

[64] Foster WA. Mosquito sugar feeding and reproductive energetics. Annual Review of Entomology 1995; 40:443-474.

[65] Beier JC. Frequent blood-feeding and restrictive sugar-feeding behavior enhance the malaria vector potential of *Anopheles gambiae* s.i. and *An. funestus* (Diptera: Culicidae) in western Kenya. Journal of Medical Entomology 1996; 33:613-618.

[66] Gary RE, Foster WA. Effects of available sugar on the reproductive fitness and vectorial capacity of the malaria vector *Anopheles gambiae* (Diptera: Culicidae). Journal of Medical Entomology 2001; 38:22-28.

[67] Gary RE, Foster WA. *Anopheles gambiae* feeding and survival on honeydew and extrafloral nectar of peridomestic plants. Medical and Veterinary Entomology 2004; 18:102-107.

[68] Gary RE, Foster WA. Diel timing and frequency of sugar feeding in the mosquito *Anopheles gambiae*, depending on sex, gonotrophic state and resource availability. Medical and Veterinary Entomology 2006; 20:308-316.

[69] Foster WA, Takken W. Nectar-related vs. human-related volatiles: behavioral response and choice by female and male *Anopheles gambiae* (Diptera: Culicidae) between emergence and first feeding. Bulletin of Entomological Research 2004; 94:145-157.

[70] Müller GC, Schlein Y. Plant tissues: the frugal diet of mosquitoes in adverse conditions. Journal of Veterinary and Medical Entomology 2005; 19:413-422.

[71] Manda H, Gouagna LC, Foster WA, Jackson RR, Beier JC, Githure JI, Hassanali A. Effect of discriminative plant-sugar feeding on the survival and fecundity of *Anopheles gambiae*. Malaria Journal 2007; 6:113.

[72] Manda H, Gouagna LC, Nyandat E, Kabiru W, Jackson RR, Foster WA, Githure JI, Beier JC, Hassanali A Discriminative feeding behavior of *Anopheles gambiae* s.s. on endemic plants in Western Kenya. Medical and Veterinary Entomology 2007; 21:103-111.

[73] Gu W, Müller G, Schlein Y, Novak RJ, Beier JC. Natural plant sugar sources of *Anopheles* mosquitoes strongly impact malaria transmission potential. PLoS One 2011; 6:e15996.

[74] Müller GC, Junnila A, Schlein Y. Effective control of adult *Culex pipiens* by spraying an attractive toxic sugar bait solution in the vegetation near larval habitats. Journal of Medical Entomology 2010; 47:63-66.

[75] Schlein Y, Müller G.C. An approach to mosquito control: Using the dominant attraction of flowering *Tamarix jordanis* trees against *Culex pipiens*. Journal of Medical Entomology 2008; 45:384-390.

[76] Müller G, Schlein Y. Sugar questing mosquitoes in arid areas gather on scarce blossoms that can be used for control. International Journal for Parasitology 2006; 36:1077-1080.

[77] Müller GC, Schlein Y. Efficacy of toxic sugar baits against adult cistern dwelling *Anopheles claviger*. Transactions of Royal Society of Tropical Medicine and Hygiene 2008; 102:480-484.

[78] Müller GC, Beier JC, Traore SF, Toure MB, Traore MM, Bah S, Doumbia S, Schlein Y. Successful field trial of attractive toxic sugar bait (ATSB) plant spraying methods against malaria vectors in the *Anopheles gambiae* complex in Mali, West Africa. Malaria Journal 2010; 9: 210.

[79] Stone CM, Taylor RM, Foster WA. An effective indoor mesocosm for studying populations of *Anopheles gambiae* in temperate climates. Journal of the American Mosquito Control Association 2009; 25:514-516.

[80] Stone CM, Jackson BT, Foster WA. Effects of bed net use, female size, and plant abundance on the first meal choice (blood vs. sugar) of the malaria mosquito *Anopheles gambiae*. Malaria Journal 2012; 11:3.

[81] Müller GC, Kravchenko VD, Schlein Y. Decline of *Anopheles sergentii* and *Aedes caspius* populations following presentation of attractive, toxic (Spinosad), sugar bait stations in an oasis. Journal of the American Mosquito Control Association 2008; 24:147-149.

[82] Sogoba N, Vounatsou P, Bagayoko MM, Doumbia S, Dolo G, Gosoniu L, Traore SF, Toure YT, Smith T. The spatial distribution of *Anopheles gambiae sensu stricto* and *An. arabiensis* (Diptera: Culicidae) in Mali. Geospat. Health 2007; 1:213-22.

[83] Müller GC, Beier JC, Traore SF, Toure MB, Traore MM, Bah S, Doumbia S, Schlein Y. Field experiments of *Anopheles gambiae* attraction to local fruit/seedpods and flowering plants in Mali to optimize strategies for malaria vector control in Africa using attractive toxic sugar bait methods. Malaria Journal 2010; 9:262.

[84] Xue RD, Barnard DR. Boric acid bait kills adult mosquitoes (Diptera:Culicidae). Journal of Economical Entomology 2003; 96:1559-1562.

[85] Xue RD, Kline D, Ali L, Barnard DR. Application of boric acid baits to plant foliage for adult mosquito control. Journal of the American Mosquito Control Association 2006; 22:497-500.

[86] WHO. Global strategic framework for integrated vector management. WHO/CDS/CPE/PVC/2004. World Health Organization, Geneva. 10:1-12. 2004.

[87] WHO. WHO position statement on integrated vector management. Wkly. Epidemiol. Rec. 83:177-181. 2008.

[88] Beier JC, Keating J, Githure JI, Macdonald MB, Impoinvil DE, Novak RJ. Integrated vector management for malaria control. Malaria Journal 2008; 7:54.

[89] Koella J. On the use of mathematical models of malaria transmission. Acta Tropica 1991; 49: 1-25.

[90] Smith D, Battle K, Hay S, Barker C, Scott T, McKenzie F. Ross, Macdonald, and a theory for the dynamics and control of mosquito-transmitted pathogens. PLoS Pathog 2012; 8: e1002588.

[91] Parham P, Pople D, Christiansen-Jucht C, Lindsay S, Hinsley W, Michael E. Modeling the role of environmental variables on the population dynamics of the malaria vector Anopheles gambiae sensu stricto. Malaria Journal 2012; 11: 271.

[92] Mandal S, Sarkar R, Sinha S. Mathematical models of malaria--a review. Malaria Journal 2011; 10: 202.

[93] Okell LC, Smith Paintain L, Webster J, Hanson K, Lines J. From intervention to impact: modeling the potential mortality impact achievable by different long lasting, insecticide-treated net delivery strategies. Malaria Journal 2012; 11(1):327.

[94] Gurarie D, Karl S, Zimmerman P, King C, St Pierre T, Davis T. Mathematical modeling of malaria infection with innate and adaptive immunity in individuals and agent-based communities. PLoS One 2012; 7: e34040.

[95] White L, Maude R, Pongtavornpinyo W, Saralamba S, Aguas R, Van Effelterre T, Day N, White N. The role of simple mathematical models in malaria elimination strategy design. Malaria Journal 2009; 8: 212.

[96] Maude R, Saralamba S, Lewis A, Sherwood D, White N, Day N, Dondorp A, White L. Modeling malaria elimination on the internet. Malaria Journal 2011; 10: 191.

[97] Committee on Strategies for the Management of Pesticide Resistant Pest Populations. Pesticide Resistance: Strategies and Tactics for Management. Washington: The National Academies Press. 1986.

[98] Chitnis N, Smith T, Steketee R. A mathematical model for the dynamics of malaria in mosquitoes feeding on a heterogeneous host population. Journal of Biological Dynamics 2008; 2: 259-285.

[99]   Koella, J, Lynch P, Thomas M, Read A. Towards evolution-proof malaria control with insecticides. Evolutionary Applications 2009; 2: 469–480.

[100]   Gourley S, Liu R, Wu J. Slowing the evolution of insecticide resistance in mosquitoes: a mathematical model. Proceedings of the Royal Society A 2011; 467: 2127–2148.

[101]   Yakob L, Dunning R, Yan G. Indoor residual spray and insecticide-treated mosquito-nets for malaria control: theoretical synergisms and antagonisms. Journal of the Royal Society Interface 2010; 8: 799–806.

[102]   Hermsen R, Hwa T. Sources and Sinks: A Stochastic Model of Evolution in Heterogeneous Environments. Physical Review Letters 2010; 105: 248104.

[103]   Ghani AC, Sutherland CJ, Riley EM, Drakeley CJ, Griffin JT, Gosling RD, Filipe JA. Loss of population levels of immunity to malaria as a result of exposure-reducing interventions: consequences for interpretation of disease trends. PLoS One 2009; 4: e4383.

[104]   Filipe J, Riley E, Drakeley C, Sutherland C, Ghani AC. Determination of the mechanisms driving the acquisition of immunity to malaria using a mathematical transmission model. PLoS Computational Biology 2007; 3: e255.

[105]   Deloron P, Chougnet P. Is immunity to malaria really short-lived? Parasitology Today 1992; 8: 375–378.

[106]   Smith R, Reynolds H. Principles, definitions and scope of integrated pest control. Proceeding of the FAO Symposium on Integrated Pest Control 1965; 1: 11-17.

[107]   Rajotte E, Kazmierczak RJ, Norton G, Lambur M, Allen W. The National Evaluation of Extension's Integrated Pest Management Programs. Virginia Cooperative Extension Publication 491-010, Blacksburg, VA. 1987.

[108]   Government of South Australia. South Australian Integrated Mosquito Management Strategy. Prepared the Environmental Health Service. Department of Health, Adelaide, Australia: 61p. 2007.

[109]   WHO, 2006. Alpha-Cypermethrin. World Health Organization, Geneva, 50p.

[110]   WHO, 2008. Bendiocarb. World Health Organization, Geneva, 33p.

[111]   WHO, 2012. Bifenthrin. World Health Organzitaion, Geneva, 45p.

[112]   USAID, 2007. Integrated Vector Management Programs for Malaria Control - Programmatic Environmental Assessment. Prepared for Bureau for Global Health by RTI International, Research Triangle Park, NC. January, 527p.

[113]   WHO, 2004. Cyfluthrin. World Health Organization, Geneva, 29p.

[114]   WHO, 1989. Environmental Health Criteria 83, DDT and its derivatives – Environmental aspects.

[115] WHO, 1990. Environmental Health Criteria 97, Deltamethrin.

[116] Yaméogo L., Traoré K., Back C., Hougard J.-M., Calamari D., 2001. Risk assessment of etofenprox (vectron®) on non-target aquatic fauna compared with other pesticides used as *Simulium* larvicide in a tropical environment. Chemosphere 42: 965-974.

[117] WHO, 1992. Environmental Health Criteria 133, Fenitrothion.

[118] WHO, 1990. Environmental Health Criteria 99, Cyhalothrin.

[119] WHO, 1986. Environmental Health Criteria 63, Organophosphorus insecticides: a general introduction.

[120] Milam C.D., Farris J. L., Wilhide J. D, 2000. Evaluating mosquito control pesticides for effect on target and non-target organisms. Archives of Environmental Contamination and Toxicology, 39: 324-328.

[121] WHO, 1983. Data sheets on pesticides n°49. Pirimiphos-methyl.

[122] WHO, 1976. Data sheets on pesticides n°25. Propoxur.

[123] Najera J, Zaim M. Malaria vector control decision making criteria and procedures for judicious use of insecticides. World Health Organization, Communicable Disease Control, Prevention and Eradication, WHO Pesticide Evaluation Scheme (WHOPES). WHO/CDS/WHOPES/2002.5. Geneva: 116p. 2003.

[124] Blom A. The effect of mosquito spraying on non-target terrestrial insects. Bachelor degree report. Faculty of the Worcester Polytechnic Institute, 33p. 2011.

[125] Davis R, Peterson R. Effects of single and multiple applications of mosquito insecticides on nontarget arthropods. Journal of the American Mosquito Control Association 2008; 24: 270-280.

[126] Boisvert, J., Lacoursière J.O., 2004. *Bacillus thuringiensis* et le contrôle des insectes piqueurs au Québec. Ministère de l'Environnement Québécois, Québec.

[127] Nasreen, A., Ashfaq, M., Mustafa, G., 2000. Intrinsic toxicity of some insecticides to egg parasitoid *Trichogramma chilonis* (Hym. Trichogrammatidae). Bulletin of the Institute of Tropical Agriculture, Kyushu University 23. 41–44.

[128] WHO, 2007. Spinosad. World Health Organization, Geneva, pp. 32.

[129] Duchet, C., Caquet, Th., Franquet, E., Lagneau, C., Lagadic, L., 2010. Influence of environmental factors on the response of a natural population of *Daphnia magna* (Crustacea: Cladocera) to spinosad and *Bacillus thuringiensis israelensis* in Mediterranean coastal wetlands. Environmental Pollution 158: 1825–1833.

[130] WHO, 1975. Data sheets on pesticides n°18. Chlorpyriphos.

[131] WHO, 1976. Data sheets on pesticides n°23. Fenthion.

[132] Thompson C. Q., Tucker J. W. Jr. 1989. Toxicity of the organophosphate insecticide fenthion, alone and with thermal fog carriers, to an estuarine copepod and young fish. Bulletin of Environmental Contamination and Toxicology 43 (5): 789-796.

[133] WHO, 1983. Data sheets on pesticides n°49. Pirimiphos-methyl.

[134] USAID, 2007. Integrated Vector Management Programs for Malaria Control - Programmatic Environmental Assessment. Prepared for Bureau for Global Health by RTI International, Research Triangle Park, NC. January, 527p.

[135] Gaines T. B., Kimbrough R., Laws ER. Jr. 1967. Toxicology of Abate in laboratory animals. Archives of Environmental Health 14: 283-288.

[136] Sinègre G., Babinot M., Vigo G., Tourenq J. N., 1990. Sensibilité de trois espèces de *Chironomus* (Diptera) à huit insecticides utilisés en démoustication. Annales de Limnologie 26: 65-71.

[137] Tomlin C.D.S. (éd.), 1997. The Pesticide Manual, 11th edition. British Crop Protection Council, Farnham, UK.

[138] Lahr J., Diallo A.O. Gadji B., Diouf P.S., Mosquitoaux J.J.M., Badji A., Ndour K.B., Andreasen J.E., van Straalen, N.M. 2000. Ecological effects of experimental insecticide applications on invertebrates in Sahelian temporary ponds. Environmental Toxicology and Chemistry 19: 1278-1289.

[139] WHO, 1996. Diflubenzuron, WHO, Geneva, 164pp.

[140] Agence de la Santé publique du Canada, 2005. Déclaration relative aux mesures de protection individuelle pour prévenir les piqûres ou morsures d'arthropodes. Relevé des maladies transmissibles au Canada, vol. XXXI, DCC-13.

[141] De Wael L., De Greef M., Van Laere O., 1995. Toxicity of pyriproxyfen and fenoxycarb to bumble bee brood using a new method for testing insect growth regulators. Journal of Agricultural Research 34: 3-8].

[142] Guillet P, Alnwick D, Cham M, Neira M, Zaim M, Heymann D, Mukelabai K. Long-lasting treated mosquito nets: a breakthrough in malaria prevention. Bulletin of the World Health Organization 2001; 79: 998.

[143] Minakawa N, Dida G, Sonye G, Futami K, Kaneko S. Unforeseen misuses of bed nets in fishing villages along Lake Victoria. Malaria Journal 2008; 7: 165-171.

[144] Sharma S, Upadhyay A, Haque M, Padhan K, Tyagi P, Ansari M, Dash A. Wash resistance and bioefficacy of Olyset net – a Long-Lasting Insecticide-Treated mosquito Net against malaria vectors and non-target household pests. Journal of Medical Entomology 2006; 43: 884-888.

[145] Dobrokotov B. Alternatives to chemical methods for vector control. Annales de la Société Belge de Médecine Tropicale 1991; 71: 27-33.

[146] Shumway C. Forgotten Waters: Freshwater and Marine Ecosystems in Africa—Strategies for Biodiversity Conservation and Sustainable Development. Biodiversity Support Program. Washington, D.C.: 167p. 1999.

[147] USAID. Integrated Vector Management Programs for Malaria Control - Programmatic Environmental Assessment. Prepared for Bureau for Global Health by RTI International, Research Triangle Park, NC. January: 527p. 2007.

[148] Calow P, Sibly R, Forbes V. Risk assessment on the basis of simplified life-history scenarios. Environmental Toxicology and Chemistry 1997; 16: 1983-1989.

[149] Caquet T, Roucaute M, LeGoff P, Lagadic L. Effects of repeated field applications of two formulations of *Bacillus thuringiensis* var. *israelensis* on non-target saltmarsh invertebrates in Atlantic coastal wetlands. Ecotoxicolog and Environmental Safety 2011; 74: 1122-1130.

[150] Poulin B, Lefebvre G, Paz L. Red flag for green spray: adverse trophic effects of Bt. on breeding birds. Journal of Applied Ecology 2010; 47: 884-889.

[151] Lundström J, Schäfer M, Petersson E, Persson Vinnersten T, Landin J, Brodinet Y. Production of wetland Chironomidae (Diptera) and the effects of using *Bacillus thuringiensis israelensis* for mosquito control. Bulletin of Entomological Research 2009; 100: 117-125.

[152] Lundström J, Brodin Y, Schäfer M, Persson Vinnersten T, Östman Ö. High species richness of Chironomidae (Diptera) in temporary flooded wetlands associated with high species turn-over rates. Bulletin of Entomological Research 2009; 100: 433-444.

[153] Lagadic L, Caquet T, Fourcy D, Heydorff M. Evaluation à long terme des effets de la démoustication dans le Morbihan: suivi de l'impact écotoxicologique des traitements sur les invertébrés aquatiques entre 1998 et 2001. Rapport Scientifique de fin de programme (Avril 2002) ; Convention de Recherche Conseil Général du Morbihan: 215p. 2002.

[154] Le Goff P, Roucaute M, Lagadic L, Caquet T. Évaluation à long terme des effets de la démoustication dans le Morbihan: suivi de l'impact écotoxicologique d'une nouvelle formulation de larvicide sur les invertébrés aquatiques : étude comparative entre Vectobac® WG et Vectobac® 12AS. Rapport de fin d'étude, Conseil Général du Morbihan, Mars 2009: 26p. 2009.

[155] EID Méditerranée. Contrôle des moustiques nuisant dans les espaces naturels méditerranéens. Proposition méthodologique pour la gestion d'un site "Ramsar" en Languedoc-Roussillon. Programme Life-Environnement n°LIFE99 ENV/F/000489. Actes du Colloque de Restitution du programme Life Environnement, Montpellier, 27 mars 2003. Rapport consultable sur le site: http://www.eid-med.org: 75 p. 2003.

[156] Lagadic L. Évaluation du risque environnemental des traitements de démoustication : harmonisation des méthodes applicables aux invertébrés non-cibles dans les

zones humides littorales méditerranéennes et atlantiques. Rapport Final, Programme PNETOX, Ministère de l'Écologie et du Développement Durable: 41 pp. 2007.

[157] Bruce-Chwatt LJ. History of malaria from prehistory to eradication. In Wernsdorfer W.H. & McGregor I., Malaria. Principles and Practice of Malariology. Churchill Livingstone, Edinburgh London Melbourne & New York. 1988.

[158] Gorgas MD, Hendrick BJ. William Crawford Gorgas: his life and work. Lea & Febiger, Philadelphia. 1924.

[159] Watson M. The Prevention of Malaria in the Federated Malay States. Murray, London. 1921.

[160] Hackett LW, Russell PF, Scharff JW, Senior White R. The present use of naturalistic measures in the control of malaria. Quaterly Bulletin of the Health Organisation of the League of Nations1938; 7: 1016-1064.

[161] Rockfeller Foundation (International Health Board). The use of fish for mosquito control. The Rockfeller Foundation New York 1924.

[162] Celli A. Storia della malaria nell'agro romano. Academia dei Lincei, Roma. 1925.

[163] Ilvento A. The reclamation of the Pontine marshes. Quaterly Bulletin of the League of Nations Health Organization. 1934; 3: 157-201.

[164] Hackett LW. Malaria in Europe. Oxford University Press, London. 1937.

[165] Sergent Ed, Vingt cinq années d'étude et de prophylaxie du paludisme en Algérie. Archives de l'Institut Pasteur d'Algérie 1928; 6: 117-434.

[166] Dedet JP. The Sergent brothers and antimalaria campaigns in Algeria (1902-1948). Parassitologia, 50 (3-4): 221-225.

[167] Blumberg L, Frean J..- Malaria Control in South Africa- challenges and successes. South African Medical Journal 2007; 91: 1193-1197.

[168] Holmstedt B, Liljestrand G. Readings in pharmacology. Pergamon Press, Oxford. 1963.

[169] Russell PF. Malaria and its influence on world health. Bulletin of the New York Academy of Medicine 1943; 1: 559-630.

[170] Müller P. Uber Zusallenhänge zwischen Konstitution und insecticide Wirkung. Helvetia Chemica Acta 1946; 29: 1560-1580.

[171] Pampana EJ. A textbook of malaria eradication. Oxford University Press, London. 1963.

[172] Pampana EJ, Russell PF. Malaria-a world problem. World Health Organization Chronicle 1955; 9: 31-96.

[173] Bruce-Chwatt LJ. Malaria and its control: present situation and future prospects. Annual Review of Public Health 1987; 8: 75-110.

Chapter 8

Perspectives on Barriers to Control of *Anopheles* Mosquitoes and Malaria

Donald R. Roberts, Richard Tren and Kimberly Hess

Additional information is available at the end of the chapter

1. Introduction

Though mankind has struggled against malaria for countless generations, it remains a major global health problem. The malaria parasite and the *Anopheles* mosquito have evolved and developed with mankind since earliest recorded history, but there is nothing inevitable about the disease. Although thousands of children die from malaria every year, the disease is preventable and entirely curable, and the history of malaria control in the 20th century demonstrates that with the right tools and funding, malaria can be controlled, or even eradicated. The key, of course, is the cost-effective use of the right tools.

2. Statement of the problem

This chapter will examine arguably the most important tool for malaria control – public health insecticides (PHIs). Insecticide opponents often mischaracterize the public health use of insecticides, to include how they are used and consequences of their use in public health programs. Common inferences are that public health use of insecticides results in broad-scale environmental contamination and harm to wildlife. It is important for the reader to understand that there are internationally accepted guidelines for public health use of insecticides and that public health use is very different from how insecticides are used for agriculture. Optimum public health use of PHIs is to spray small quantities on inside walls of houses. In the case of DDT, it is approved only for use in public health programs. Applying it to inside walls leverages DDT's powerful repellent actions, giving continual protection from malaria-infected mosquitoes, for months on end, to those living inside the sprayed house. It should be obvious that a small amount of an insecticide on house walls is a far cry from spraying insecticides on vast acreages of cropland, as one might envisage for insecticides used in agriculture. Thus we emphasize that the subject of this chapter is public health use of insecticides, with no conno-tations whatsoever for the use of insecticides in agriculture.

We will summarize, with specific examples, the way that modern PHIs, and DDT in particular, have saved millions of lives since the 1940s. Despite this remarkable achievement, popular campaigns by activists, some scientists and even United Nations (UN) agencies, have stigma-tized and often demonized PHIs. Instead of regarding insecticides in the same light as medicines and diagnostics, essential elements of a malaria control program, insecticide opponents have mounted vocal campaigns to halt their use. Frequently these campaigns avoid or ignore the scientific process and rely on the flimsiest of evidence to make great claims about human health or ecological effects of PHIs. We will characterize examples of studies and claims against PHIs used by the activist communities and we will describe the major failings of each as they relate to the use of PHIs.

The claims by those who oppose PHIs, as we will explain and demonstrate with specific examples, do not comply with even the most basic epidemiologic criteria to prove a cause and effect relationship – yet those claims drive public opinion and policy. We will also document how UN bureaucrats have made outrageous claims that malaria can be controlled without PHIs. At the same time, the UN has set grand goals of achieving near-zero deaths from malaria by 2015. There is a valid debate to be had about whether or not this goal can be met, or even properly defined and measured; however, what is clear, is that progress against malaria cannot be achieved and sustained without access to PHIs. For access to be secured, the malaria community, including program managers, researchers, advocates and others, must defend PHIs rigorously and emphatically. The overarching goal of this chapter is to help with that defense. Without it, the lives of men, women and children living at risk of malaria will be greatly imperiled. However, for proper defense of PHIs, there must be a clear understanding about how insecticide opponents have succeeded in past anti-insecticide campaigns, and that influential groups and UN organizations actively oppose the use of PHIs. As anti-insecticide campaigners employ distinct strategies and tactics, it is important to know what they are and how they are used.

3. Malaria control today versus the early years of PHI use

Today there is great enthusiasm and substantial funding to advance global efforts to control and, in some regions, eradicate malaria. Indeed, and as suggested by recent outcomes of control programs, we are beginning to see promising results [1,2]. The necessary change for refocusing efforts to control malaria started in 1998, when, faced with mounting evidence that the global burden of malaria was increasing, and had been for some time, the World Health Organization (WHO) formed a new malaria control partnership, Roll Back Malaria (RBM). The RBM Partnership is made up of WHO and several UN agencies, such as UNICEF and UNDP, and development agencies, such as the World Bank and the US Agency for International Devel-opment (USAID), along with the private sector and NGOs. RBM's stated goal in 1998 was to halve the burden of malaria by 2010 [3].

RBM began with limited funding and an apparent disdain for scientific evidence. The early efforts were disappointing. Far from achieving any reduction in malaria cases, by 2004 there was evidence that malaria cases were in fact increasing. RBM was described in a stinging editorial in the *British Medical Journal* as a 'failing public health campaign [4].' One of the main reasons for this was the Partnership's dogged support for the use of insecticide treated bednets (ITNs) over other vector control interventions, e.g., indoor residual spraying (IRS) with insecticides such as DDT. The limited and controlled spraying of insecticides inside houses has long been known to rapidly reduce malaria cases and deaths, yet in the early years of the RBM Partnership was roundly ignored. In addition RBM's Partners failed to support any change in treatment policy away from failing drug therapies to the new artemisinin-based combination therapies (ACTs).

It was not until 2006 that progress against malaria finally started to be made. To its credit RBM acknowledged some of the problems it faced and set about restructuring and reforming. Much of impetus for these reforms came from a newly appointed head of the WHO's Global Malaria Program, Dr. Arata Kochi. Dr. Kochi had little history in malaria control and perhaps because of this had no need to defend any misguided previous policy decisions. One of Kochi's first acts was to re-issue WHO's treatment guidelines, recommending ACTs.

Shortly thereafter Kochi re-addressed WHO's policy on both DDT and IRS, and in a public and, for WHO, aggressive gesture issued a statement strongly endorsing the use of DDT. At the same time the US global malaria control program run by USAID underwent a major reform, creating the President's Malaria Initiative (PMI). A distinguishing feature of the PMI, which sets it apart from other major bi-lateral donor funded malaria control programs, is its support for IRS and its willingness to pay for use of DDT [5].

Together these reforms marked a change in global malaria control and as a result, malaria cases began to decline. As described below, malaria funding increased by more than 20 fold in a decade and malaria deaths, according to WHO modeling data, have fallen.

Malaria funding for the PMI and the Global Fund to Fight AIDS, TB and Malaria (Global Fund) through 2011 is estimated at $1,858,370,500 for the PMI [6], and $6,156,000,000 in malaria grants through 2011 for the Global Fund (based on $22.8b value of grant portfolio as of December 31, 2011, of which 27% is for malaria) [7].

International funding for malaria control has gone from less than $100 million in 2000 to $2 billion in 2011 [8]. Likewise, the estimated changes in global malaria burden since 2000 are compliant with improved funding of control efforts after 2005. For example, estimated numbers of malaria cases and malaria deaths in 2000 were 223 million and 755,000 respectively. In 2005 the values were 237 million cases and 801,000 deaths, whereas in 2011, the values were 216 million cases and 655,000 deaths [8].

Clearly progress is being made in the renewed focus on malaria. The positive changes with regard to funding IRS and DDT's place in malaria control are obviously welcomed. However these advances can be reversed at any time and as we explain in this chapter, the forces opposing the careful and effective use of PHIs are well-funded, organized, and aggressive. The malaria control community should remember, and learn from history, that we have been at this stage before. We can get a sense of this by looking back to what was happening in 1959. At this time DDT was used widely in agriculture and for pest management around the world. Aerial spraying of DDT was common as farmers sought to protect their crops, but in malaria control DDT use was entirely different. Most malaria vectors enter houses in search of blood meals, and so protecting people while they are at home, often asleep, is crucial. Soon after the Allied forces first used DDT during World War II, scientists discovered that DDT acts primarily as a spatial repellent. In other words, if the interior of a house is sprayed with DDT, mosquitoes are driven away and are unlikely to enter. DDT will also act as a contact irritant, so if a mosquito lands on a sprayed surface, it is likely to exit the house rapidly, often before feeding. Of course DDT will also act as a toxicant, killing the mosquito. However it is a relatively weak toxicant and its spatial repellency is the insecticide's most important mode of action by far. Widespread area spraying of DDT would have been pointless for malaria control.

In 1959 malaria was in rapid retreat in many endemic countries as a consequence of effective DDT use. The global malaria eradication program was just barely underway. By that time, the malaria control community had already used DDT to free 300 million people from the burdens of endemic disease. By the program's end in 1969, the lives of almost one billion people would be equally improved. In 1959 there was a wealth of malaria control expertise, substantial funding, and programmatic emphasis on malaria prevention; there were powerful and successful national programs, goal-oriented malaria control policies, and great enthusiasm for the goals of the global program. We suggest that few, if any workers of that time could, in their wildest imaginings, have predicted what was to come. In just 20 years from that auspicious beginning most highly effective national control programs would begin grinding to a halt. Their malaria control expertise would be frittered away, their funding would be gone, the price of DDT would be up and its availability down, and the international policies for malaria control would be changed from disease prevention to case detection and treatment. The declining population of malaria control workers would begin seeing the disease they had worked so hard to control expanding back into malaria-free areas. Malaria would once again be inflicting ever-greater harm on the people they had tried to help. We should pause and consider how that happened, how our community failed to recognize the threat, and why it failed to respond.

The answers to these questions are perhaps more simple than one might think. During the 1960s, and into the 1970s, our community was committed, and had its nose to the grindstone, so to speak. From the initial use of DDT in the mid-1940s, our community had been in a position to observe any adverse effects from insecticides, if they were to occur. The community had close and continuous contact with the populations living in sprayed houses, and they saw no meaningful adverse effects. In brief, it had no evidence of any problems that appeared suddenly or gradually with the public health use of insecticides. Simultaneously the community saw great improvements in health when DDT was used to prevent the diseases it sought to eliminate. It was, perhaps, beyond the community's ability to think that anyone would work against a worthy and effective public health program; but the community was wrong. Additionally, the community had not focused on diverging malaria control interests of developed and developing countries. Divergences occurred because the developed countries had used DDT to eliminate malaria and no longer needed it. Meanwhile the developing countries still needed DDT to help with their disease control problems. Last but not least, the community had no prior experience with the ruthless and scientifically indefensible fear tactics that were being unleashed against its disease control programs.

Threats to the old malaria eradication effort evolved from two ideologies within the environmental movement. One was that there are too many people on planet earth and malaria elimination allowed excessive population growth of poor people in developing countries. The second theme was that man-made chemicals endangered wildlife and human health. In 1970, George Woodwell, a prominent and entrenched anti-insecticide campaigner, captured the two ideologies in a paper he published in *Science* magazine. He concluded that the answer to the problem of environmental pollution was "Fewer people, unpopular but increasing restrictions on technology (making it more and more expensive) [9]." His concluding comment captured the thinking of major stakeholders within the environmental movement at that time. Through the careful use of fear tactics, global campaigns grew up around each ideology. Eventually the ideologies became established at the highest levels of the UN and national governments of developed countries. Those campaigns eventually destroyed effective disease control programs. The campaigns against PHIs achieved success through misrepresentations of science, by dragging companies and public organizations into courts in order to grab headlines for their fear-invoking claims, by using smear tactics against those who spoke in defense of insecticides, and, lastly, through extremely well-funded anti-insecticide advocacy. Through it all, anti-insecticide campaigners were supported by a popular press that fed off the fear invoked by the movement's predictions of insecticides causing catastrophic harm to wildlife and human health.

Naysayers will claim this is an exaggeration and that the old disease eradication programs were eliminated for a slew of reasons not mentioned here. Indeed there were other factors; but the overwhelming factors, as documented in annual proceedings of the WHO's Executive Board, discussions of the World Health Assembly (WHA), internal documents of UNICEF, and other published and unpublished reports, were those delineated above. Those who choose to believe current programs are not at risk of a similar fate may venture the opinion that regardless of past events, circumstances are entirely different now. They might even conclude movements that brought down the old programs are no longer active. For certain, the people, the claims, and the organizations have changed; but the themes and the scare tactics are the same. Nevertheless we will concede one point. The circumstances facing disease control programs today are entirely different from those that confronted the old disease eradication programs. Chief among the differences are that the old programs were not confronted by:

• Global networks of well-funded anti-insecticide advocacy,

• A WHO that, aside from its support for DDT under Dr. Kochi's brief leadership of the Global Malaria Program, frequently prioritizes the agenda of environmentalist groups over public health interests,

• Educational systems seeded with anti-insecticide propaganda,

• A Conference of the Parties to the Stockholm Convention on persistent organic pollutants that has independent authority to select insecticides for global elimination,

- Large national and international bureaucracies for regulatory control of insecticides,

- A vast, and largely anti-insecticide, research establishment functioning in universities and research institutes around the world,

- Billions of dollars for regulatory control and research against insecticides,

- A declining arsenal of insecticides for malaria control, and

- Regulatory controls that are major impediments to the research and development of new PHIs.

4. Environmentalism over public health policies

With an annual caseload estimated at 216 million and 655,000 deaths, malaria continues as one of the most important insect-borne diseases [10]. Yet, it is just one of many insect-borne diseases that collectively claim millions of lives and stifle economic growth and development in disease endemic countries. PHIs and other public health chemicals are vital to the global struggle to control these diseases. Where PHIs are removed or their use restricted, disease rates increase. For example, two large eradication programs that were based almost entirely on public health use of DDT, freed Bolivia of malaria, dengue fever, and risk of urban yellow fever from the 1950s to the mid-1970s. The WHO acknowledges the importance of one program as follows: "Historically, mosquito control campaigns [that employed DDT] successfully eliminated *Aedes aegypti*, the urban yellow fever vector, from most mainland countries of central and South America. However, this mosquito species has re-colonized urban areas [with cessation of the *Aedes aegypti* eradication program] in the region and poses a renewed risk of urban yellow fever [11]." In spite of marvelous improvements in human health that were achieved by use of PHIs, international anti-insecticide pressures were brought to bear on those programs.

Bolivia abandoned *Aedes aegypti* eradication in the 1970s. This occurred because Bolivia, as with many countries of the Americas, ramped down eradication efforts once the US buckled to anti-DDT pressures in 1969 and ended use of DDT for *Aedes aegypti* eradication. Almost all countries of the Americas followed the US example in the 1970s. Years later Bolivia abandoned use of DDT for malaria control. As a consequence, malaria and threats of urban yellow fever are once again commonplace in Bolivia [12], and in 2009 Bolivia was savaged by a major dengue epidemic.

India is another case study. In the early 1950s, India had an estimated 75 million malaria infections, with roughly 800,000 deaths each year. Spraying DDT brought numbers of cases down to 49,151 by 1961. Today, the number of malaria cases each year is in doubt. What seems certain however is that the number of cases is huge and the number of deaths is on an order of hundreds of thousands. Estimates for cases vary from a few million to tens of millions of cases per year [13].

Despite the considerable human and economic toll caused by past increases in diseases like malaria and dengue, the current arsenal of PHIs for spraying on house walls is limited to just

12 compounds from four chemical classes, namely pyrethroids, organophosphates, carba-mates and organochlorines. Most PHIs are pyrethroids. DDT, the only organochlorine permitted for use, is one of the 12 approved compounds.

Even though production and use of DDT has declined continuously during the last four decades, DDT has grown as a convenient target of environmental science research. A recent PubMed search (in early 2011) for research papers on insecticides uncovered almost 60,000 papers, and about one sixth (9,459) were on DDT. These are remarkable statistics considering that DDT is hardly in use anymore. The decline in usage was sudden and corresponds to precipitous drops in human body burdens of DDT residues. Today, for example, the amount of DDT in human breast milk, based on serial surveys in many countries, is an infinitesimal fraction of what it was in the 1960s—and even those exceedingly low levels are declining [14]. Along with precipitous reductions in DDT use, one could reasonably expect that research on DDT would decline. However, as revealed in Figure 1, the numbers of published papers on DDT have actually increased, and more so in recent years than in the past. Furthermore, papers on DDT and malaria account for only a minor proportion (2.6 to 14.8% per year) of those published papers. So, why is the research effort on DDT increasing even as the use of DDT fades to inconsequential levels? To answer this question we will delve more into the modern themes of environmental research and anti-insecticide advocacy.

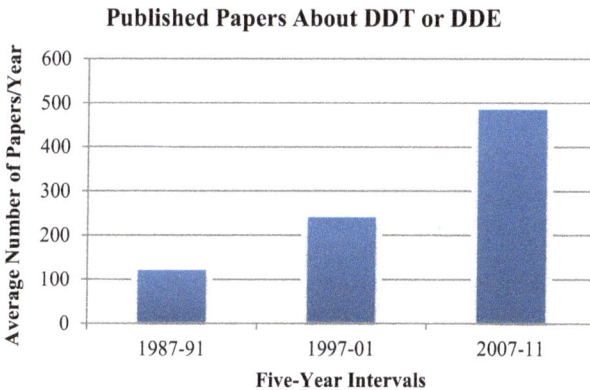

Figure 1. Average number of papers published per year on DDT or DDE. Data based on PubMed searches on key words--DDT and/or DDE. Counts summed for five-year intervals of 1987-1991, 1997-2001, and 2007-2011.

5. Why increased research on insecticides?

A 2005 paper by Dr. Stephen Safe, a Distinguished Professor and recipient of the Distinguished Lifetime Toxicology Scholar Award from the Society of Toxicology, explains much about the modern trend of increased funding and research on DDT [15]. Professor Safe is a professor at

Texas A&M and is a specialist in toxicology and molecular biology of estrogenic and anti-estrogenic compounds. To summarize introductory comments in his 2005 paper, modern emphasis on DDT is linked to a series of 1990 papers and the concept of the precautionary principle. The papers proposed that endocrine disrupting chemicals (EDCs), which include both man-made (synthetic) and naturally occurring chemicals, were contributing to diverse health problems worldwide. The diverse harms include decreased male sperm counts, increased birth defects, decreased fertility, increased incidence of breast and testicular cancers, etc. As Dr. Safe states, the role of synthetic EDCs as a cause of diverse health problems has been subjected to multiple challenges, to include a lack of biological plausibility for some responses and failure to consider that people are more heavily exposed to natural or dietary EDCs compared to relatively low exposures to the synthetic EDCs. Additionally, the natural compounds are often far more potent endocrine disruptors than synthetic EDCs.

The 1990s papers and the concept of the precautionary principle resulted in new funding and renewed interests in insecticides. As described by Dr. Safe, "Regulatory and research funding agencies have taken the endocrine disruptor hypothesis seriously [15]." Funds for research grew and, as a result, "... numerous laboratory animal and clinical studies have been initiated to test the validity of the hypothesis and to determine the association between health problems and exposure to EDCs [15]." This, in large part, seems to explain the huge growth in research and numbers of publications about potential harms from DDT and other insecticides. It is worth noting that extremely sensitive assays are available for DDT and other synthetic EDCs; but assays are often not available for more abundant and more diverse populations of natural EDCs. Thus it seems that the selection of DDT as a research topic is more closely related to availability and familiarity with quantitative assays opposed to some understanding of what the real threats are from synthetic versus natural EDCs.

In his 2005 paper Dr. Safe reviews many recent studies, and we refer the reader to his paper for more in-depth analyses. He comments on the synthetic EDCs as casual agents in breast cancer and male reproductive track anomalies. For the former, he reviews several studies, to include a meta-analysis, and concludes that the evidence does not support the hypothesis that DDE causes breast cancer. He concludes further that "If organochlorines do not significantly impact on this disease [breast cancer], it is now time to generate new hypotheses and focus on identifying other etiological factors that are linked to the high incidence of sporadic breast cancer in women [15]."

Dr. Safe reviewed numerous studies on DDT and other synthetic organochlorines (OCs) reportedly causing diseases of the male reproductive tract. The claim that sperm counts are declining is central to the thesis of many alarmists who propose that synthetic OCs are causing declining male sexual function. Dr. Safe reviews past reports and concludes, "results from various clinics are not sufficient to support a global decrease or increase [15]" in sperm counts. He also concludes "the hypothesized role of *in utero* exposure to estrogens as a factor in regulating sperm count in adult males is also questionable [15]." Dr. Safe goes on to review studies on possible associations between levels of synthetic EDCs with urogenital birth defects and increasing trends of testicular cancer. For the former, he found that both the evidence of increasing rate of birth defects and the hypothetical associations between those rates and exposures to synthetic EDCs were not persuasive. Additionally, evidence of multiple studies did not support the hypothesis that synthetic EDCs were a cause of testicular cancer.

In this brief section we have described the major themes of research that will be the source of future claims against PHIs. Dr. Safe sounded a warning in his comments about EDCs and breast cancer. He pointed out that our abilities to detect EDCs and a wealth of other variables (for example, biomarkers, genotypes, and a wealth of other biological, biochemical, environmental, and sociological variables) "increases the probability of 'chance' correlations, and there are several examples of these associations that are not consistent across all studies [15]." So, it seems clear that we should expect a greater frequency of claims against PHIs in the future. That said, anti-insecticide advocacy more so than research poses the greatest threat to the future of effective disease control programs. As we observed in the negotiations for the Stockholm Convention on Persistent Organic Pollutants (POPs) described below, well-funded anti-insecticide advocacy is the operational arm of the environmental movement. But unlike the careful deliberations of most environmental scientists, anti-insecticide groups are not constrained by subtle considerations of consistent and meaningful evidence and other criteria for cause-effect relationships, or by considerations of harm versus benefits of insecticide use.

6. Renewed malaria control programs beset by opposition to PHIs

As stated in an earlier section, today there is great enthusiasm and considerable funding to advance the goals of global control of malaria. We arrive at this period of enthusiasm only because we lived through many years of almost no hope at all.

The steady increase in malaria cases that led to RBM's formation had several underlying causes. Among them was the spread of drug resistance around the world. Since the 1940s chloroquine had been a mainstay of malaria treatment programs, but resistance by the *Plasmodium falciparum* parasite to the drug first appeared in the 1950s and slowly spread worldwide. Chloroquine was duly replaced by sulphadoxine-pyrimethamine (SP) in the 1980s, but resistance soon emerged to this drug as well.

Another cause of the growing burden of malaria was the lack of interest in malaria control by major donor agencies and malarial country governments. Enthusiasm for malaria dissipated when the great push against malaria - the global malaria eradication campaign of the 1950s and 60s – was called off. Malaria control is expensive, requiring the employment of trained personnel, logistics specialists, scientists and large quantities of drugs and vector control products. Continuing to pay for malaria control year in and year out when it was clear that global eradication was not feasible was a tough sell. Concurrently the focus for many development agencies was away from disease control and towards population control, as we touch on in this chapter and explain in more detail in *The Excellent Powder, DDT's Political and Scientific History* [16]. Few newly independent and highly malarial African countries sustained malaria control programs that had been run by colonial rulers. In Zambia, for instance, malaria control programs that had been set up when the country was ruled by Great Britain as Northern Rhodesia collapsed along with the Zambian economy in the 1980s.

However, as illustrated in the examples of disease control history in Bolivia and India, arguably one of the greatest obstacles to sustained malaria control was the growing campaign against PHIs, and DDT in particular. DDT had been used in malaria control since World War II. The effectiveness of this insecticide in controlling malaria was unprecedented. As we explain above, DDT, when sprayed on the inside walls of houses, acts to repel mosquitoes, but it will also irritate mosquitoes so they exit houses sooner than they otherwise would and will kill mosquitoes that rest on a sprayed surface long enough.

Through these multiple modes of action, and thanks to the dedicated work of thousands of hard working malaria control program officers, DDT saved around one billion people from malaria during the eradication era. But what some people heralded as a great savior, others decried as a harbinger of doom. Chief among the anti-DDT crusaders was Rachel Carson whose 1962 book, *Silent Spring*, is a florid and grossly exaggerated attack on the chemical for its supposed impact on wildlife and human health [17]. There were, and are, no shortages of Carson acolytes who have joined in with their own attacks on DDT, as we explain later in this chapter.

Following the banning of DDT for most uses in the US and Western Europe in the 1970s, production fell dramatically. Although DDT was still permitted for use in disease control, supplies dwindled and predictably the cost began to rise. It mattered little that the WHO's malaria control advisers still supported the use of DDT, when the reality was that fewer countries could obtain it. In 1969, Scandinavian countries, Canada and the US started to place 'severe' restrictions on the use of DDT [18]. Thus, it was no coincidence that global malaria eradication and the United State's *Aedes aegypti* eradication programs were both stopped in 1969—just as it was no coincidence that both relied on use of DDT [16]. Unsurprisingly, within just a few years, malarial countries were complaining to the WHO of their inability to obtain the chemical and use it to save lives [19]. Along with the growing campaigns against DDT, donor agencies like USAID, under pressure of legal actions, began to withdraw funding for DDT and malaria control in the 1970s.

In the following section we will detail, with a specific example, how the bio-politics of environmental activism against DDT and other PHIs translated into real world harm to human health. For this example we have chosen a country that has a strong tradition in science and a long and proud history of combating malaria.

7. Public health insecticides and malaria

The value of PHIs in controlling malaria is best evidenced by historical data on DDT sprayed houses. Brazil, as with other countries with territory within the Amazon Basin, struggles with difficult malaria control issues. The Amazon Basin is the most enduring environment in the Americas for the persistence of endemic malaria. Populated with many rural, poorly housed and mobile inhabitants, the Amazon Basin covers a vast geographical area of warm, humid environments. More importantly, it is populated with the Hemisphere's most dangerous vector of human malaria, *Anopheles darlingi*. In the absence of this species or in regions of the

Americas where it is less common, the chain of malaria transmission is weaker and more easily interrupted. For this reason, malaria often declines to low levels in the face of organized control programs in regions outside the Amazon Basin. In contrast, within the Amazon Basin, malaria exhibited some refractoriness to control measures even during years of the global malaria eradication program. As a consequence, eradication was not achieved. Nevertheless the spraying of DDT on house walls greatly reduced malaria infections and lifted a large part of the burden of malaria from the backs of people in the Amazon Basin.

Successful malaria control by spraying DDT was maintained for many years. Yet, the succession of bio-political events described in the previous section and elsewhere eventually destroyed Brazil's well-orchestrated malaria control program. Malaria cases began to increase when the numbers of houses being sprayed were progressively reduced in the 1980s. The many years of successful control followed by years when the spray program withered away are detailed in Figure 2.

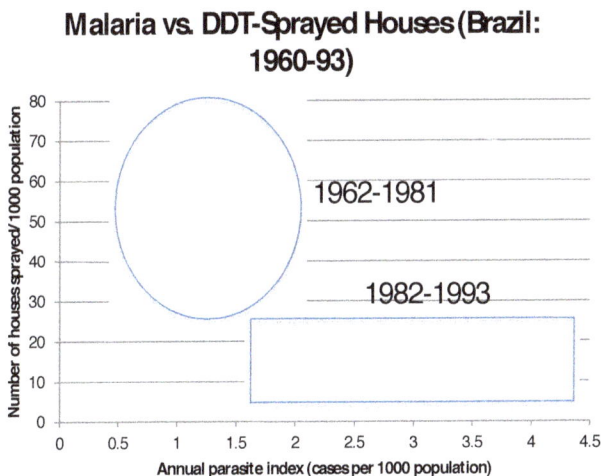

Figure 2. Number of houses sprayed per 1000 population versus the annual parasite index (cases per 1000 population) in Brazil during the years 1962 to 1993. Data for these years were collected under uniform data collection methods (see Roberts et al. 1997. for data sources [34]).

The graph presents annual parasite indices (APIs) and house spray rates (HSRs) from 1962 to 1993. Two clusters of data points are identified. One group represents the years from 1962 to 1981 when house spray rates were high and malaria indices were low. The API is a standard malaria control index, calculated as the annual number of diagnosed malaria cases X 1000/ population size. The HSR represents the number of houses sprayed per 1000 population. As shown in this graph, APIs in years after 1981 increased in response to reductions in numbers of houses being sprayed.

To bring Brazil's story up to date, Figure 3 presents statistics on malaria cases through 2010. As described in the previous section, there has been a global renewal in efforts to control malaria. Thus, in recent years, Brazil expanded its malaria control efforts. But even with increased financial support and availability of new malaria control technologies (e.g., case treatment with the new and effective ACTs, insecticide treated nets and so-called long-lasting nets), the accomplishments of recent years are less than what is needed and certainly far less than what was achieved and sustained during 20 years of spraying houses with DDT. As demonstrated in Figure 3, there was an average of 100,000 cases per year during those 20 years of major reliance on DDT. As DDT use declined in the 1980s, the average number of cases/year increased to 450,000. In the next decade, DDT use was abandoned completely and cases increased to over 500,000 per year. Today, even with an expanded program of control, the average number of cases per year is well over 400,000. The differences in results of the last 30 years over what was achieved with DDT roughly sums to 10.5 million cases that might have been prevented if DDT had not been abandoned. While population growth as an independent variable might account for some growth in numbers of cases, the increased number of cases corresponds, over time, to changes in slide positivity rates. The slide positivity rate is neutral in terms of population size. As a reminder, the estimate of 10.5 million excess malaria cases is for Brazil alone.

Numbers of Malaria Cases In Brazil

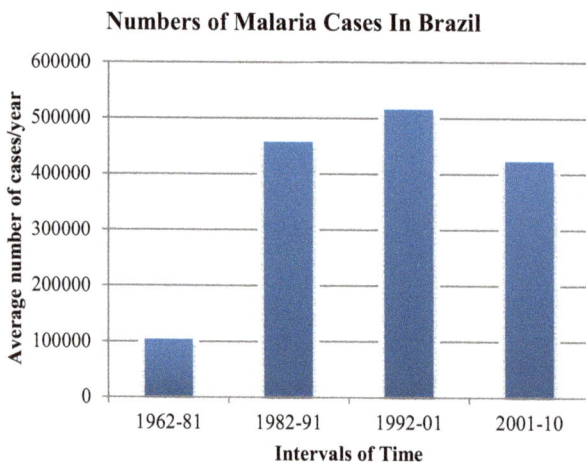

Figure 3. Average number of cases per year in Brazil across defined blocks of years (x-axis). Data for these years were collected under uniform data collection methods (see Roberts et al. 1997 for data sources [34] and PAHO malaria data [57]).

Clearly the great reductions of malaria from 1962 to 1981 compared to later blocks of years reveals the enormous benefit of DDT and other insecticides.

One of the most compelling examples of the usefulness of DDT in malaria control comes from recent experience in South Africa. This country had successfully used DDT in malaria control since the late 1940s and in so doing had dramatically reduced the malarial areas to the regions bordering Mozambique to the east and Zimbabwe to the north. In 1996 South Africa's Malaria Advisory Group (MAG) advised the national malaria control program to begin phasing out DDT. This advice was based on two main factors. First, DDT is best applied to the mud and dung walls of traditional African houses rather than on the plastered and painted walls of western style houses where the DDT can stain the walls. Given the staining, homeowners were often reluctant to allow the spray teams to enter their houses. As the rural areas of South Africa have developed and become wealthier, more and more people have built western style houses, requiring alternative insecticides. Second, the MAG had taken note of the political pressure against the use of DDT and anticipating greater restrictions on the use of DDT, decided to transition over to other chemicals. In the late 1990s therefore the provincial malaria programs began replacing DDT with pyrethroids. The first province to do so was KwaZulu Natal, which borders Mozambique and at the time was the most malarial of the countries three malarial provinces [16].

Almost as soon as the KwaZulu Natal malaria control program changed over to pyrethroids, malaria cases started to rise. By 2000, malaria cases had increased five fold from just over 8,500 cases to almost 42,000 cases. Malaria deaths increased from just 22 in 1996 to 320 in 2000 as malaria patients overwhelmed clinics and hospitals [20].

Research showed that a major driver of the epidemic was resistance to pyrethroid insecticides. In addition, evidence was rising that malaria parasite resistance had grown to SP, or Fansidar. The Department of Health took the decision to reintroduce DDT and change treatment regimen from Fansidar to the newly-available ACT, artemether-lumefantrine, or Coartem. Within a year malaria cases plummeted by around 80 percent [21]. The combination of a proven and effective PHI along with effective treatment reduced malaria transmission so dramatically that within just a few years, malaria elimination was within sight.

Given the benefit and usefulness of DDT and other PHIs in the control of malaria, as described above, how is it possible that PHIs have been so effectively demonized? In the next section we will describe strategies and tactics that have been employed to paralyze malaria control programs in countries around the world. As an aside, it is worth noting that those who ruthlessly campaign against DDT and other PHIs shamelessly deny any responsibility whatsoever for the increasing burdens of disease that inevitably occur when their campaigns succeed.

8. Goals, strategies, and tactics of anti-insecticide campaigns

The goal for environmental campaigns is to reduce or eliminate use of PHIs for the presumed but ambiguous purpose of better environmental health. Another goal, at least for some, appears to be stopping the use of chemicals that protect health and save lives in order to slow growth of human populations.

In the 1960s, the goal of halting or reducing the use of man-made insecticides was laid out in Rachel Carson's unscientific writings in *Silent Spring*. In 1968, the Malthusian rantings of Paul

Ehrlich in *The Population Bomb* focused attention on the contributions of DDT to growth of human populations in malaria-endemic countries. The goal of reducing human populations was never silenced; and it is once again a topic of heated debate, with some claiming billions of people must be eliminated [22].

The goal of today's anti-insecticide activists is still to reduce or eliminate synthetic insecticides. Achieving such a goal requires strategies and tactics. There are three visible strategies for achieving the goal of reducing or eliminating PHIs. The first is to convince people that PHIs are harmful. The second is to claim the chemicals are not needed in order to control diseases. The third strategy is to predict that grave harm will occur if the PHIs continue to be used. In this section we will give background information and three examples of the first strategy. In most cases we will focus on issues of DDT, but the same strategies and tactics are employed against other PHIs.

In a historical context, anti-insecticide advocates used propaganda and emotional arguments to convince people insecticides were dangerous and their use should be stopped. They were helped by science writers of the popular press and their efforts led to public health programs being abandoned around the world – and a resurgence of malaria infections. We have already presented one example of such an outcome (see Figures 2 and 3).

Anti-insecticide activism is an even stronger force today, and anti-insecticide advocates are even more determined to deny developing countries the protections from disease and death that only insecticides can provide. Because of environmental and anti-insecticide advocacy, the WHA adopted a resolution (WHA 50.13) in May 1997 that calls on countries to reduce reliance on use of insecticides for disease control [23]. Then, in 1998, the United Nations Environment Programme (UNEP) began negotiations for a POPs treaty targeting DDT and 11 other chemicals for global elimination [24]. The beginning of those negotiations stimulated malaria scientists and other public health professionals to mount a global campaign to defend the use of DDT in disease control programs. The public health campaign was successful and DDT was listed on Annex B of the Stockholm Convention on Persistent Organic Pollutants, which allowed its continued use. Yet, and despite the public health campaign's success, anti-DDT and anti-insecticide advocacy is unabated in UNEP, the US Environmental Protection Agency, the European Union, and, to lesser extent, in public agencies financing disease control programs. As a result, DDT factories closed their doors. Today, only one in India is still in operation. Also, environmental campaigners have erected formidable international barriers to the purchase and supply of DDT. Countries are under continual pressure from anti-DDT advocacy groups, and they are being enticed by financial mechanisms of Global Environment Facility (GEF) to stop using DDT.

WHA resolution 50.13 and the Stockholm Convention on Persistent Organic Pollutants, described above, are only the most recent in 50 years of efforts to eliminate DDT and other PHIs. Success in anti-PHI campaigns has been achieved by scaring people with false claims. Anti-DDT propaganda typically claims DDT causes all manner of harm to human health. Readily embraced and trumpeted by the popular press, the claims, in reality, never satisfy even the most minimal cause-effect criteria [25]. These internationally accepted criteria are:

- Strength of the association. The stronger an observed association appears over a series of different studies, the less likely this association is spurious because of bias.

- Dose-response effect. The value of the response variable changes in a meaningful way with the dose (or level) of the suspected causal agent.

- Lack of temporal ambiguity. The hypothesized cause precedes the occurrence of the effect.

- Consistency of the findings. Most, or all, studies concerned with a given causal hypothesis produce similar findings.

- Biological or theoretical plausibility. The hypothesized causal relationship is consistent with current biological or theoretical knowledge.

- Coherence of the evidence. The findings do not seriously conflict with accepted facts about the outcome variable being studied.

- Specificity of the association. The observed effect is associated with only the suspected cause (or few other causes that can be ruled out).

In the case of a true cause-effect relationship we can reasonably expect measurable levels of harm as a result of human exposures. Levels of harm will be proportional to harmfulness of the agent and to durations and characteristics of exposures. The more harmful an agent, the more likely it is to produce obvious levels of harm. Harm from weaker agents, on the other hand, will probably not be obvious and be definable only through population-based statistics. Regardless, ending use of a weak, but truly harmful, agent will reduce exposure to the chemical, reduce chemical concentration in the environment, and reduce the levels of harm. This is true even if the chemical is characterized as persistent, as is DDT. Persistence does not mean the chemical does not degrade. It just means that in certain compartments of the environment or living organisms it will degrade or be eliminated more slowly. Levels of DDT in the environment generally decline rapidly after its use is stopped. It is precisely because DDT does degrade that house walls are re-sprayed once or twice a year in order to achieve effective levels of malaria control.

Here, with the example of cigarette smoke and cancer, we illustrate application of cause-effect criteria. The link between smoking and human cancer has been validated through experimentation and vital statistics. In general, the argument that cigarette smoke caused cancer was convincing because patterns of low or high cancer rates consistently correlated with patterns of low or high smoking rates and duration of smoking. Furthermore, as people stopped smoking their risk of cancer actually declined. Consistent and persuasive evidence of cause-effect relationships between cigarette smoking and cancers formed the basis of public health campaigns to reduce or stop cigarette smoking. Unlike those public health campaigns, however, the environmental campaigns against PHIs are not based on persuasive and, certainly not, consistent, scientific evidence. The occasional observational study that suggests use of a public health insecticide harms health is countered by many other studies that suggest otherwise. Nevertheless, and as illustrated below, environmental campaigners readily ignore essential criteria for establishing a cause-effect relationship and greedily grab any new study that suggests some association between PHIs and human disease. The activist community has shown itself to be highly adept at getting such studies widespread national and international media coverage, often with headlines and messages designed to strike fear into people's hearts. These headlines are also very useful in advancing careers and ensuring ongoing research funding. We will describe three examples of how environmental advocates, and in some cases the environmental scientists themselves, ignore the criteria for establishing cause-effect relationships and use preliminary studies to push their anti-PHI agenda, or, more selfishly, their personal research agenda. The three examples are illustrations of the first strategy to convince people that DDT is a public health threat.

Example 1:

Mary Wolff and co-authors (1993) published a paper in which they claimed a statistical association of DDE (a major DDT metabolite) with breast cancer [26]. DDT opponents then used this paper to gain public attention and convince people that DDT caused breast cancer. To be specific, we are talking about anti-insecticide activists, not Dr. Wolff. Years later, with completion of many other studies, and without fanfare or wide publicity, researchers concluded DDE was not a cause of breast cancer. The WHO reassessment of DDT exposures from indoor spray programs states, "Overall, the association between DDT and breast cancer is inconclusive [27]." Regardless, for many years, anti-DDT activists heralded the 1993 paper as final proof of DDT harm and used it to generate funds and recruit new members to campaigns for DDT elimination [28].

Example 2:

Following a different thread of research, Rogan and coauthors reported that DDE was associated with reduced duration of lactation [29,30]. As with the reported association of DDT and breast cancer, this claim was grabbed by the WWF in 1998 and used in the propaganda campaign leading up to the Stockholm Convention on Persistent Organic Pollutants. The stated goal of the WWF campaign was a phase out of DDT by 2007 [28]. In their coverage of this topic, the WWF stated that studies "showed that the duration of lactation was inversely related to the concentration of DDE in milk." Separate from the WWF's use of these claims, the claims were, in part, also the basis for two high-profile publications by Rogan and coauthors in the journals, *Emerging Infectious Diseases* [31] and *The Lancet* [32]. They proposed that the benefits of spraying DDT on house walls to control malaria in Africa would be cancelled out by lowered child survival due to reduced durations of lactation and potential increases in premature births. The claims were used in campaigns against DDT and used to justify more research support.

Once published, the claims became tools for anti-DDT advocacy. For example, the claim is part of a 2005 Physicians for Social Responsibility (PSR) document about DDT and its use in Kenya. The PSR author states, "DDT may have a substantial impact on infant mortality, by increasing the risk of pre-term birth and by decreasing the duration of breast-feeding after birth. In this paper, Chen and Rogan conclude that DDT may cause comparable increase in infant mortality through these mechanisms compared to the decrease in infant mortality it causes by killing mosquitoes and thus reducing malaria cases [33]."

Without doubt the papers had great value for the anti-DDT advocacy community, yet the background studies for those claims did not fulfill the criteria for establishing DDT as the cause of reduced lactation or of pre-term births. In fact, even Chen and Rogan [31] stated the reported associations did not prove DDT caused any of the illnesses they discussed. Regardless, the claims were used as if they proved, beyond any doubt, that DDT was the cause of harm. This was illustrated in an exchange of letters to the Editor of the journal, *Emerging Infectious Diseases*. The exchange was between Roberts [34,35] and the WWF (written by Matteson) [36]. Matteson stated in her letter, "DDT also is associated with reduced lactation, premature births..." Naturally, Matteson used those reported associations to demonize DDT as part of WWF's push for global elimination of DDT by 2007. Misuse of those claims is further illustrated by an article defending Rachel Carson by the Rachel Carson Council. As with the PSR author, this writer used both claims plus the assertions included in the two papers by Rogan and coauthors about the benefits of DDT being canceled out by increased deaths of newborns in Africa. As stated in this very recent online article: "...significant shortening of the lactation cycle-time that human mothers can produce milk for their babies linked to DDT exposure. Based on reports for both premature births and reduced lactation cycles, scientists have predicted that regular DDT exposure could increase the possibility of higher levels of infant mortality for women in Africa who live in treated environments [37]."

There are many other examples of how these claims have been used and continue to be used in anti-insecticide propaganda. As stated in a 2006 article advocating against the use of DDT by the Pesticide Action Network in the UK, "Other studies have linked DDT to reduced breastmilk production, premature delivery and reduced infant birthweights [sic] [38]." Last but not least, Wikipedia includes the following statement:

Human epidemiological studies suggest that exposure is a risk factor for premature birth and low birth weight, and may harm a mother's ability to breast feed. Some 21st-century researchers argue that these effects may increase infant deaths, offsetting any anti-malarial benefits. A 2008 study, however, failed to confirm the association between exposure and difficulty breastfeeding [39].

Mention of the 2008 study is perhaps helpful; but it is not sufficient. Given that DDT produces great benefit in control of malaria, Wikipedia contributors should be careful in comments about DDT lest their written assessments inflict grave harm on poor people in malaria endemic countries. Point of fact, the Wikipedia assessment leaves the reader thinking that DDT causes premature births and reduced duration of lactation, when the weight of scientific evidence shows it does not.

Example 3:

Unfortunately, the false claims against DDT are unabated. One of the more recent and truly tragic examples of a false public image for PHIs occurred in 2009 when researchers in South Africa reported DDT was associated with urogenital birth defects in boys in a region where houses are sprayed with DDT to control malaria [40]. Although the authors, led by Prof. Riana Bornman of the University of Pretoria, suggest that DDT may not have caused the birth defects, the authors still state people should be informed about risks of birth defects if DDT is used.

Their interpretations and claims were aired broadly in the print and electronic media in South Africa. The public's concern over the researcher's claims created difficulties for the malaria control program. DDT, through decades of use in South Africa, had already proven its disease preventing capabilities. Given its proven record of performance, it is hardly reasonable to alarm people unless DDT is proven to be seriously harmful. In this case, the weaknesses of the researcher's claims had been addressed in the journal where the paper was published. Richard Grady addressed this issue in the editorial comment that accompanied the Bornman *et al.* paper [40]. Grady stated that issues of association and causality could not be distinguished in the paper. Grady was right; Bornman and coauthor's claims that DDT caused birth defects did not fulfill criteria for establishing a cause-effect relationship. As point of published fact, there were no statistically significant differences in the proportions of malformed genitalia among boys in sprayed and unsprayed villages. Given this fundamental failing, their pronouncements should not have been published and certainly should not have been used to scare the public away from having their houses sprayed. However, attempts in South Africa to scare people about DDT continue even now.

One of the researchers behind the urogenital birth defects claims recently reported on the levels of DDT in breast milk in sprayed villages in South Africa compared to results of an unsprayed village [41]. During the 70+ years of DDT use, many studies of DDT in breast milk have been performed. Based on those reports, it is expected that residents of DDT sprayed houses will have higher quantities of DDT in breast milk than residents of unsprayed villages. It is expected that intake by some infants will exceed the Provisional Tolerable Daily Intake (PTDI) and, in some cases, the residue levels will exceed the Maximum Residue Limit (MRL). In order to exaggerate the importance of their study, the authors emphasized the outlier measurements beyond confidence limits of mean values, e.g., in the abstract they report their statistics include "the highest ΣDDT level ever reported for breast milk from South Africa." Their control village was not sprayed and had no history of ever being sprayed. Yet the authors fail to mention that mean values of residues were at or above the MRL in the unsprayed village. They fail to mention that outlier data points in the control village, as with sprayed villages, exceeded the PTDI. They fail to mention that confidence limits for measurements from the control village overlap those of some sprayed villages. Authors emphasize gender differences in infants and associated levels of DDT in breast milk even though the differences were not statistically significant. They suggest the results require further research. Additionally, authors [41] report that mean levels of DDT had no impact on duration of lactation.

In press coverage of this paper the headlines read, "Researchers measure highest DDT levels in breast milk from South African nursing mothers [42]." In fact, outlier data points can result from erroneous dilutions, tests, conversions, or other parts of the experimental process, or just uncommon natural variation. For these reasons most researchers give outlier data points little weight. Yet the authors of this study used an outlier data point as a hook for grabbing headlines in the popular media. Media coverage went on to state, "In the region where the measurements were carried out, malformed genitalia among boys was significantly more common in areas treated with DDT compared with untreated areas." The assertion that DDT affects male urogenital development is mentioned in the paper, e.g., referring to the 2009 study they state,

"Research...identified DDT-associated effects on male urogenital parameters...[41]." However, the statement is misleading because, as described above, there were no statistically significant differences in the proportions of malformed genitalia among boys in sprayed and unsprayed villages.

Presented in three examples above is clear and unambiguous demonstration of orchestrated and non-scientific campaigns against PHIs, and DDT in particular. Claims that DDT causes one sort of harm or another are repeated in anti-insecticide propaganda even after published studies show the claims are false, or published rebuttals draw attention to errors in data analyses or research interpretations. A common part of these campaigns is how activists use the term "association" or "associated" as meaning there is a cause-effect relationship between an exposure and disease. In fact, these terms relate only to a statistical association that is often an artifact of study design or a product of systematic bias. Such issues as bias are of particular concern, and are discussed at length in David Savitz's book *Interpreting epidemiologic evidence* [43].

In the history of efforts to preserve use of DDT for public health programs, this chain of events has been repeated over and over, with claims of causation eventually being disproven, but not before they were used to generate funds, recruit new members to anti-insecticide campaigns, and change public health policies. Last but not least, each change in disease control policy has weakened global capacities to control malaria and other diseases. Almost every change is a result of anti-insecticide propaganda that misrepresents the scientific process, as revealed for the three examples described above:

- The breast cancer example reveals a general trend of anti-DDT campaigners railing against DDT while failing to meet minimal evidentiary standards for proof of cause-effect relationships (as defined by the principles of causation [25]). In brief, those who campaign against DDT have failed to show, through replicated and confirmatory studies, that a specific type of public health harm from DDT was a consistent finding across studies, and that it was consistent with current biological or theoretical knowledge of the type of harm and its known risk factors; for example:

  o More common with higher DDT exposure and less common with lower exposure,

  o Less common prior to DDT exposure and appeared or increased in frequency with onset of DDT exposure, and

  o More common with DDT exposure and less common once DDT use was stopped.

- The example of DDT as a reputed cause of reduced duration of lactation illustrates how an unproven claim can be used in scientific literature to assert that an unintended consequence of DDT might cause as much harm as benefit. Also it shows how the claim can continue to appear in anti-insecticide propaganda long after it is disproven.

- The example of malformed male genitalia illustrates how false associations can be used in attempts to scare people away from allowing their houses to be sprayed. Also the example illustrates how tangential studies (a survey of DDT in breast milk) can be used to exaggerate dangers of DDT and to cast further attention on the results of weak studies. Sadly, the two studies are being used to scare people who live in malarious regions.

9. Dichotomies in patterns/trends of human disease with/without DDT

Decades ago, developed countries used extraordinary quantities of DDT. The richer countries placed DDT in the human food chain through its heavy agricultural use at that time. More explicitly, DDT was used in the environment, around houses, and intensively inside homes. It is now 40 years since being banned for most uses in the US and other developed countries. Yet, recent claims of DDT causing disease or birth defects are not reflected in the historical medical reports and vital statistics for regions and years of broad and heavy DDT usage. The lack of proof that DDT caused harm to human health back in the days of intense exposures goes far in explaining why, to this day, there is no evidence that human health has been improved in any way by stopping public health uses of DDT.

There is a dichotomy in the huge benefit from use of DDT to prevent diseases and deaths versus no definable benefit from stopping its use. For slightly more than three decades (1945-1979) many malaria endemic countries maintained house spray programs. That era was followed by decades, from 1979 through to present time, when most of the same countries phased house spraying out of national programs. The result is a historical record of years when DDT and other insecticides were sprayed in houses followed by almost as many years when spraying was greatly decreased or stopped entirely. An even more drastic stoppage of DDT spraying occurred in agriculture. The dichotomies of outcomes are listed in Table 1.

Benefits versus harms of public health insecticides	1946-79 (period of DDT spraying in houses)	1980-present (period when DDT spraying was reduced or stopped)
Harm from insecticide exposures	Increases in poisonings and deaths from insecticide exposures in houses	Reductions in poisonings and deaths as house spraying is eliminated
Benefits from using insecticides to control malaria and other diseases	Reductions in malaria infections and deaths as a consequence of DDT on house walls	Increases in malaria infections and deaths as house spraying of DDT is eliminated

Table 1. Grid of cause-effect relationships for public health outcomes during periods of use and non-use of DDT in public health programs.

As explained for smoking and human cancers, the relationship of declining risk with reduced exposure attests to a true and meaningful causal relationship. An inverse finding of increasing risk with increasing exposure to a causative agent also attests to a true and meaningful causal relationship. These indicators of causation make it all the more amazing that through decades of anti-insecticide advocacy, insecticide opponents have documented no obvious public health harm as a result of DDT residues on house walls. Likewise, they have documented no meaningful improvements in health or reduced deaths as a direct result of having eliminated

DDT exposure by ending house spray programs. These failings suggest DDT opponents have not been challenged to balance an equation of measurable benefits from preventing the use of DDT and other public health insecticides versus the measurable increases in human deaths and diseases, like malaria, as consequence of stopping use of public health insecticides.

10. Models for modern advocacy against PHIs

Now, on the fiftieth anniversary of *Silent Spring*, the goal of reducing or eliminating DDT and other PHIs is, and has been for decades, entrenched in environmental advocacy literature and in bureaucracies of the UN. In the case of DDT, this goal was clearly enunciated by UNEP in 2000:

WHO and UNEP have joined forces to protect both human health and the environment by promoting strategies to reduce malaria

with reduced reliance on DDT. An important first step was taken in March 2000 through a WHO-convened Regional Consultation

to Prepare African Countries Towards Reduction of Reliance on DDT for Malaria Control, with UNEP support. [44]

For UNEP bureaucrats, the statement codifies the environmentalist's belief that small quantities of DDT sprayed on house walls harms the environment. Also it codifies the belief that DDT is not needed in malaria control programs. In both cases, the bureaucrats are wrong.

Information presented in Figures 2 and 3 illustrate the enormous danger of forcing countries to abandon DDT and other PHIs. Since the early 1980s over 10.5 million preventable malaria cases were recorded above and beyond what might have occurred if Brazil had not abandoned DDT. There were no DDT resistance issues that caused malaria program managers to abandon DDT, there were no important studies showing DDT repellent properties did not work, there were no malaria trend analyses showing a lack of efficacious control with DDT sprayed walls, and there were no cost-effective insecticides that could be used instead. DDT was abandoned in Brazil and in other countries of South America as a consequence of global environmental policies and anti-insecticide campaigns. DDT was not eliminated from Peru's malaria program until the late 1980s. Peru's malaria problems grew exponentially worse immediately after the country dispensed with DDT spraying. These disastrous outcomes were repeated in many countries.

With the beginning of the 21st Century and infused with renewed support and improved targeting in application of control efforts, malaria control programs are beginning to make some progress. But further progress is needed and malaria continues as a huge public health problem. Meanwhile, as in the 1960s, insecticide opponents are poised to counter the recent progress against malaria. We will now focus on specific tactics that are and will continue to be used in the anti-insecticide campaigns.

As we have described, the first strategy of insecticide opposition is to convince people that DDT or other PHIs are harmful. An important tactic for achieving success is to develop and broadcast widely and repeatedly a list of diverse claims of chemical harm. We have already described examples of how this tactic is implemented. A list of diverse sources of harm is not easy to counter. When an authoritative rebuttal of one claim occurs, the other claims are still in play. Additionally, a broad list of claims allows campaigners to tailor platforms for constituencies, advancing one set of claims with one constituency and a different combination for another. Another tactic is to focus on the most recent study hinting at some health impact of the chemical. It is easier to get the popular media interested in a study that can be presented as a new and sensational finding--a favorite theme of science writers. Regardless, a list of multiple claims of harm is hardly sufficient to achieve a ban of a truly useful PHI. Thus, the second strategy of convincing people the chemical is not needed becomes extraordinarily important. The tactic behind this goal is to argue that alternative chemicals or methods can be used as replacements. We will present two examples of tactics employed in support of this strategy. The third strategy is to predict that grave harm will occur if the chemical continues to be used.

The success of Rachel Carson's *Silent Spring* serves as a model for the three strategies. In *Silent Spring*, Rachel Carson used the strategies on her primary target, DDT. She described a very large list of potential adverse effects of insecticides, including human health and ecological effects. She argued that insecticides were not really needed because their use selected for super bugs that were resistant to the insecticides and that the chemicals only made problems worse. Last but not least, she described scary scenarios of severe harm with continued use of DDT and other insecticides.

Carson focused attention on examples of overuse or misuse of DDT and other insecticides and described the effects of their misuse. Nevertheless, the misuse of chemicals is not a valid reason for banning an insecticide. In the case of DDT, a successful campaign to eliminate it requires that even its proper use will cause a large and systematic adverse effect. However, the proper public health uses of DDT yield no large and systematic adverse effects. Absent such adverse actions, the activists must then rely on claims about insidious effects, particularly insidious effects that scientists will find difficult to prove one way or the other, and that activists can use to predict a future catastrophe.

Rachel Carson relied heavily on possible insidious chemical actions as a means of alarming and scaring the public. Many of those who joined the resulting campaign to ban DDT and other insecticides made extensive use of claims of insidious effects. In particular Carson alluded to insidious effects on reproduction. Her assertions were amplified by the popular press and became part of the public perception about insecticides. Although those perceptions are wrong, they are firmly entrenched in anti-insecticide propaganda.

The three strategies, while largely bogus in terms of their scientific underpinnings, were very effective in anti-insecticide campaigns. The strategies are still used today. Rogan and Chen used these strategies in their two papers against DDT [31,32]. The authors presented strategy number two in the form of a superficial review of the role of DDT in malaria control. They strove to cast doubt on DDT's value in modern malaria control programs. They admitted that

DDT had been very effective in the past, but then argued that malaria control programs no longer needed it and alternative methods of control should be used. Rogan and Chen also employed the first strategy of environmentalism [32]. Their list of potential harms from DDT exposures included toxic effects, neurobehavioral effects, cancers, decrements in various facets of reproductive health, decrements in infant and child development, and immunology and DNA damage. To get the paper past reviewers they presented balanced coverage of their diverse claims of harm, and, as consequence, had to conclude they could not prove that DDT caused any harm at all. Amazingly, they promptly negated this honest conclusion by asserting that if DDT is used for malaria control then great harm might occur. So, while not proving DDT causes harm, the authors still predict severe harm if it is used.

Rogan and Chen end their paper with a call for more research. One could conclude that the intent of the whole paper is merely to lobby for research dollars to better define DDT harm, and what's the harm in that? Surely increasing knowledge is a fine goal. However, having engaged issues of malaria control and what should or should not be done to control the disease, specifying more research funds for research on potential harms of insecticide exposures is unjustified. Large numbers of children and pregnant women die from malaria every year, and the disease sickens hundreds of millions more. Yet, not one death or illness can be attributed to an exposure to the public health use of DDT. Figure 1 illustrates growth in DDT research, with numbers of published papers doubling from one decade to the next. Almost all papers are in environmental literature and many are on potential adverse effects of DDT. Only a small proportion of papers deal with malaria and DDT. It bears repeating that DDT is a spatial repellent, and hardly an insecticide at all, but a search on DDT and repellents will produce even fewer papers. This disparity represents an egregiously disproportionate emphasis on non-sources of harm compared to the enormous harm of malaria.

The US used DDT to eradicate malaria. After malaria disappeared as an endemic disease people in the US became richer. They built better and more enclosed houses. They screened their windows and doors. They air-conditioned their homes. Also, during those early years, the US developed an immense arsenal of mosquito control tools and chemicals. Today, when there is a risk of mosquito borne disease, urban and rural areas can bring this arsenal to bear and quickly eliminate risks. And, as illustrated by aerial spray missions in the aftermath of hurricane Katrina, they can afford to do so. Yet, those modern and very expensive chemicals are not what protect the US from introductions of the old diseases. Use of those chemicals can only respond to a threat; it cannot prevent the old diseases from being reintroduced. What protects US populations is their enclosed, screened, air-conditioned housing, the physical representation of their wealth. Their wealth and living standards stop dengue at the border with Mexico, not the use of insecticides. Stopping mosquitoes from entering and biting people inside their homes is critical in the prevention of malaria and many other insect-borne diseases. This is what DDT does for poor people in poor countries. It stops large proportions of mosquitoes from entering houses. It is, in fact, a form of chemical screening, and until people in disease endemic countries can afford properly enclosed houses and physical screening, or it is provided for them, chemical screening is the only kind they have.

DDT is a protective tool that has been taken away from countries around the world, mostly due to governments acceding to the whims of the anti-pesticide wing of environmentalism, but it is not only the anti-pesticide wing that lobbies against DDT. The activists have a sympathetic lobbying ally in the pesticide industry. DDT opposition was made clear in writings of those within the insecticide industry; a Bayer official stated:

[I speak] Not only as the responsible manager for the vector control business in Bayer, being the market leader in vector control and pointing out by that we know what we are talking about and have decades of experiences in the evolution of this very particular market. [but] Also as one of the private sector representatives in the RBM Partnership Board and being confronted with that discussion about DDT in the various WHO, RBM et al circles. So you can take it as a view from the field, from the operational commercial level - but our companies [sic] point of view. I know that all of my colleagues from other primary manufacturers and internationally operating companies are sharing my view. [45]

The official goes on to say that,

DDT use is for us a commercial threat (which is clear, but it is not that dramatical [sic] because of limited use), it is mainly a public image threat.

However the most damming part of this message was the statement that,

---

...we fully support EU to ban imports of agricultural products coming from countries using DDT...

This email message from Bayer, one of the largest global manufacturers of alternatives to DDT, provides clear evidence of industry applying international and developed country pressures to stop poor countries from using DDT to control malaria. This message also shows the complicity of the insecticide industry in those internationally orchestrated efforts.

The environmental movement lobbied for a WHA resolution that required countries to move away from using insecticides in disease control altogether [23]. The WHA is the premier policy-setting forum for all health issues and is the governing body of the WHO. At that time, 1997, there was no evidence that vector-borne diseases could be controlled without man-made insecticides. The same is true today. The resolution was adopted by the WHA in 1997. Essentially, the lobbying of environmental groups elevated politics and anti-insecticide sentiment above scientific evidence and left hundreds of millions at high risk of death and illness from entirely preventable diseases. As we will show in the next section, UNEP has a particularly odious history of elevating environmental politics over science.

11. UNEP's war against PHIs

The UN Stockholm Convention on POPs, which came into force in 2004, governs the use of DDT. DDT is the only chemical under the POPs Convention that is granted an exemption for use in public health. It is against this background that the Stockholm Convention Secretariat (the Secretariat) and the financial mechanism of the Convention, the GEF, the UNEP, and groups within the Pan American Health Organization (PAHO) and WHO, have engaged in scientific malfeasance to achieve political goals. UNEP's target goal in 2007, now removed from the UNEP website, was DDT elimination by 2020.[1]

The GEF was established in 1991 and is a partnership of 10 agencies, including the World Bank, which houses the GEF. The GEF has allocated over $9bn in funds for projects with the aim of improving the environment and has raised over $40bn from other partners for its projects. At stake is not only increased power over the use of chemicals for the control of diseases but also the reputational benefits of achieving a goal deemed desirable by environmental groups. In addition, one cannot discount the fact that many millions of dollars are programmed by numerous governments via the UN system to rid the world of POPs and find alternatives to DDT. Control over the use of insecticides for public health also gives agencies control over, and benefit from, these funds.

UNEP's and GEF's misrepresentations of scientific records against the use of DDT and other PHIs were exposed in a peer-reviewed paper in *Research and Reports in Tropical Medicine* [46]. The paper exposed the false claims about an insecticide-free malaria control project managed by UNEP and financed by GEF in Mexico and Central America (Mexico/CA). The project was designed to demonstrate successful control of malaria through use of "environmentally sound" methods without DDT and other insecticides. Almost inevitably, the projects' backers claimed it achieved this objective. A proper analysis of epidemiologic data, however, revealed no such success; reductions in malaria cases and deaths in the region were achieved primarily through pharmacosuppression (therapeutic and prophylactic use of anti-malarial drugs). Claims that UNEP's environmental interventions were effective were invalid.

The project, Regional Program of Action and Demonstration of Sustainable Alternatives to DDT for Malaria Vector Control in Mexico and Central America (Mexico/CA Project), was conducted in eight countries (Belize, Costa Rica, Guatemala, Honduras, Mexico, Nicaragua, Panama and El Salvador). It was executed by PAHO's Sustainable Development and Environmental Health Program and implemented by UNEP. It was co-financed by the GEF with additional support from the Commission for Environmental Cooperation of North America (CEC), PAHO, and participating country governments. The project's aim was to improve coordination and national capacity so that new, integrated disease vector (mosquito) control techniques could be implemented, thereby eliminating the need for DDT reintroduction [47]. The objectives of the project (as stated by UNEP) were to: "Demonstrate feasibility of integrated

---

1 The Stockholm Convention is a UN Convention that arose from UN Environment Program efforts to control and/or ban the production and use of certain persistent organic pollutants. PAHO is an international public health agency and is the Regional Office for the Americas of the WHO and part of the UN.

and environment-friendly methods for malaria vector control without the use of DDT," and "assess the effects of these methods on malaria occurrence [48]."

According to UNEP, the key interventions in the project were as follows: 1) Reduction of contact between mosquitoes and people via treated bed nets; meshes on doors and windows; the planting of repellent trees like neem and oak; and the liming of households. 2) Control of breeding sites by clearing vegetation; draining stagnant water, ditches and channels; and the use of biological controls such as fish and bacteria in some countries. 3) Elimination of places near houses that attract and shelter mosquitoes through, for example, the cleaning and tidying up of areas in and around homes, alongside the promotion of personal hygiene [49].

The project's final evaluation, published in November 2009, mentions various pharmaceutical methods of prophylaxis and treatment within human populations [50]. However, those methods were ongoing components of malaria control in each country prior to the Mexico/CA Project, operating nationally in each country before and during the project. The available evidence suggests national malaria control programs (NMCPs) functioned regardless of the presence or absence of UNEP's project personnel. Thus, anti-malarial treatment (the major component of the NMCPs) in demonstration areas was not part of the epidemiological evaluation of the Mexico/CA Project [51]. Likewise, use of ITNs had no obvious definable role in the Mexico/CA Project. Project successes are therefore advertised as having been achieved without mention of the accompanying use of insecticides.

The project included demonstration areas, where the GEF environmental interventions would be implemented, as well as control areas within epidemiologically similar areas, where the interventions would be excluded, for proper comparisons [51]. As stated by Cesar Chelala, medical consultant affiliated with the Mexico/CA Project, demonstration areas were selected "based on the high incidence of transmission and the persistence of malaria in those places [52]."

An epidemiological evaluation identified 202 demonstration areas and 51 control areas [51]. The former included a total population of 159,018 and the latter 50,834.

The public statements regarding the Mexico/CA Project proclaimed dramatic and very impressive reductions in malaria cases for its environmentally benign interventions. The final report of the Mexico/CA Project, published by the environmental sector of PAHO in December 2008, claims "a 63% reduction in the number of people with the disease without using DDT or any other type of pesticide [53]."

These statistics and claims of success were repeated in an official press release issued by UNEP, WHO and GEF in May 2009 [54]. UNEP Executive Director, Achim Steiner, also repeated these claims and characterized the project as "calculated and tested science [49]." Similar claims have been made in the popular media [52] and used by anti-insecticide activist groups as evidence that malaria control is possible without insecticides [55].

Regrettably, the claims of malaria control through application of GEF interventions were incorrect and fundamentally misleading.

Countries in Latin America were forced away from using DDT in compliance with the North American Free Trade Agreement (NAFTA), wherein the CEC pressured Mexico in the mid-1990s to stop production and use of DDT [56]. Without DDT, countries used more expensive insecticides, which had to be sprayed more frequently, creating problems for malaria control [57]. Over time, the countries in Central America moved to greater use of pharmacosuppression. Malaria cases have fallen as a result of this widespread use of malaria treatments, but not through the environmental controls touted by the UN. Officials of GEF, UNEP and the Secretariat, however, ignored the use of pharmacosuppression in their discussion of successful malaria control in Mexico/CA. Furthermore, these officials falsely attribute changes in malaria burdens to GEF's environmental interventions. A separate epidemiological evaluation which was designed to measure any changes in disease rates, found no statistical differences in malaria rates in demonstration areas versus rates in control areas, and this was consistent across all eight countries [51]. Malaria rates in most countries were falling, but with no difference between the demonstration areas and controls, the decline cannot be attributed to the environmental interventions. But UNEP, GEF, the Secretariat and other officials ignored those findings. Furthermore, despite the fact that the control areas were a crucially important part of the project, they were not even mentioned in the 2008 final report [53]. Ultimately, the successful reduction of malaria was most likely entirely due to pharmacosuppression.

One might wonder why a control program would require insecticides and vector control if pharmacosuppression is such a powerful method of malaria control. This is a complex issue, but it is important to note that even though reductions in malaria cases have been achieved in Mexico and Central America, their model of widespread distribution of the anti-malarial drugs chloroquine and primaquine is not transferable elsewhere and may not be sustainable over the long-term. As a model for malaria control, it is not transferable for several reasons. First, widespread drug resistance to chloroquine in Africa and Southeast Asia would mean the intervention would be largely useless. Second, primaquine is a radical treatment for vivax malaria, whereas in Africa over 90 percent of malaria cases are caused by falciparum malaria, the more deadly form of the disease.[2] Third, pharmacosuppression is expensive and requires more sophisticated health systems than exist in most of Africa, where the greatest burden of malaria lies. So even if UNEP, GEF and their partners were straightforward about the real reasons for the declines in malaria in the project areas, there would be no reasonable argument to claim that pharmacosuppression has any application in most other endemic areas.

Global malaria control policy gives scant notice to pharmacosuppression. In fact, it appears that global leaders are intent on ignoring how countries of the Americas are making use of pharmacosuppression. Yet, and as commonly observed in reports from South America, the only cost-effective insecticides (pyrethroids) they have must be sprayed so frequently as to be of limited value. Thus, countries of the Americas really have no viable cost-effective options for use of PHIs. In absence of an insecticidal solution then, pharmacosuppression becomes the best option for effectively reducing malaria caseloads.

---

2 In addition, there are concerns about the side effects of using primaquine among people with G6PD deficiency. See Baird K. Eliminating malaria – all of them.Lancet 2010;376(9756): 1883-5. http://www.thelancet.com/journals/lancet/article/PIIS0140-6736%2810%2961494-8/fulltext (accessed 19 September 2012).

If we assume there is a decision to keep quiet on how malaria is being controlled in absence of insecticides, then it is easier to understand why there is less transparency in malaria data for the Americas. Historically PAHO openly reported statistics on the numbers and types of curative treatments dispensed per year in each country. However, transparency of malaria control statistics is down from just two or three years ago. A visit to PAHO's website on interactive malaria control data for the Americas will reveal no data on numbers of treatments with chloroquine or primaquine. Indeed, the only data that is readily available is on use of ACTs for treating cases of falciparum malaria.

12. Conclusion

We have described the systematic and often coordinated campaigns by activists, scientists and UN agencies against essential tools for disease control. We will conclude here with statements that bring our analyses full circle. Rachel Carson started broad scale unscientific attacks on DDT in 1962, with publication of her book, *Silent Spring*. The claims of harm by exposures to DDT, as we describe in this chapter, were not and are not true. In other words, the attributed harms are not caused by DDT exposures. Yet, presented in a 2012 article titled "Critisism [sic] of Carson over DDT unfounded" is a denial of any responsibility whatsoever for the reductions and eliminations of DDT in disease control programs as legacy of her book. In their article the Rachel Carson Council makes the following claims: "DDT has been associated with serious adverse effects in humans, including reduced sperm production in men, shorter lactation times and increasing numbers of pre-term births in women,… breast cancer...[58]."

We ask the reader to compare their claims with those we describe as not meeting even minimal criteria for cause-effect relationships. So the Rachel Carson Council denies responsibility for harm inflicted by Carson's anti-DDT rhetoric, while, at the same time, it continues to implement her strategies for DDT elimination and employs her tactics of falsifying the scientific record to scare the public. Amazingly, when the false statements and fear tactics employed by anti-DDT campaigners succeed in stopping use of DDT to protect health and save lives, the anti-PHI advocacy community, as revealed in the Rachel Carson Council's denial of responsibilities, expects the public to think they had no role in such inhumanely disastrous changes in public health policies. As we have shown, they are, in fact, the very cause of those changes in policy.

We have shown that vast sums of money, mostly from taxpayers, have been spent over many decades undermining and often directly attacking the use of DDT in life-saving disease control programs. These vast expenditures have not delivered alternative strategies or tools to replace DDT. The few alternatives that disease control programs do have for some malaria-endemic regions pale in comparison to the powerful life-saving properties of DDT. It almost goes without saying that if the disease control tool in question were not DDT but were a vaccine or a medicine, there would be a sense of outrage in the general public along with well-funded advocacy to preserve and protect a tool that has the power to save lives. Yet such is the power of the environmental movement, that aside from a few outspoken scientists and individuals, there has been almost no response from the malaria community or the wider public health community. The strategies employed by anti-DDT activists are anti-science and rely on distortions, half-truths and sometimes outright lies. Ordinarily such behavior would be roundly criticized, yet because DDT is being attacked, such actions are given a free pass.

We are greatly concerned that the majority of private insecticide companies far from opposing the unscientific agenda of the anti-DDT campaigns, support them. These companies may be merely motivated to sell more of their own product, but this is surely one of the most short-sighted strategies imaginable. We already see a growing number of studies finding associations between alternatives to DDT and possible human health harm. As with DDT, the anti-insecticide activists are starting to hype and spread fear about these associations. As the Stockholm Convention adds more and more chemicals to its list of banned or controlled substances, and as the UNEP flexes its regulatory muscles, we fully expect it will become more and more difficult to produce, trade, transport and use all PHIs. It is precisely because of such restrictions that countries of the Americas have had to adopt programs of mass drug distributions (pharmacosuppression) to control vivax malaria. Basically those countries have no cost-effective options for use of PHIs. Continuation of these anti-PHI practices, as we have learned from history, will inflict great harm on disease control efforts and eventually exact a heavy cost in lives from some of the poorest and most vulnerable communities on earth.

We hope this chapter has shed some light on the strategies and tactics of environmental groups, activists, scientists and UN agencies. Well-established patterns of behavior have been set with these groups and individuals and we hope that the malaria community and the wider public health community begin to recognize these patterns and begin to more effectively investigate and respond to claims against PHIs long before the claims become the basis for further restrictions on the efficacy of disease control programs.

List of the acronyms used in the text

ACT-- artemisinin-based combination therapies

API—annual parasite index

CEC—Commission for Environmental Cooperation (The full title is North Americas Commission for Environmental Cooperation. Created as a side agreement of the North American Free Trade Agreement.)

DDT/DDE—Diethyl dichloro trichloroethelene. DDE is a metabolic product of DDT.

EDC-- endocrine disrupting chemicals

GEF—Global Environment Facility

HSR—house spray rate

IRS—indoor residual spray

ITN—insecticide treated net

MRL—maximum residue limit

NAFTA—North American Free Trade Agreement

NGO—Nongovernmental organization

NMCP—National Malaria Control Program

OC—organochlorine compound

PAHO—Pan American Health Organization

PHI—public health insecticide

PMI—President's Malaria Initiative

POP—persistent organic pollutant

PTDI—provisional tolerable daily intake

RBM—Roll Back Malaria

SP-- sulphadoxine-pyrimethamine

UN—United Nations

UNDP—United Nations Development Programme

UNEP—United Nations Environment Programme

UNICEF—United Nations Children's Fund

USAID—United States Agency for International Development

WHA—World Health Assembly

WHO—World Health Organization

WWF—World Wildlife Fund

Author details

Donald R. Roberts[1,2*], Richard Tren[3] and Kimberly Hess[3]

*Address all correspondence to: drdonaldroberts42@gmail.com

1 Uniformed Services University of the Health Sciences, Bethesda, MD, USA

2 Retired, Professor Emeritus, Clifton Forge, VA, USA

3 Africa Fighting Malaria, Washington, DC, USA

References

[1] Roll Back Malaria Partnership: RBM Vision. http://www.rbm.who.int/rbmvision.html (accessed 4 December 2012).

[2] The President's Malaria Initiative: PMI Results. http://www.fightingmalaria.gov/about/results.html (accessed 4 December 2012).

[3] World Health Organization: What is Roll Back Malaria? https://apps.who.int/inf-fs/en/InformationSheet02.pdf (accessed 19 September 2012).

[4] Yamey G. Roll Back Malaria: a failing global health campaign. BMJ 2004;328: 1086. http://www.bmj.com/content/328/7448/1086 (accessed 19 September 2012).

[5] World Health Organization: WHO gives indoor use of DDT a clean bill of health for controlling malaria. http://www.who.int/mediacentre/news/releases/2006/pr50/en/ (accessed 19 September 2012).

[6] The President's Malaria Initiative: Sixth Annual Report to Congress: April 2012. http://www.fightingmalaria.gov/resources/reports/pmi_annual_report12.pdf (accessed 19 September 2012).

[7] The Global Fund to Fight AIDS, TB and Malaria: The Global Fund Annual Report 2011. http://www.theglobalfund.org/en/library/publications/annualreports/ (accessed 19 September 2012).

[8] World Health Organization: World Malaria Report 2011. http://www.who.int/malaria/world_malaria_report_2011/en/index.html (accessed 19 September 2012).

[9] Woodwell GM. Effects of pollution on the structure and physiology of ecosystems. Science 1970;168(3930) 429-433.

[10] World Health Organization: Malaria Fact sheet No. 94: April 2012. http://www.who.int/mediacentre/factsheets/fs094/en/ (accessed 19 September 2012).

[11] World Health Organization: Yellow fever Fact sheet No. 100: January 2011. http://www.who.int/mediacentre/factsheets/fs100/en/ (accessed 19 September 2012).

[12] World Health Organization: World Malaria Report 2009. http://www.who.int/malaria/world_malaria_report_2009/en/index.html (accessed 19 September 2012).

[13] Malaria Site: Malaria in India. http://www.malariasite.com/malaria/MalariaInIndia.htm (accessed 19 September 2012).

[14] Smith D. Worldwide trends in DDT levels in human breast milk. Int J Epidemiol 1999;28(2) 179-88.

[15] Safe S. Clinical correlates of environmental endocrine disruptors. Trends Endocrinol Metab 2005;16(4) 139-44.

[16]   Roberts D, Tren R, Bate R, Zambone J. The Excellent Powder, DDT's Political and Scientific History. Indianapolis, IN: Dog Ear Publishing; 2010.

[17]   Carson R. Silent Spring. New York: Houghton Mifflin Company; 1962.

[18]   World Health Organization. Executive Board, 47th Session, Part II, Appendix 14. "The place of DDT in operations against malaria and other vector borne diseases." Geneva, 1971, p. 176.

[19]   World Health Organization. Official Records, 1972, no. 198. Executive Board, 49th Session, Part II. Chapter II, page 23. Under section titled "Report on the Proposed Programme and Budget Estimates for 1973."

[20]   South African Department of Health. "Malaria Updates, May 2000." Pretoria.

[21]   Barnes KI, Durrheim DN, Little F, et al. Effect of artemether-lumefantrine policy and improved vector control on malaria burden in KwaZulu-Natal, South Africa. PLoS Med 2005;2(11) e330.

[22]   Navarro M. Breaking a long silence on population control. The New York Times 2011. http://www.nytimes.com/2011/11/01/science/earth/bringing-up-the-issue-of-population-growth.html?pagewanted=all (accessed 19 September 2012).

[23]   World Health Organization: World Health Assembly Resolution 50.13: Promotion of chemical safety, with special attention to persistent organic pollutants: May 1997. http://www.who.int/ipcs/publications/wha/whares_53_13/en/index.html (accessed 19 September 2012).

[24]   United Nations Environment Programme: Proceedings of the Governing Council at its Nineteenth Session: Nairobi, 27 January - 7 February 1997. http://www.unep.org/resources/gov/prev_docs/97_GC19_proceedings.pdf (accessed 19 September 2012).

[25]   Hill AB. Principles of medical statistics. 9th edition. New York: Oxford University Press; 1971.

[26]   Wolff MS, Toniolo PG, Lee EW, Rivera M, Dubin N. Blood levels of organochlorine residues and risk of breast cancer. J Natl Cancer Inst 1993;85(8) 648-52.

[27]   World Health Organization: International Programme on Chemical Safety: Environmental Health Criteria 241: DDT in Indoor Residual Spraying: Human Health Aspects. http://whqlibdoc.who.int/publications/2011/9789241572415_eng.pdf (accessed 19 September 2012).

[28]   World Wildlife Fund: Resolving the DDT Dilemma: Protecting Biodiversity and Human Health. http://awsassets.panda.org/downloads/resolvingddt.pdf (accessed 19 September 2012).

[29]   Rogan WJ, Gladen BC, McKinney JD, et al. Polychlorinated biphenyls (PCBs) and dichlorodiphenyl dichloroethene (DDE) in human milk: effects on growth, morbidity, and duration of lactation. Am J Public Health 1987;77(10) 1294-7.

[30] Gladen BC, Rogan WJ. DDE and shortened duration of lactation in a northern Mexican town. Am J Public Health 1995;85(4) 504-08.

[31] Chen A, Rogan WJ. Nonmalarial infant deaths and DDT use for malaria control. Emerg Infect Dis 2003;9(8): 960-4. http://wwwnc.cdc.gov/eid/article/9/8/03-0082_article.htm (accessed 19 September 2012).

[32] Rogan WJ, Chen A. Health risks and benefits of bis(4-chlorophenyl)-1,1,1-trichloroethane (DDT). Lancet 2005;366(9487): 763-73. http://www.thelancet.com/journals/lancet/article/PIIS0140-6736%2805%2967182-6/fulltext (accessed 19 September 2012).

[33] Physicians for Social Responsibility (PSR) - Kenya: Kenya POPs situation report: DDT, pesticides and polychlorinated biphenyls. http://www.ipen.org/ipepweb1/library/ipep_pdf_reports/1ken%20kenya%20country%20situation%20report.pdf (accessed 19 September 2012).

[34] Roberts DR, Laughlin LL, Hsheih P, Legters LJ. DDT, Global Strategies, and a Malaria Control Crisis in South America. Emerg Infect Dis 1997;3(3): 295–302. http://wwwnc.cdc.gov/eid/article/3/3/97-0305_article.htm (accessed 19 September 2012).

[35] Roberts DR, Laughlin LL. Malaria control in South America-response to P.C. Matteson. Emerg Infect Dis 1999;5(2): 310–311. http://wwwnc.cdc.gov/eid/article/5/2/99-0230_article.htm (accessed 19 September 2012).

[36] Matteson PC. Malaria control in South America. Emerg Infect Dis 1999;5(2): 309–311. http://wwwnc.cdc.gov/eid/article/5/2/99-0229_article.htm (accessed 19 September 2012).

[37] Post D (Rachel Carson Council): DDT, Political Pesticide. http://www.rachelcarsoncouncil.org/uploads/brochures/DDT%20Political%20Pesticide.PDF (accessed 19 September 2012).

[38] Schafer K (Pesticide Action Network North America): What's behind the 'DDT comeback'? http://www.pan-uk.org/pestnews/Issue/pn74/pn74p4.pdf (accessed 19 September 2012).

[39] Wikipedia: DDT. http://en.wikipedia.org/wiki/DDT#Chronic_toxicity (accessed 19 September 2012).

[40] Bornman R, de Jager C, Worku Z, Farias P, Reif S. DDT and urogenital malformations in newborn boys in a malarial area. BJU Int 2010;106(3): 405-11. http://onlinelibrary.wiley.com/doi/10.1111/j.1464-410X.2009.09003.x/full (accessed 19 September 2012).

[41] Bouwman H, Kylin H, Sereda B, Bornman R. High levels of DDT in breast milk: Intake, risk, lactation duration, and involvement of gender. Environ Pollut 2012;170 63-70.

[42] Linköping Universitet. Researchers measure highest DDT levels in breast milk from South African nursing mothers. News-Medical.Net 2012. http://www.news-medi-

cal.net/news/20120903/Researchers-measure-highest-DDT-levels-in-breast-milk-from-South-African-nursing-mothers.aspx (accessed 19 September 2012).

[43] Savitz DA. Interpreting epidemiologic evidence. Strategies for study design and analysis. New York, NY: Oxford University Press; 2003.

[44] United Nations Environment Programme: Contribution of the United Nations Environment Programme to the Implementation of Agenda 21 and the Programme for the Further implementation of Agenda 21: 16 June 2000. http://www.unep.org/malmo/Agenda21.pdf (accessed 19 September 2012).

[45] Email correspondence on file with authors and available upon request.

[46] Roberts DR, Tren R. International advocacy against DDT and other public health insecticides for malaria control. Research and Reports in Tropical Medicine 2011;2011(2): 23-30. http://www.dovepress.com/international-advocacy-against-ddt-and-other-public-health-insecticide-peer-reviewed-article-RRTM (accessed 19 September 2012).

[47] Global Environment Facility: Detail of GEF Project #1591: Regional Program of Action and Demonstration of Sustainable Alternatives to DDT for Malaria Vector Control in Mexico and Central America. http://www.gefonline.org/projectDetailsSQL.cfm?projID=1591 (accessed 19 September 2012).

[48] Betlem J (UNEP), Neira M (WHO), Whyllie P (SSC). Demonstrating and Scaling-up of Sustainable Alternatives to DDT in Vector Management (DSSA - Global Programme). A program implemented by United Nations Environment Program- UNEP and executed by World Health Organization – WHO (Regional Offices) and the governments of participating countries. Approved by GEF Council on 23 April 2008. Presentation on file with authors.

[49] United Nations Environment Programme: Speech by Achim Steiner, UN Environment Programme (UNEP) Executive Director at the Helsinki Chemicals Forum 2009. http://www.unep.org/Documents.Multilingual/Default.asp?DocumentID=588&ArticleID=6191&l=en (accessed 19 September 2012).

[50] Narváez Olalla A: United Nations Environment Programme: Final Evaluation of the UNEP GEF project "Regional Program of Action and Demonstration of Sustainable Alternatives to DDT for Malaria Vector Control in Mexico and Central America". http://www.iwlearn.net/iw-projects/Fsp_112799467892/evaluations/DDT%20Final%20Evaluation%20Report.pdf (accessed 19 September 2012).

[51] Arbeláez Montoya MP. Control de la malaria sin DDT en Mesoamérica: control focalizado y manejo de criaderos como estrategias básicas Aspectos Epidemiológicos. Programa Regional de Acción y Demostración de Alternativas de Control de Vectores de la Malaria sin el Uso de DDT (Proyecto DDT/PNUMA/GEF/OPS). Presentation on file with authors.

[52] Chelala C. Taking a bite out of malaria. Americas 2008; 38-45.

[53] PAHO/WHO, UNEP, GEF: Regional program of action and demonstration of sustainable alternative to DDT for malaria vector control in Mexico and Central America (Project DDT/UNEP/GEF/PAHO): Final Report from September 2003 to December 2008. http://www.paho.org/english/ad/sde/DDT_GEF_Final_Report%282008%29.pdf (accessed 19 September 2012).

[54] UNEP/WHO/GEF: Countries move toward more sustainable ways to roll back malaria. http://www.who.int/mediacentre/news/releases/2009/malaria_ddt_20090506/en/index.html (accessed 19 September 2012).

[55] Pesticide Action Network: Global network calls for safe malaria solutions. http://panna.org/media-center/press-release/global-network-calls-safe-malaria-solutions (accessed 19 September 2012).

[56] North American Commission on Environmental Cooperation: North American Regional Action Plan on DDT: June 1997: Appendix-Presentation by the Mexican Ministry of Health. http://www.cec.org/Page.asp?PageID=924&ContentID=1262#mexhealth (accessed 19 September 2012).

[57] Pan American Health Organization: Report on the situation of malaria in the Americas, 2008: Regional section. http://new.paho.org/hq/index.php?option=com_content&task=view&id=2459&Itemid=2000 (accessed 19 September 2012).

[58] Rachel Carson Council: Critisism of Carson over DDT Unfounded. http://www.rachelcarsoncouncil.org/index.php?page=critisism-of-carson-over-ddt-unfounded (19 September 2012).

Chapter 9

New Salivary Biomarkers of Human Exposure to Malaria Vector Bites

Papa M. Drame, Anne Poinsignon, Alexandra Marie,
Herbert Noukpo, Souleymane Doucoure,
Sylvie Cornelie and Franck Remoue

Additional information is available at the end of the chapter

1. Introduction

Mosquitoes are the most menacing worldwide arthropod disease vectors. They transmit a broad range of viral, protozoan and metazoan pathogens responsible of the most devastating human and animal diseases [1]. Among the main frequent mosquito-borne diseases, malaria represents the most widespread and serious infection in terms of heavy burden on health and economic development throughout the world. Despite substantial efforts and increasing international funding to eliminate it, malaria is still a major public health problem with nearly a million of deaths per year, especially in children younger than 5 years old (86%) [2]. Approximately two thirds of the world's population live in areas at risk for malaria [3, 4]. Understanding mechanisms that govern its transmission remains therefore a major scientific challenge, but also an essential step in the design and the evaluation of effective control programs [5, 6].

Entomological, parasitological and clinical assessments are routinely used to evaluate the exposure of human populations to *Anopheles* vector bites and the risk of malaria transmission. However, these methods are labor intensive and difficult to sustain on large scales, especially when transmission and exposure levels are low (dry season, high altitude, urban settings or after vector control) [7, 8]. In particular, the entomological inoculation rate (EIR), the gold standard measure for mosquito–human transmission intensity of *Plasmodium*, is highly dependent on the density of human-biting *Anopheles* [9]. This latter is estimated by using trapping methods such as human-landing catches (HLC) of adult mosquitoes, the commonly used for sampling host-seeking mosquitoes and then for assessing the human exposure level.

HLC may be limited because of ethical and logistical constraints to relevantly apply it to children [10]. Transmission estimates based on the prevalence or density of human infection are susceptible to micro-heterogeneity caused by climatic factors and the socioeconomic determinants of the host-seeking behavior [8]. Incidence of disease may be the closest logical correlate of the burden of disease on health systems. However, it can be subject to variability between sites and may not be appropriate for the evaluation of early phase studies of vector control or reliable for epidemic prediction [10]. More recently, serological correlates of transmission intensity have been described, yet they represent long-term rather than short-term exposure data [8]. They are not then suitable in evaluating the short-term impact of vector control programs. Therefore, it is currently emphasized the need to develop new tools assessing reliably human malaria risk and control interventions, and monitoring changes over time at both population and individual levels [5, 6].

Malaria is a parasitic disease caused by protozoan agents of the genus *Plasmodium* (*Aplicomplexa*; *Haemosporida*). Five *Plasmodium* species are pathogen for humans: *P. falciparum*, *P. vivax*, *P. ovale*, *P. malariae* and *P. knowlesi*. During their complex life cycle in the female *Anopheles* mosquito (*Insecta*; *Diptera*), *Plasmodium* parasites go through several developmental transitions, traverse the midgut and reach the salivary gland (SG) epithelium. They acquire their maturity within SGs of the vector and can be then transmitted by the bite of the female mosquito. This latter needs, during the first days after emergence, to feed on sugar to meet the energy demands of basic metabolism and flight, but also to feed on vertebrate blood for its eggs' development and maturation [11], and therefore to keep perennial its life cycle and indirectly malaria transmission cycle.

Anopheles mouthparts comprise six pieces that form a long stylus allowing to perforate human tissues and to suck the internal liquid. However, it is clear that *Anopheles* mosquito acts not only as syringe injecting parasites during the bite. When taking a blood meal, it also injects into human skin avascular tissue [12] a cocktail of bioactive molecules including enzymes that are injected in human skin by saliva [13, 14]. Some of these salivary compounds are essential to the *Plasmodium* life cycle [15]. They have substantial anti-hemostatic, anti-inflammatory, and immunomodulatory activities that assist the mosquito in the blood-feeding process by inhibiting several defense mechanisms of the human host [16]. Furthermore, many of them are immunogenic and elicit strong immune responses, evidenced by the swelling and itching that accompany a mosquito bite [17]. Specific acquired cellular [18, 19] or/and humoral responses are developed by human individuals when exposed to bites of *Anopheles* mosquitoes [20-23]. These immune responses may play several roles in the pathogen transmission ability and the disease outcomes [24]. In addition, recent studies have demonstrated that the intensity of the antibody response specific to salivary proteins could be a biomarker of the exposure level of human to *Anopheles* bites [22, 25]. Therefore, studying *Anopheles*-human immunological relationships can provide new promising tools for monitoring the real human-*Anopheles* contact and identifying individuals at risk of malaria transmission. It can also allow the development of novel methods for monitoring control and mosquito-release programmes' effectiveness.

However, whole saliva could be inadequate as a biomarker tool, because it is a cocktail of various molecular components with different nature and biological functions. Some of these elements are ubiquitous and may potentially cause cross-reactivities with common salivary epitopes of other haematophagous arthropods [26]. In addition, a lack of reproducibility between collected whole *Anopheles* saliva batches has been observed and difficulties to obtain sufficient quantities needed for large-scale studies were highlighted [26]. Therefore, specific and antigenic proteins have been identified in the secretome of *Anopheles* mosquitoes and a specific biomarker of *Anopheles* bites was developed by coupling bioinformatic and immuno-epidemiological approaches. This promising candidate, namely, the gSG6-P1 (*An. gambiae* Salivary Gland Protein-6 peptide 1), has been described to be highly antigenic [26]. It has been then validated as a pertinent biomarker assessing specifically and reliably the exposure level to *Anopheles* bites [27-29] and/or the effectiveness of malaria vector control [30] in all age-classes of human populations (newborns, infants, children and adults) from several malaria epidemiological settings (rural, semi-urban and urban areas...) throughout sub-Saharan Africa countries (Senegal, Angola and Benin).

The present chapter contributes therefore to a better understanding of the human-mosquito immunological relationship. It resumes most of the studies highlighting the roles of mosquito saliva on the human physiology and immunology, approaches, techniques, and methods used to develop and validate specific candidate-biomarkers of exposure to *Anopheles* bites and their applications on malaria control in several different epidemiological settings. Effects of various explanatory variables (age, sex, seasonality, differential use of vector control...) on human antibody responses to *Anopheles* salivary antigens are also discussed in the aim to optimize their use in epidemiological and vector-borne disease (VBD) control studies. Finally, different ways of application of such salivary biomarker of exposure of *Anopheles* vector bites in the field of operational research by National Malaria Control Programmes (NMCP) are highlighted.

2. Human host-mosquito relationship: Roles of mosquito saliva

Arthropods represent the vast majority of described metazoan life forms throughout the world, with species' richness estimated between 5 to 10 million [31]. The blood feeding habit has arisen and evolved independently in more than 14,000 species from 400 genera in the arthropod taxonomy [32]. In mosquitoes, only the adult female is hematophagous, whereas both male and female take sugar meals [33]. During the probing and the feeding stages, like all blood-sucking arthropods, female *Anopheles* must circumvent the highly sophisticated barriers represented by human defense systems (Fig. 1): haemostatic and inflammatory reactions, innate and adaptive immune system defenses. Therefore, they express in their saliva potent pharmacological and immunogenic components.

2.1. Pharmacological properties of mosquito saliva

The first-line of the human host non-specific defense to the insect bite is the haemostatic reaction. It provides an immediate response to the vascular injury caused by the intrusion of

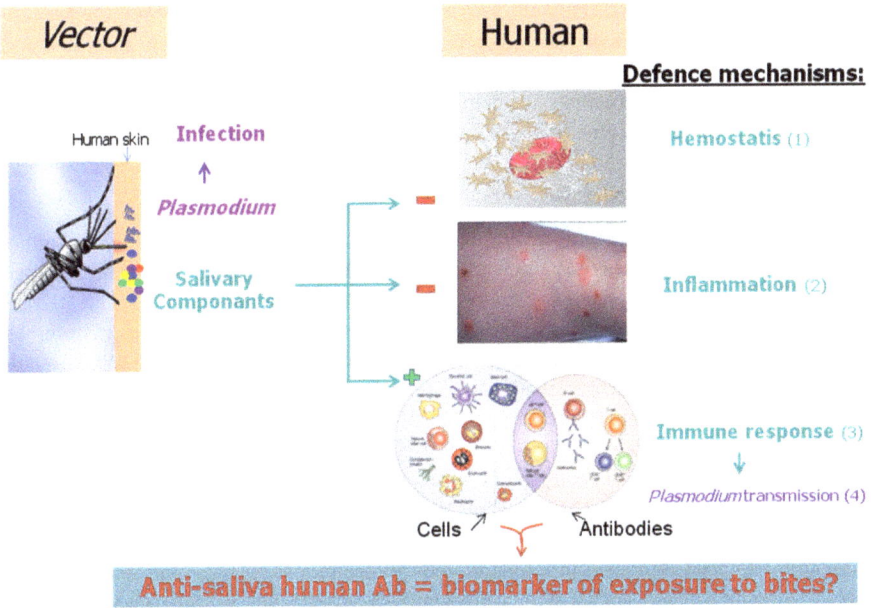

Figure 1. Effects of *Anopheles* saliva on hemostatic, inflammatory and immune reactions of the human to the vector bites.

the mosquito mouthparts in host vessels, thus preventing the extensive loss of host blood [32, 34]. The haemostatic reaction consists of three not physiologically distinct mechanisms: i) the blood coagulation that leads to the production of fibrin clots, ii) the thrombus formation and wound healing mediated by platelet aggregation, and iii) the vasoconstriction that leads to restricted influx of blood to the injured site. Each mechanism is activated by several pathways, in response to different exogenous and endogenous stimuli. Platelet aggregation is the first step in the haemostatic cascade and follows the interaction between blood platelets and the exposed extracellular matrix. This latter contains a large number of adhesive macromolecules such as collagen which is abundant underneath endothelial cells (not found in blood). This interaction results to the activation of platelets by mainly collagen and adenosine diphosphate (ADP, released by damaged cells and by activated platelets), the primary agonists of platelet aggregation. Platelets can be also activated by other agonists such as thrombin (produced by the coagulation cascade) and thromboxane A2 (TXA_2, produced by activated platelets) [35]. Activated platelets release endogeneous secretions such as serotonin and TXA_2, two potent vasoconstrictors. In parallel, the blood coagulation mechanism is getting underway. The main task of the coagulation cascade is to produce fibrin that supports aggregated platelets in a thrombus formation. The coagulation process consists of an enzymatic cascade with two ways of activation, the exogenous and the endogenous, where several amplification points and regulatory mechanisms are known.

However, mosquitoes can successfully engorge on their hosts within a half-minute because antihemostatic components of their saliva facilitate location of blood vessels and the blood sampling [36]. These salivary secretions, named sialogenins (from the Greek *sialo*, saliva; *gen*, origin, source; and *ins* for proteins), are mainly an array of potent anticoagulants, anti-platelets, vasodilators and anti-inflammatory substances [16, 32, 37, 38].

2.1.1. Inhibition of platelet aggregation

Compared to other blood-sucking arthropods like ticks and sand flies, only a limited number of *Anopheles* mosquito sialogenins involved in the inhibition of platelet aggregation have been characterized. *Apyrase* (Adenosine triphosphate (ATP)-diphosphohydrolase EC 3.6.1.5) is ubiquitous for hematophagous arthropods (mosquitoes, bugs, sand flies, fleas, triatomines, and ticks) and hydrolyses ATP and ADP into adenosine monophosphate (AMP) and inorganic phosphate (P_i), thus inhibiting platelet aggregation [16]. Three classes of apyrase have been characterized at the molecular level in different blood-sucking arthropods (reviewed by [39]). One named 5'-nucleotidase family is highly expressed in the salivary gland of *Anopheles gambiae* [40]. The *D7 protein family* is one of the most abundantly expressed sialogenins of mosquitoes. Two classes have been described in the saliva of mosquitoes: long (28–30 kDa) and short (15–20 kDa) forms [41-43]. The D7-related proteins may inhibit activation of host plasma. It has been described in *Anopheles* mosquitoes in a short form and may block the platelet activation by scavenging serotonin (agonist-positive feedback loop to increase platelet aggregation), while it principal function is reported to modulate tonus of vessels (vasocon-striction) [44]. *Anophelin* from *An. stephensi* saliva is a 30-kDa protein that directly binds to immobilized collagen and specifically inhibits collagen-induced platelet aggregation and the intracellular Ca^{2+} increase [45]. It can also act by inhibiting the activity of thrombin which plays a role in concentration of platelet aggregation [46].

2.1.2. Inhibition of blood coagulation cascade

Arthropod anticoagulants mostly target factor X-active (fXa), which plays a central role at the nexus of the intrinsic and extrinsic pathways, as well as an ultimate role of thrombin in driving production of fibrin from fibrinogen. However, *Anopheles* mosquitoes produce an anti-thrombin [38]. In *An. albimanus* for example, *Anophelin* protein has been shown to be a potent anticoagulant that acts as a specific and tight-binding thrombin inhibitor [46], blocking or delaying then the clot formation process until blood meal completion [34]. In addition, a D7-related protein of *An. stephensi* saliva has been characterized as an inhibitor of fXII [47].

2.1.3. Vasodilator effect on host blood vessels

In human, various types of endogenous vasoconstrictors (serotonin, TXA_2, noradrenalin...) are released few seconds after tissue injury in order to stop the blood flow locally at the bite site. Diverse types of vasodilators have been characterized in the saliva of hematophagous arthropods. *Aedes* mosquitoes use sialokinins that mimic the endogenous tachykinin substance P which stimulate the production of nitric oxide (NO), a potent dilator of blood vessels [48, 49]. In contrast, the saliva of the adult female *Anopheles* mosquito has been shown to contain a myeloperoxidase with a vasodilator activity associated with a catechol oxidase/peroxidase activity [50]. This latter drives the H_2O_2-dependent destruction of noradrenalin and serotonin, two important endogenous vasoconstrictors [50]. In addition, some D7 proteins of *Anopheles* have been described to bind to biogenic amines such as serotonin, histamine, and norepinephrine [44]. These strategies remove the human host's ability to maintain vascular tone at the bite site, resulting to a weak but persistent local vasodilatation [14].

2.2. Immunological effects of mosquito saliva

The tissue injury causes an immediate onset of acute inflammation and innate immunity, which promote tissue repair, prevent colonization of the damaged tissues by opportunistic pathogens and initiates adaptive immunity, which is more specific [51]. These responses mobilize multiple elements such as phagocytes and antigen-presenting cells, cytokine-producing cells, T and B lymphocytes (TL and BL) and complement (classical and alternative pathways). It may result to the development of strong cell and humoral immune reactions, thereby altering physiologically the environment at the bite site and leading to the rejection of the blood-sucker [52]. The saliva of *Anopheles* mosquitoes (like blood-feeding arthropods in general) has selected, during evolution, compounds that can counter these host responses by modulating immune cells and cytokines' production [52, 53]. This certainly allows mosquitoes to complete successfully a blood meal in only few seconds. Immunomodulatory effects of *Anopheles* mosquito saliva can therefore affect the transmission of pathogens and the development of associated pathologies [54]. Understanding the mechanisms which govern this immunomodulation could then allow the development of new prevention tools or strategies against malaria transmission [54-56].

2.2.1. Inhibition of host inflammatory reaction

The host inflammatory reaction following tissue injury consists of the triple response of Lewis: redness, heat and pain, triggering the awareness of the host to the blood sucker action [16]. If redness and heat are ones of the direct consequences of the dilatation of blood vessels, pain is induced by an increased vascular permeability under the effect of ADP, serotonin and histamine released by platelets and mast cells, following activation of the fXII by tissue-exposed collagen [16]. The fXIIa converts prekallikrein to kallikrein, which hydrolyzes blood kininogen to produce the vasodilator peptide, bradykinin. This latter induces TNF-α (Tumor Necrosis Factor alpha) release by neutrophils [57], which in turn stimulates the release of IL (interleukin)-1β and IL-6 from various cell types. These cytokines contribute to the phenomenon of hyperalgesia (increased sensitivity to pain) that accompanies inflammation. Host inflammatory reaction to bites has been described as mast cells-dependent in individuals bitten by *Anopheles* mosquitoes [58]. In contrast to ticks which need to be attached to their host for several hours (tick *Argasidæ*) or weeks (tick *Ixodidæ*), mosquitoes take just few seconds for a successful blood meal. This certainly explains the poverty of anti-inflammatory components in their saliva in contrast to the ticks' one. Nevertheless, some salivary components of *Anopheles* mosquitoes can inhibit the human inflammatory reaction. In particular, a 16kDa D7 family proteins of *An. stephensi* (Hamadarin) inhibits the contact system by preventing the mutual activation between the fXIIa and the kallikrein in the presence of Zn^{2+} [47].

2.2.2. Modulation of host immune response

A role for arthropod saliva in modifying the outcome of transmission and infection is not a novel idea introduced in the context of mosquitoes and malaria parasites. The increased pathogen infectivity in association with ticks, sand flies, and mosquitoes saliva has been described previously [54]. If ticks that take a long time to engorge must additionally necessitate in their saliva anti-inflammatory and immunosuppressive factors, rapidly feeding dipterans, in particular mosquitoes and sand flies, clearly have evolved salivary factors that directly modulate host immune defenses [52]. One possible explanation is that these molecules have evolved because they have long-term beneficial effects for the populations rather than to the individual at the time of feeding [24]. Although the molecular mechanisms by which mosquito saliva induces alteration of the host immune response are unclear [59, 60], data evidently demonstrate that effects depend on the global regulation of the Th1/Th2 cytokines' balance, as it has been described in sand flies/*Leishmania* model, the most studied striking host-parasite vector system [61]. The Th1 response has been described to lead to a protective immunity and the resistance of the host to intracellular pathogens, while the Th2 response might favor the survivor of pathogens (parasites, virus...) and then the disease transmission and evolution [24]. For mosquitoes, studies have globally shown an enhancement of transmission and disease when pathogens are introduced in the presence of vector saliva. Mosquito saliva is commonly associated with a downregulation of the expression of Th1 and an upregulation of the Th2-type cytokines. In mouse models, mosquito saliva can potentiate the infection of arboviruses [24, 62, 63]. The co-inoculation of Sindbis virus with *Aedes aegypti* salivary gland extract resulted on a reduced interferon- gamma (IFN-γ) expression, when compared to injection of virus alone [64]. It has been also shown that *Ae. aegypti* saliva contains multiple factors that can affect various components of the host immune response [65]. For example, factor Xa inhibitor may inhibit complement activation and leukocyte migration to the bite site [24] and other factors inhibit TNF-α release from activated mast cells [66]. Chickens subcutaneously infected with *P. gallinaceum* sporozoites in the presence of *Aedes fluviatillis* salivary gland homogenates showed a higher level of parasitaemia when compared to those that received only sporozoites [67]. For *Anopheles*, mice exposed to mosquito feeding in tandem with the inoculation of sporozoites had higher parasitemia and an elevated progression to cerebral malaria. This was associated with, in particular, elevated levels of IL-4 and IL-10, suppression of overall transcription in response to infection, and decreased mobility of dendritic cells and monocytes [19]. It was also described that *Anopheles stephensi* saliva downregulates specific antibody (Ab) immune responses by a mechanism that is mast cell and IL-10 -dependent [60]. IL-10, by inhibiting pro-inflammatory and Th1 cytokines, stimulates certain T, mast and B cells and has pleiotropic effects in immunoregulation and inflammation, while IL-4 is the prototypical Th2 cytokine (it differentiates CD4+ T-cells and up-regulates MHC class II production). The enhancement of IL-10 expression could account for reduction in secretion of other cytokines because it inhibits antigen presentation, IFN–γ expression, and macrophage activation [68]. However, some data have suggested a paradoxical protective role of mosquito saliva against pathogen transmission and disease infection. *Ae. aegypti* saliva can inhibit infection of dendritic cells by dengue virus, and the pre-sensitization of dendritic cells with saliva prior to infection enhanced this inhibition. Moreover, the proportion of dead cells was also reduced in virus-infected dendritic cell cultures exposed to mosquito saliva, and an enhanced production of IL-12 and TNF-α was detected in these cultures [69]. In addition to these effects on cellular immunity, *Anopheles* saliva can also acts on humoral host immune response. Indeed, specific antibodies (immunoglobulins [Ig] G, M and E) to salivary antigens have been described in several studies [20, 22, 23, 25, 56, 70]. However, the implication of these Ab responses in disease pathogenesis or protection is not yet elucidated.

Therefore, future studies are needed for an overall understanding of mosquito saliva effect, especially *Anopheles* mosquito saliva, in pathogen transmission, disease development and pathogenesis.

2.2.3. Human host-Anopheles *vector immune relationship and applications*

The study of immunological properties of salivary proteins of *Anopheles* mosquitoes represents a new research thematic which can significantly improve the understanding of *Plasmodium* transmission mechanisms and therefore help for the effective prevention and control of malaria. It can notably lead to major applications in three areas: i) development of vaccines, diagnosis, treatment, ii) prevention of allergies, and iii) development of biomarkers of exposure to bites and malaria disease risk.

The development of parasite transmission-blocking vaccines, by stimulating the immune response against the vector is an attractive alternative way for malaria control. Several studies targeted the effect of Abs specific to the mosquito midgut antigens have shown promising results [71-73]. The study of the immune response induced by vector saliva at the biting site and its potential effect on the transmission and the development of pathogens suggests the possibility to control parasite transmission by vaccinating the host with immunogenic salivary compounds [54, 74]. In a mouse model, it has been shown that two salivary proteins (29 and 100 kDa) of the female *An. gambiae* can induce production of Ab which can block about 75% of the invasion of *An. stephensi* salivary glands by *P. yoelii* sporozoites [75]. In addition, the prior exposition to non infective *An. stephensi* bites induces a Th1 immune response with increased production of IL-12 and IFN-γ. Its effect can subsequently limit future *P. yoelii* infection (reduced rate of liver and blood parasites) and the development of cerebral malaria in mouse [18]. In this context, saliva can be thought as a non-specific "adjuvant" which could be effective at inducing a Th1-biased environment that is known to be protective against malaria infection. However, the development of such vaccines is complex. For example, Ab produced by immunization (with salivary proteins) must be ingested by the mosquito during a bite, cross it midgut and digestive enzymes, migrate to the salivary glands, before they can block the invasion by sporozoites. Nevertheless, the possibility to develop a pan-arthropod vaccine has been recently demonstrated by another mechanism. Indeed, an immune response directed to salivary proteins that adsorb to pathogens can turn the microorganism into an innocent bystander of anti-salivary immunity as it has been recently reported in a salivary protein (Salp15) from the hard tick *Ixodes scapularis* [76] and vaccine candidate for the control of Lyme disease [77]. Unfortunately, any hematophagous arthropod saliva-based vaccine has not yet been tested on humans.

In the field of allergic reactions to salivary proteins of mosquitoes, the first studies were mainly conducted in Canada and Finland. They concerned *Aedes* and *Culex* mosquitoes which express a panel of allergens in their saliva during the blood feeding time [17, 56, 78]. These proteins can thus be used in recombinant form, as diagnostic tool of the level of human exposure to allergens or in immunotherapy injections for desensitization of human [56, 70, 79]. It exists yet no study highlighting the presence and effect of allergens in the *Anopheles* mosquitoes' saliva.

The study of immunological relationship between human-vector by quantifying specific Ab responses to salivary proteins may also allow the identification and characterization of biological markers for epidemiological assessment of the exposure of individuals and populations to the *Anopheles* bites and thus to the risk of malaria transmission [22]. The development of such biomarkers or indicators (see next chapter) can be a complementary alternative to current referent entomological and parasitological methods which present several limitations especially in low exposure/transmission contexts.

3. Development of biomarkers of human exposure to *Anopheles* bites and indicators of malaria vector control effectiveness

3.1. Validation of concept with whole *Anopheles* saliva

To improve the fight against malaria and regarding numerous limitations described with current entomological and parasitological tools, the World Health Organization (WHO) has emphasized the need of new indicators and methods to evaluate, at individual and population levels, the exposure level to *Anopheles* vectors and the effectiveness of vector control strategies. One promising concept is based on the fact that mosquito saliva injected to the human host during the vector bite is antigenic and can induce an adaptive humoral host response (see Figure 1). Therefore, a logical positive correlation between the human exposure level to *Anopheles* bites and human anti-mosquito saliva Ab level can be expected. In this way, anti-mosquito saliva Ab response can be a pertinent epidemiological biomarker of human exposure to vector bites.

The epidemiological importance of human exposure to the saliva of vectors has been firstly described in Lyme disease [80, 81], leishmaniasis [82] and Chagas disease [83]. During the last decade, studies have provided data on human exposure to anopheline saliva and its interaction with malaria transmission. In particular, Remoue *et al.* [22] have shown that children living in a seasonal malaria transmission region of Senegal developed IgG responses to *An. gambiae* whole saliva (WS). Interestingly, these specific IgG levels were positively associated with an increased rainfall and the *Anopheles* mosquito density, measured by referent entomological methods. Indeed, an increase in the level of IgG was observed according to the *Anopheles* aggressiveness and density in September (Figure 2), the peak of malaria transmission.

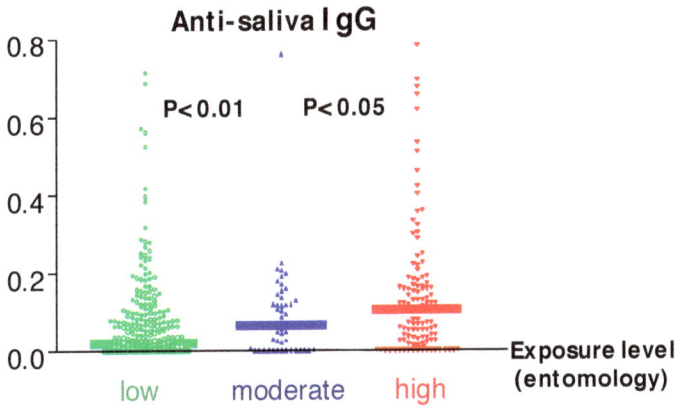

Figure 2. Anti-saliva IgG according to the intensity of exposure [22]. Individual absorbance (OD) values in September are shown for the three groups with different levels of exposure. Bars indicate the median value for each group. Statistical significances between each group by non-parametric Mann–Whitney U-test are indicated.

Importantly, IgG response to *An. gambiae* WS can predict clinical malaria cases. Indeed, children who developed a malaria attack in December had higher levels of anti-WS IgG in September of the same year, i.e. three months before they develop the disease (Figure 3) [22].

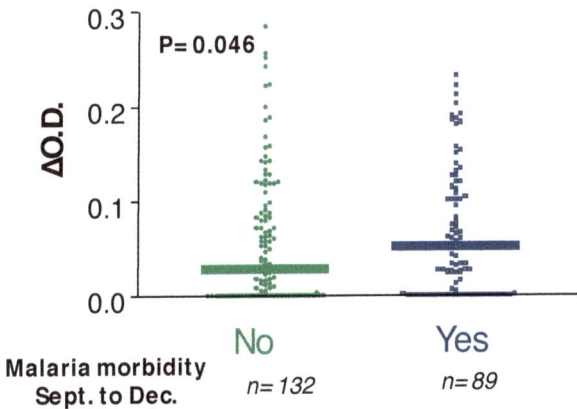

Figure 3. Anti-salivary IgG according to malaria morbidity. The results of individual absorbance (OD) values in September are shown according to subsequent detection of clinical malaria for the age ≥1 year. Bars indicate the median value for each group. Statistical significance between groups is indicated by a non-parametric Mann–Whitney U-test).

Anti-mosquito saliva Ab appeared transitional. Soldier travelers transiently exposed to *An. gambiae* bites in endemic areas of Africa (especially Ivory Coast and Gabon) developed specific

IgG responses to anti-*An. gambiae* WS which strongly decreased several weeks after the end of their trip [21]. In addition, anti-*An. gambiae* saliva IgG levels waned rapidly after 6 weeks of Insecticide-Treated Nets (ITNs) well-use in a semi-urban population in Angola, before a new significant increase two months later following the stop of ITN use [84]. Data on human exposure to anopheline saliva and its interaction with malaria were also provided by studies from other none African areas. In South-eastern Asia, it has been described that anti-*An. dirus* salivary protein Ab occur predominantly in patients with acute *P. falciparum* or *P. vivax* malaria; people from non-endemic areas do not carry such Abs [23]. In the Americas, the presence of anti-*Anopheles* saliva Ab has been also described. In adult volunteers from Brazil, anti-*An. darlingi* WS Ab levels increased with *P. vivax* infections [20]. The presence of anti-*An. albimanus* WS Ab with exposure to mosquito bite has been recently described in Haiti [25]. Specific IgG response to *An. gambiae* WS has also been described as an immunological indicator evaluating the efficacy of malaria vector control strategies. Indeed, Drame *et al.* have recently shown in a semi-urban area (Lobito, Provence Benguela) in Angola that specific IgG levels drastically decreased after the introduction of ITNs and this was associated with a drop in parasite load (Figure 4) [84].

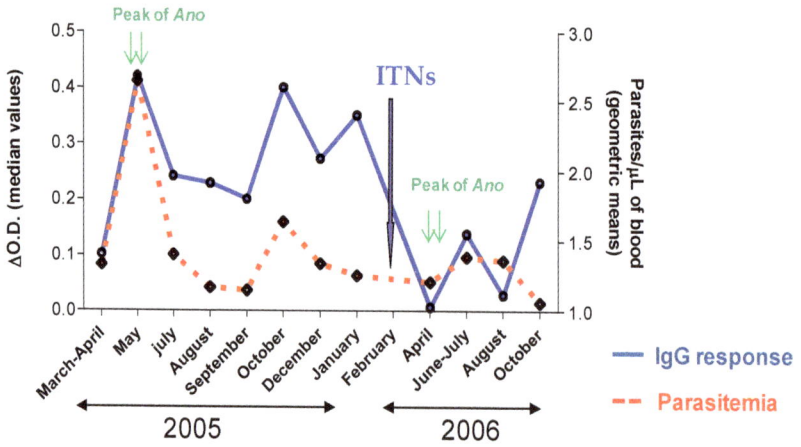

Figure 4. Evolution of anti-*Anopheles* gambiae saliva IgG and *Plasmodium falciparum* infections before and after ITN implementation, (Ano=*Anopheles*).

Anti-*Anopheles* saliva IgG response has also been recently used to evaluate and compare the effectiveness of three malaria vector control strategies in another area (Balombo) of Angola [85]. Indeed, Brosseau *et al.* [85] have investigated over a period of two years (2008-2009) Ab response to *An. gambiae* WS in children between 2 to 9 years old, before and after the introduction of three different malaria vector control methods: deltamethrin treated long lasting impregnated nets (LLIN) and insecticide treated plastic sheeting (ITPS) - Zero Fly®) (ITPS-ZF), deltamethrin impregnated Durable (Wall) Lining (ITPS-DL-Zerovector®) alone, and indoor residual spraying

(IRS) with lambdacyhalothrin alone. They observed considerable decreases in entomological (82.4%), parasitological (54.8%) and immunological criteria analyzed. In particular, the immunological data based on the level of anti-saliva IgG Ab in children of all villages significantly dropped from 2008 to 2009, especially with LLIN+ZF and with IRS (Figure 5).

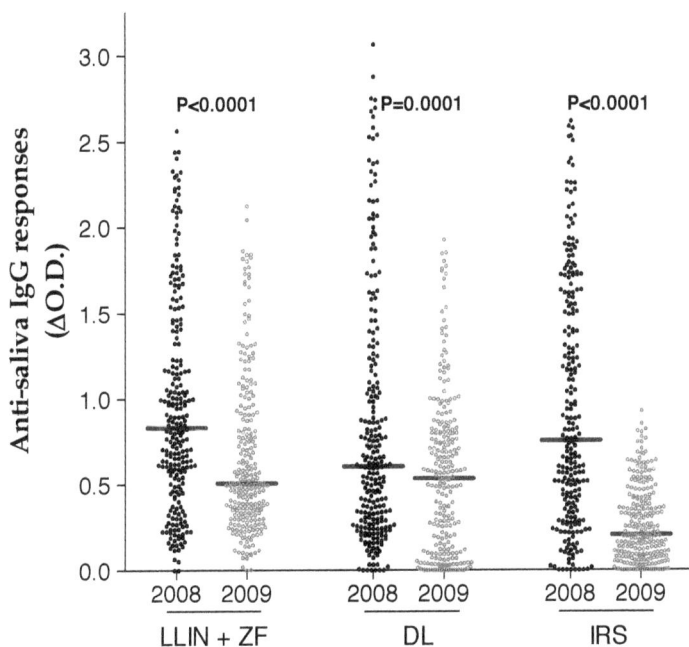

Figure 5. Comparison of median values of the IgG antibody response to *Anopheles* saliva obtained before and after implementation of each vector control method [85].

Taken together, these studies indicated that the estimation of human IgG Ab responses specific to *Anopheles* WS could provide a reliable biomarker for evaluating the *Anopheles* exposure level, the risk of malaria transmission, the disease outcomes and the effectiveness of vector control strategies. However, the pertinence and the practical large-scale application of serological tests for epidemiological purposes have been hampered by several limitations. First, WS is a cocktail of various molecular components with different nature and biological functions. Some components are *Anopheles*-specific and other widely distributed within genus, families, orders or classes of bloodsucking *Diptera* or Arthropods [16]. Therefore, the evaluation of *Anopheles* exposure or vector control effectiveness based on the immunogenicity of WS could be skewed and over or underestimated by possible cross-reactivities between common epitopes between mosquito species or other organisms [26]. Second, the collection of saliva or salivary gland extracts is tedious and time-consuming; therefore it will be difficult or impossible to have an adequate production of mosquito saliva needed for large-scale epidemiological studies [26].

Third, saliva composition can be affected by several ecological parameters such as age, feeding status or infectivity of *Anopheles* [86],which in turn may influence the anti-saliva immune response measured and may cause a lack of reproducibility between saliva batches. An alternative for optimizing the specificity of this immunological test would thus be to identify *Anopheles* genus-specific proteins [87].

3.2. Methods for the identification of specific *Anopheles* salivary proteins

The isolation of salivary components has been a challenge for many years. Many functional active salivary proteins have been isolated following classical biochemical and molecular biology approaches [88]. Protocols mainly consisted of the isolation of salivary components from hundreds of salivary gland pairs, obtaining amino-terminal or internal peptide sequence of the purified component, screening of a salivary gland library with the information obtained, and isolation of the cDNA or gene of interest (Fig. 6).

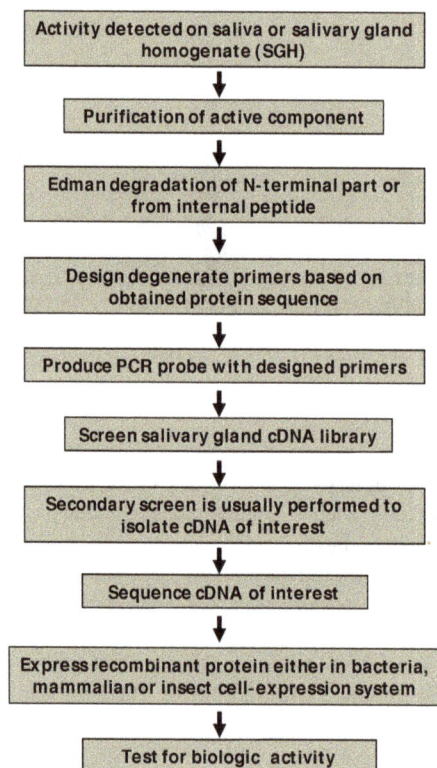

Figure 6. Classical biochemical and molecular biology protocol used for isolation and characterisation of salivary proteins and cDNA from vectors of disease [90].

During the last decade, technical advances in molecular biology have allowed the sequencing of the genome, including transcripts of salivary glands [89], of most disease vectors, comprising *Anopheles* mosquitoes [90]. However, protocols do not allow to obtain entire sequences [89]. Nowadays, researchers have switched from testing one salivary molecule at a time to studying the whole complex of genes and secreted proteins in blood-feeding arthropods using transcriptomic and/or proteomic approaches. The transcriptomic is the complete set of transcripts in an organism for a specific developmental stage or physiological condition. Transcriptomic techniques help to interpret the functional elements of the genome, and to understand the transmission and development of diseases [91]. They aim to catalogue transcript of major *Anopheles* species, including mRNAs, non-coding RNAs and small RNAs; to determine the transcriptional structure of genes and to quantify the changing expression levels of each transcript during development and under different conditions [91]. Proteomic is a large-scale study of the gene expression at the protein level, which ultimately provides direct measurement of protein expression levels [92]. The proteomic revolution is hitting the vector biology field as well as many other fields. The isolation and sequencing of all the proteins from SGs of disease vectors and, more specifically, secreted salivary proteins, is clarifying the complexity of proteins present in the saliva of various blood-feeding arthropods [93]. During the last years, a comprehensive high-throughput approach has been developed (Figure 7) [88]. It combines massive sequencing protocol of high quality full-length salivary gland cDNA libraries, a proteomic approach to isolate a large set of salivary proteins, and high-throughput computational biology and functional assays to analyze and test the biologic activities of these novel molecules. It is a powerful tool which can help easily and rapidly to identify and characterize genes or transcripts encoding for various proteins of SGs (the sialome) of blood-sucking arthropods. This high-throughput approach has then allowed an unprecedented insight into the complexity of salivary gland compounds of mosquito vectors of disease agents, indicating that the diversity of their targets is still larger than previously thought [16].

3.3. Salivary proteins (sialome) of *Anopheles* mosquitoes

The increasing power of large-scale genomic, transcriptomic and proteomic analyses allowed the accumulation of a considerable amount of information on the salivary secretions of blood-sucking arthropods [86]. As far as mosquitoes are concerned, the analysis of salivary transcriptomes of a number of *Anopheles* have allowed the discovery of a variety of genes that matched the sequence of various protein families, providing some clues on the evolution of blood feeding [15, 41-43, 92, 94-100]. Many of the salivary protein sequences are coded by genes related to intrinsic functions of the cell (housekeeping genes). However, the large number of salivary proteins is secreted during plant or blood feeding. Finally, a little number has no similarities to sequences deposited in databases, representing unknown and novel sequences [41, 94, 101]. This emphasizes how much still need to be learned concerning the biological functions of salivary proteins in blood feeding, pathogen transmission and manipulation of host responses.

The analysis of the adult *Anopheles* sialome has shown that secreted proteins and/or peptides (secretome) can be ubiquitous or specific to arthropod classes, orders, families, genus or species

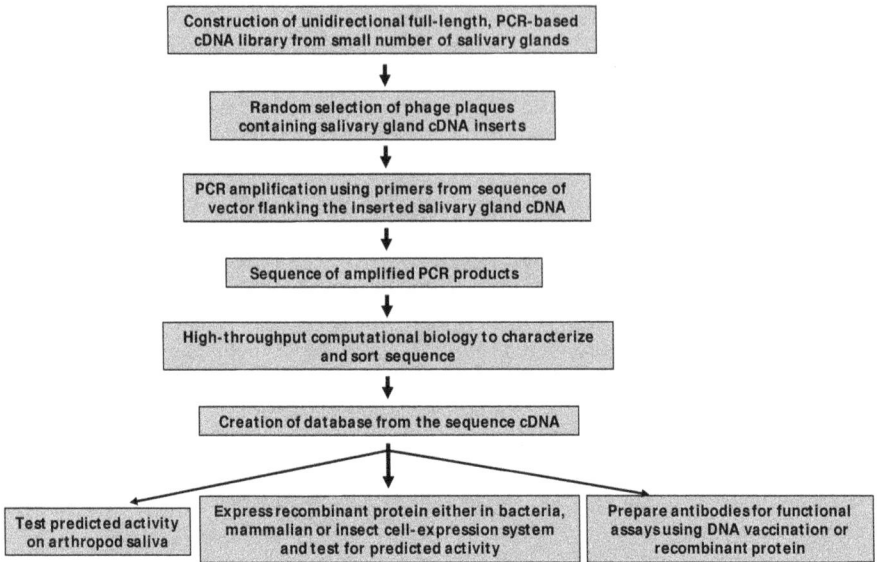

Figure 7. Current high-throughput strategies used for the isolation and characterisation of salivary cDNA and proteins from disease vectors [90].

[44, 101, 102]. In *An. gambiae* salivary gland females over 70 putative secreted salivary proteins have been identified [94].

3.3.1. Ubiquitous salivary proteins

AG5 family proteins are found in the salivary glands of many blood-sucking insects and ticks [102, 103]. In *An. gambiae*, four proteins belonging to this family were identified, but only one (putative gVAG protein precursor) was coding for transcripts enriched in the adult female SGs [94]. A precursor of gVAG protein was also described in *An. funestus* (84% sequence identity) and *An. stephensi* (85% sequence identity) sialome [95, 100]. The function of any AG5 protein in the saliva of any blood-sucking arthropod is still unknown.

Enzymes such as maltase, apyrase, 5′ nucleotidase, and adenosine deaminase, are also secreted during the bite of many blood-sucking arthropods, including *Anopheles* mosquitoes [95]. They generally assist in sugar feeding (maltase) or in degradation of purinergic mediators of platelet aggregation (apyrase, 5′ nucleotidases) and inflammation (adenosine deaminase).

3.3.2. Salivary proteins found exclusively in Diptera

D7 family proteins are specific to SGs of blood-sucking Nematocera, including mosquitoes and sand flies [104, 105]. They are highly represented in the sialome of *Anopheles* mosquitoes in short and long forms [95, 96, 101, 104, 105]. *An. funestus* D7 proteins vary between 64% and

75% identity with their *An. gambiae* closest match [105]. D7 proteins could act as anti-hemostatic factors by trapping agonists of hemostasis [44, 47]. However, further investigations are needed to clearly describe their function.

Other Diptera-specific protein families or peptides have also been described in the sialome of blood-feeding mosquitoes [95]. However their function is still unknown, even if some were known to play a role in antimicrobial property of mosquito saliva.

3.3.3. Protein families found exclusively in mosquitoes

The 30-kDa antigen family found exclusively in the SGs of adult female mosquitoes has been found in both culicine and anopheline mosquitoes [95, 100, 101, 106-108]. Only one gene enriched in SGs of adult females is known in *An. gambiae*. The *An. funestus* homologue is also abundantly expressed and shares 63% identity with the *An. gambiae* orthologue. The function of this protein family is still unknown [95].

The *gSG (An. gambiae Salivary Gland)-5 family* was first discovered in the SGs of *An. gambiae* and shown to be exclusively expressed in the adult female [94, 109]. This protein shows a high similarity to *Aedes* and *Culex* proteins [101]. Transcripts coding for this family were found in the sialotranscriptome of *An. darlingi* with 46% identical to the *An. gambiae* orthologue and only 26% and 23% identical to the culicine proteins [101]. The function of this mosquito-specific protein remains unknown, but its tissue- and sex-specific expression profile suggests it is possibly related to blood feeding.

The *gSG8 family* is highly divergent with members only found in *An. gambiae* and *Ae. aegypti*. In *An. gambiae*, this protein is specifically expressed in female SGs [109], suggesting a likely role in blood feeding.

Various types of *mucins* have been described in the saliva of adult mosquitoes and may function/act as a lubricant of their mouthparts [15, 41, 94, 102]. Three mucins encoding transcripts have been identified in the *An. gambiae* larval SG [110], suggesting the importance of mucins at multiple developmental stages. Mucins may also play a crucial role in *Anopheles* salivary gland invasion by *P. berghei* sporozoites [111]. Several protein families are also represented in this group, including gSG-3, gSG-10, and 13.5-kDa families [101]. These families were also found abundantly expressed in the sialotranscriptome of *An. gambiae* adult male [112], indicating their function is not related specifically to blood feeding.

3.3.4. Protein families found exclusively in Anophelines

Anophelin was described as a short acidic peptide with strong thrombin inhibitory activity in *An. albimanus* [46]. *An. funestus* anophelin is 59% identical to the *An. gambiae* orthologue [95], and *An. darlingi* anophelin is 86% identical to *An. albimanus* [101].

The 8.2-kDa family is represented in several *Anopheles* species. In *An. funestus* the peptide have 42% identity with the 8.2-kDa salivary peptide of *An. stephensi* and similar proteins from *An. gambiae* and *An. darlingi* [95]. In *An. gambiae*, this peptide was found enriched in adult female SGs, suggesting a role in blood feeding.

The 6.2-kDa family was first described in a sialotranscriptome of *An. gambiae* [94], where it was found enriched in adult female SGs compared to other tissues. The *An. funestus* member of this family is 61% identical to the *An. gambiae* [95], and 53% to an *An. darlingi* [101] homologues.

The SG-1 family proteins appear to be exclusively expressed in the female SGs of *Anopheles* mosquitoes and not observed in other tissues [94, 101]. However, their function remains to be determined.

The SG-2 family proteins were identified from *An. gambiae* saliva and shown to be expressed in female SGs and adult males but not in other tissues [113]. Related, but very divergent, sequences were obtained from salivary transcriptomes of other anopheline species [95, 101]. Because this protein family is expressed in both male and female *An. gambiae*, and due to its relatively small size, it may display antimicrobial function [101].

The *hyp 8.2* and *hyp 6.2 proteins* are similarly enriched in *An. gambiae* adult female SGs [94]. *An. stephensi* and *An. funestus* also have members of these protein families.

The *SG-7/Anophensin family* is also unique to anophelines. In *An. gambiae*, it is highly enriched in female SGs [94]. More recently, the *An. stephensi* homologue was determined to inhibit kallikrein and production of bradykinin, a pain-producing substance [114]. Four putative alleles representing the homologue(s) of gSG7 in *An. darlingi* were identified. These *An. darlingi* transcripts have no more than 45% identity to the *An. gambiae* gSG7 and *An. stephensi* anophensin [101].

The *SG6 protein* is a small protein first described in *An. gambiae* [109] and a unique sequence codes for a mature peptide/protein of ~10 kDa (116 amino-acids) with ten cysteine residues making probably five disulphide bonds. A homologue was later found in the sialotranscrip-tome of *An. stephensi* [100] and *An. funestus* [95]. *An. funestus* SG6/fSG6 (f for funestus) has 81% and 76% identities with *An. stephensi* and *An. gambiae* polypeptides, respectively. It is not found in the transcriptomes of the Culicinae subfamily members analyzed so far, i.e. *C. pipiens quinquefasciatus*, *Ae. aegypti* and *Ae. albopictus* [108, 115, 116]. In *An. gambiae*, the transcript coding for gSG6 (g for *gambiae*) was found to be 16 times more expressed in SGs of adult females than in males [94]. The gSG6 protein plays some essential blood feeding role and was recruited in the anopheline subfamily most probably after the separation of the lineage which gave origin to *Cellia* and *Anopheles* subgenera [99]. The gSG6 protein, because immunogenic, can be therefore a reliable indicator of human exposure specific to *Anopheles* mosquito bites [99], vectors of malaria.

3.4. Specific salivary biomarker of exposure to *Anopheles* bites: The gSG6-P1 peptide candidate

The SG6 salivary protein has been reported to be immunogenic in travelers exposed for short periods to *Anopheles* bites [21], and in Senegalese children living in a malaria endemic area by an immuno-proteomic, coupling 2D immunoblot and mass spectrometry [117], and by an ELISA [26] approaches. Recently, its immunogenicity has been confirmed in individuals from a malaria hyperendemic area of Burkina Faso [118, 119], by using a recombinant form expressed as purified N-terminal His-tagged recombinant protein in the *E. coli* vector pET28b(+) (Novagen) [99, 119].

A

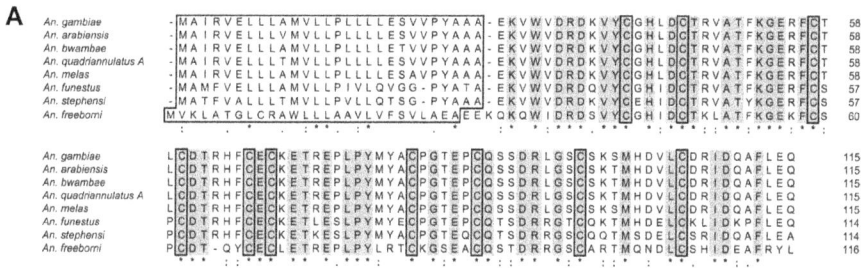

B

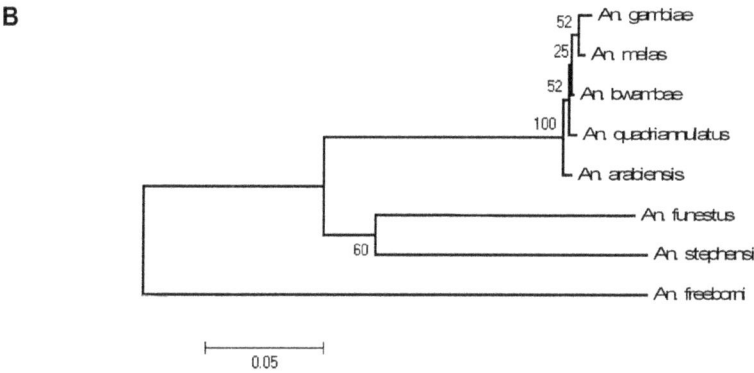

Figure 8. Sequences of the anopheline gSG6 proteins [99]. (A) Clustal alignment of anopheline gSG6 proteins. Signal peptides and conserved Cysteines are boxed. Conserved sites are shaded. (B) Phylogenetic tree (NJ algorithm, boot-strapped 10,000 times) constructed from the alignment of the nucleotide sequence encoding the mature gSG6 poly-peptides.

In particular, increased anti-gSG6 IgG levels were observed in exposed individuals during the malaria transmission/rainy season [119]. In addition, anti-gSG6 IgG response appeared to be a reliable serological indicator of exposure to bites of the main African malaria vectors (*An. gambiae*, *An. arabiensis* and *An. funestus*) in the same area [119]. However, gSG6 recombinant protein has been described to relatively generate a high background in control sera from individuals not exposed to *Anopheles* bites, and considerable variations in specific Ab response between children supposed to be similarly exposed to *Anopheles* bites [26]. Therefore, with the objective of optimizing *Anopheles* specificity and reproducibility of the immunological assay, a peptide design approach was undertaken using bioinformatic tools [26].

3.4.1. Identification and sequence of gSG6-P1 peptide

Several algorithms were employed for prediction of potential immunogenic sites of the gSG6 protein by using bioinformatics. The prediction of immunogenicity was based on the deter-mination of physico-chemical properties of the amino-acid (AA) sequences with BcePred and FIMM databases and on the identification of MHC class 2 binding regions using the ProPred-2 online service. This led to define five gSG6 peptides (gSG6-P1 to gSG6-P5) of 20 to 27 AA residues in length (Fig. 9), overlapping by at least 3 residues and spanning the entire sequence of the mature gSG6 protein. Both predictive methods for putative linear B-cell epitopes (FIMM and BcePred) assigned the highest immunogenicity to gSG6-P1, gSG6-P2, gSG6-P3, and then gSG6-P4.

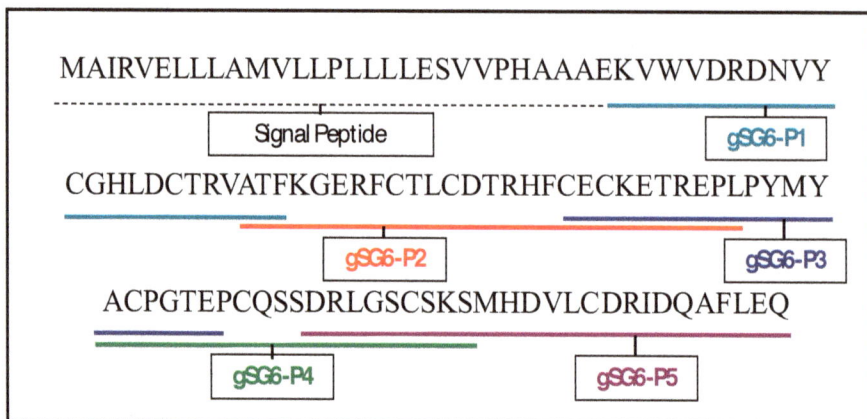

Figure 9. Amino-acid sequence of gSG6 Peptides. Amino-acid sequence of the SG6 protein of *Anopheles gambiae* (gi: 13537666) is presented and sequences of the selected peptides, gSG6-P1 to gSG6-P5, are underlined. Signal peptide (SP) sequence is indicating by dotted underline [26].

Similarities were also searched using the Blast family programs, including both the genome/EST libraries of other vector arthropods available in Vectorbase and of pathogens/ organisms in non-redundant GenBank CDS databases. No relevant identity was found with proteins of other blood-sucking arthropods. Indeed, the longest perfect match was 6 AAs between a putative protein from *Pediculus humanus* and gSG6-P2 and gSG6-P3 peptides. In the case of gSG6-P1, the best match was 4 AAs in length with *Culex pipiens quinquefasciatus* salivary adenosine deaminase. Moreover, no relevant similarity was found with sequences from pathogens or other organisms. The highest hits of gSG6-P1 were with the cyanobacterium *Microcystis aeruginosa* (3 AAs) and with *Ostreococcus* OsV5 virus (4 AAs). Altogether, this analysis confirmed the *bona fide* high specificity of the five selected gSG6 peptides for the *Anopheles* species. Peptides were then synthesized.

3.4.2. Antigenicity of gSG6 peptides

IgG Ab responses to the five gSG6 peptides were evaluated by ELISA in a randomly selected subsample of children (n<30) living in a rural area of Senegal. All peptides were immunogenic, but the intensity of the IgG level was clearly peptide-dependent; weak immunogenicity was observed for gSG6-P3, gSG6-P4 and gSG6-P5, whereas gSG6-P1 and gSG6-P2 appeared highly immunogenic (Fig. 10).

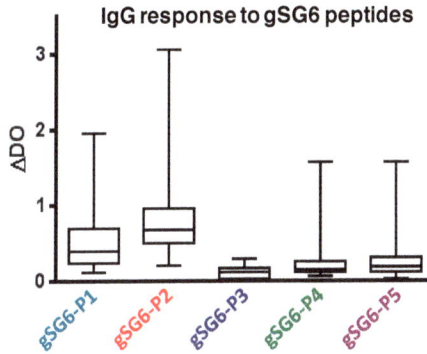

Figure 10. IgG antibody response according to gSG6 peptides [26]. For each peptide, the IgG Ab level was evaluated in a subsample of exposed children. Results at the peak of the season of *Anopheles* exposure are reported according to gSG6 peptides. Results are presented by box plot graph where lines of the boxes represent the 75th percentile, median and 25th percentile of individual average ΔOD values; whiskers represent the lower and upper adjacent values.

3.4.3. Validation as a biomarker of exposure in several epidemiological settings

The specific IgG level to the two most antigenic gSG6 peptides (gSG6-P1 et gSG6-P2) was then evaluated according to the level of exposure (estimated by entomological data) in a larger sample (n=241) of children living in a malaria seasonal area [26]. A positive trend was found for both peptides, but only significant for gSG6-P1 (Figure 11). Altogether, these results indicated that only the IgG response to gSG6-P1 is suitable to be a pertinent biomarker of exposure to *Anopheles* bites and thus to risk of malaria.

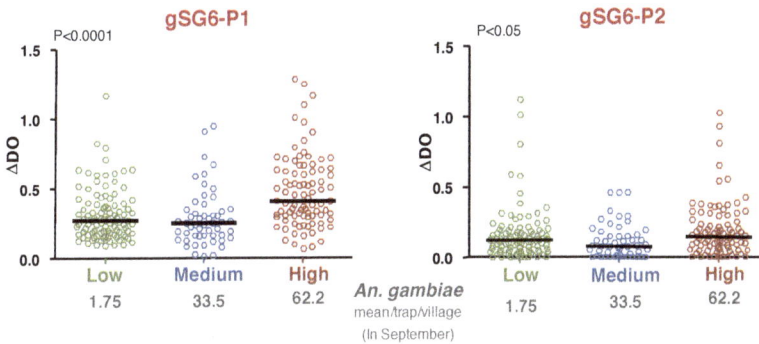

Figure 11. IgG response to gSG6-P1 and gSG6-P2 according to intensity of exposure to *Anopheles* gambiae bites [26]. Individual ΔOD (Optical Density) values in September (peak of the season of *Anopheles* exposure) are shown for the three different exposure groups. Results are presented for the same children (n=241) for gSG6-P1 (A) and gSG6-P2 (B). Exposure groups were defined by entomological data. Bars indicate median value for each exposure group. Statistical significance between the 3 groups is indicated (non-parametric Mann-Whitney U-test).

Therefore, the gSG6-P1 was selected as the most pertinent candidate as marker of exposure. Indeed, this peptide appeared to satisfy several requirements that an exposure biomarker should fulfill. First, it thus far appears to be specific to *Anopheles* genus and therefore, no relevant cross-reactivity phenomena with epitopes from other proteins of arthropods or pathogens would be expected. Second, because it is of a synthetic nature, it guarantees high reproducibility of the immunological assay. Third, it elicits a specific Ab response which correlates well with the level of exposure to *An. gambiae* bites.

3.4.3.1. Biomarker of Anopheles *vector bites*

As previously suggested, anti-gSG6-P1 IgG response was described as a biomarker of *An. gambiae* bites in children living in Senegalese villages where malaria transmission seasonally and moderately occurred [26]. In the same area, a specific IgG response to the peptide has been detected in 36% of children living in villages where very few *An. gambiae*, or none, were collected by classical entomological methods [28]. This deals with a high sensitivity and specificity of the gSG6-P1 epitope(s) after a low immunological boost induced by weak bites exposure. This result points to the potential use of such serological tool as an epidemiological biomarker of *An. gambiae* bites in very low exposure areas, where the sensitivity of current entomological methods of malaria risk assessment is weak.

One study aimed to evaluate the risk of malaria transmission in children and adults living in urban area of Senegal (Dakar region) by using the gSG6-P1 peptide biomarker. Results showed considerable individual variations in anti-gSG6-P1 IgG levels between and within districts, in spite of a context of a global low *Anopheles* exposure level and malaria transmission [27]. Despite this individual heterogeneity, the median level of specific IgG and the percentage of immune responders differed significantly between districts. In addition, a positive association was observed between the exposure levels to *An. gambiae* bites, estimated by classical entomological methods, and the median IgG levels or the percentage of immune responders reflecting the real contact between human populations and *Anopheles* mosquitoes [27]. Differences in exposure levels to *An. gambiae* bites could then partly explain district and/or group-variations in anti-gSG6-P1 IgG Ab response as previously described in a low-exposure rural area of Senegal [28]. Interestingly, in urban Dakar area, immunological parameters seemed to better discriminate the *Anopheles* exposure level between different groups compared to referent entomological data. Moreover, in this study, some discrepancies were observed in the correlation between immunological parameters and the exposure level to *An. gambiae* bites assessed by entomological data in districts. This suggests the main role of the human behavior influencing the contact with vectors. A differential use of Vector Control Measures (ITNs, sprays, curtains) can for example drastically reduce human-vector contact. Many household characteristics (height, type, use of air conditioning, well-closed windows), which can differ between districts, could also be crucial factors. Importantly, the effect of these factors may be not taken into account by assessing the mosquito exposure level and malaria risk with classical entomological tools. This strengthens the usefulness of such biomarker as an alternative tool in the evaluation of exposure levels to *Anopheles* bites, especially in low/very low exposure, where current entomological methods can give inaccurate estimations of the human-mosquito contact [27].

In a population from a malaria hyperendemic area of Burkina Faso, the use of gSG6 recombinant protein as reliable indicator of exposure to the 3 main African malaria vectors (*An. gambiae s.s.*, *An. arabiensis* and *An. funestus*) has been suggested [119]. This probably could be relied to a wide cross-reactivity between SG6 sequences of principal *Anopheles* vectors, which highly share identical epitopes between species. Moreover, the gSG6-P1 peptide has been used to accurately evaluate the exposure level to *An. funestus* bites in a rural area in Senegal [29]. Indeed, two-thirds of 2-9 years old children from this area developed an IgG response to gSG6-P1, in an area where *An. funestus* only was reported. In addition, IgG response increased during the *An. funestus* exposure season, and a positive association was observed with the level of exposure to *An. funestus* bites [29]. This result deals with the cross-reactivity between *An. gambiae* gSG6-P1 and *An. funestus* fSG6-P1 sequences which share a high level of identity. Indeed, these sequences differ only by the substitution of two AAs: asparagine by glutamine (position 9) and leucine by isoleucine (position 15) (Fig. 12).

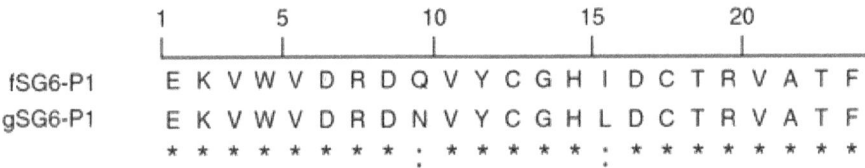

```
     1        5        10       15       20
     |        |        |        |        |
     └────────┴────────┴────────┴────────┴──────

fSG6-P1    E  K  V  W  V  D  R  D  Q  V  Y  C  G  H  I  D  C  T  R  V  A  T  F
gSG6-P1    E  K  V  W  V  D  R  D  N  V  Y  C  G  H  L  D  C  T  R  V  A  T  F
           *  *  *  *  *  *  *  *  :  *  *  *  *  *  :  *  *  *  *  *  *  *  *
```

Figure 12. Sequences of the SG6-P1 salivary peptide [29]. Sequences are shown for *An. funestus* (fSG6-P1), for *An. gambiae* (gSG6-P1). Identities are marked with '*' and strong AA conservations with ':'.

AAs from fSG6-P1 are close in terms of polarity and charge to those from *An. gambiae* gSG6-P1. The main consequence is that individuals exposed to *An. funestus* bites can sufficiently develop a specific Ab response against gSG6-P1 *An. gambiae* antigen. This observation, in conjunction with present results, suggests that these substitutions do not alter the synthesis and the recognition of specific Ab because epitope appears to be conserved.

All mentioned studies were conducted on subjects older than 1 year. However, to be more relevant in epidemiological surveys and studies on malaria, such biomarker tool must pertinently be applicable to all human age-classes, including newborns and young infants (<1 year old) who can be also bitten by *Anopheles* and at high risk of malaria transmission [120]. In this way, a recent study has indicated that human Ab responses to gSG6-P1 biomarker help to assess *Anopheles* exposure level and the risk of malaria in younger than 1 year old infants living in moderate to high transmission area of Benin (Drame *et al.*, submitted).

Indeed, the presence of anti-gSG6-P1 IgG and IgM in the blood of respectively 93.28 and 41.79% of 3-months old infants (the majority of infants) and their gradual increasing levels until 12 months (Fig. 13), whatever the *Anopheles* exposure level or the season. These observations are consistent with the development and maturation patterns of the newborn immune system during the first months of life. Indeed, the immature human immune system completes its maturation during infancy following exposition to antigens. Therefore, newborns are naive and increasingly susceptible to infectious agents; their immune system is not or insufficiently

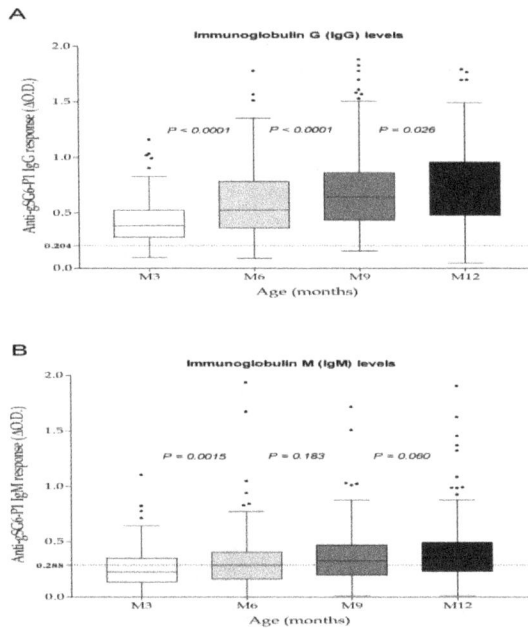

Figure 13. IgG and IgM responses to *Anopheles* gSG6-P1 salivary peptide in the first year-life. Individual IgG (A) and IgM (B) responses to the *Anopheles* gSG6-P1 are represented for infants in months 3 (white), 6 (light-gray), 9 (dark-gray) and 12 (black box) after their birth. Horizontal lines in the boxes indicate medians of the individual data. Horizontal black dotted lines represent the cut-off of IgG (0.204) and IgM (0.288) responder. Statistical significant differences between all age groups (multivariate linear mixed model analysis) are indicated.

stimulated by antigens. In endemic malaria transmission area, they are progressively exposed to salivary antigens of *Anopheles* [121], probably explaining the progressive increase of anti-gSG6-P1 IgG and IgM from 3 to 12 months-old. Individual or population factors and behaviors enhancing the level of the human-*Anopheles* contact with age can play a crucial role on accelerating this gradual acquisition [122, 123].

3.4.3.2. Factors of variation of antibody response to gSG6-P1 and their consequences

Specific gSG6-P1 Ab responses can be influenced by several determinant factors in their variations between individuals, districts, villages, regions... Therefore, identifying effects of human intrinsic (gender, age...) and extrinsic (period of sampling, use of vector control measure...) factors will be useful to the application of the gSG6-P1 biomarker in epidemiological studies or monitoring, evaluation and surveillance of risk of malaria programmes.

Effect of age

Studies have globally reported an increasing anti-gSG6-P1 Ab level according to individual age. In a moderate transmission semi-urban area in Angola, the lowest and highest specific

IgG levels have been described in young children (0-7 years old) and in teenagers/ adults (>14 years old) respectively [30]. In a low malaria transmission urban area (Dakar region) in Senegal, specific IgG levels were significantly higher in adults (>18 years old) compared to 6-10 years old children and in this latter group compared to those aged from 2 to 5 years [27] [124]. In Tori Bossito, moderate-high rural transmission area of Benin, both anti-gSG6-P1 IgG and IgM levels were low at 3 months of age and gradually increased until 12 months after birth (Drame et al., submitted). The increase of specific IgG response with age is consistent with the gradual acquired immunity against Anopheles mosquito saliva [30] following the development of individual factors and behaviors enhancing the probability of human-vector contact [122, 123]. However, few data have reported a decrease of IgG levels to gSG6-P1 peptide [28] or to SG6 protein [118] with age. In particular, in Senegalese children (0 to 60 months old), the highest specific IgG levels were reported in the youngest children in spite of a probable very weak exposure to An. gambiae [30]. It can be explained by a passive IgG transfer from mother to child during pregnancy or breastfeeding as recently reported in young infants from Benin (Drame et al., submitted). This represents a way of overestimation of the assessment of human-Anopheles contact level and the risk of malaria in young infants by using anti-gSG6-P1 IgG Ab. Therefore, the evaluation of specific IgM Ab levels could be a relevant solution to bias in IgG measurements. Indeed, IgM Ab, in a form of polymers (usually pentamers) in the human organism, could not cross the maternal-foetal barrier [125] and are the first Ab to appear in response to initial or primary exposure to antigen [126]. Interestingly, in Tori Bossito, specific IgM levels seemed to be a serological marker only during the first 6-months of exposure. In infants older to 6 months, the assessment of gSG6-P1-specific IgG showed a more pertinent evaluation of exposure level.

Effect of sex

Some studies have reported higher levels of anti-gSG6-P1 in female individuals (children and women) compared to males (children and men) [27, 30] ([124]; Drame et al., submitted). However, this difference was not significant, suggesting that it might be only physiological.

The season of Anopheles exposure

The season of individual sampling may be also a factor of confusion in the use gSG6-P1 biomarker in epidemiological studies on malaria risk assessment or control. Indeed, significant seasonal-ly variations in anti-gSG6-P1 IgG or/and IgM levels have been reported in studies conducted in newborns, children or/and adults from endemic malaria areas in Senegal [27-29, 124], Angola [30] and Benin (Drame et al., submitted). In Senegal, in particular, specific gSG6-P1 in urban children and adults steadily waned from the beginning (October) to the end (December) of the study, due to an important drop in human exposure level to An. gambiae s. l. bites from the end of rainfalls (October) to the beginning of the dry season (December) [127, 128].

One direct application of a salivary biomarker of exposure could serve in the elaboration of maps representing the risk of exposure to Anopheles bites. Such immuno-epidemiological marker might represent a quantitative tool applied to field conditions and a complementary tool to those currently available, such as entomological, ecological and environmental data [59, 129]. It could represent a geographic indicator of the risks of malaria transmission and thus a useful tool for predicting malaria morbidity risk as previously described [22]. Furthermore, it may represent a powerful tool for evaluation of vector control strategies (impregnated bednet, intradomiciliary aspersion, etc.) and could here constitute a direct criterion for effectiveness and appropriate use (malaria control program) [84].

3.4.3.3. Indicator of malaria vector control effectiveness

Long and short-term evaluation of ITN efficacy

A longitudinal study associating parasitological, entomological and immunological assessments of the efficacy of ITN-based strategies using the gSG6-P1 biomarker has been conducted in a malaria-endemic area in Angola. Human IgG responses to gSG6-P1 peptide were evaluated in 105 individuals (adults and children) before and after the introduction of ITNs and compared to entomo-parasitological data. A significant decrease of anti-gSG6-P1 IgG response was observed just after the effective use of ITNs (Fig. 14). The drop in gSG6-P1 IgG levels was associated with a considerable decrease of *P. falciparum* parasitaemia, the current WHO criterion for vector control efficacy [130]. It was particularly marked in April-August 2006, corresponding to the season peak of *An. gambiae* exposure. Interestingly, the entomological data indicated that this season-dependent peak was of similar intensity before (2005) and after (2006) ITN use, suggesting ITN installation had no impact on *An. gambiae* density, probably because of the low percentage of the overall human population covered in the studied area [131]. This study indicated also that the drop of anti-gSG6-P1 IgG response was associated with correct ITN use and not due to low *Anopheles* density. In addition, this was observed in all age groups studied (<7 years, 7–14 years, and >14 years), suggesting that this biomarker is relevant for ITN evaluation in all age groups. This rapid decrease after correct ITN usage appears to be a special property of anti-gSG6-P1 IgG which is short-lived (4-6 weeks) in the absence of ongoing antigenic stimulation, at/for all age classes.

The response does not seem to build up but wanes rapidly, when exposure failed. This property represents a major strength when using such salivary biomarker of exposure for evaluating the efficacy of vector control. In addition, using a response threshold (ΔOD=0.204) combined with ΔOD$_{ITNs}$ - the difference between April (after ITNs) and January 2006 (before) - makes possible the use of this operational biomarker at individual level (Fig. 15). The threshold response (TR) represents the non-specific background IgG response (the cut-off of immune response) and was calculated in non-*Anopheles* exposed individuals (n= 14- neg; North of France) by using this formula: TR= mean (ΔDO$_{neg}$) + 3SD = 0.204. An exposed individual was then classified as an immune responder if its ΔOD> 0.204. If the ΔOD$_{ITNs}$ value is comprised between -0.204 and +0.204, no clear difference in exposure level to *Anopheles* bites can be defined.

In contrast, if the individual ΔOD$_{ITNs}$ value <−0.204, it could be concluded with a high level of confidence that this individual is benefiting from ITN installation. The ΔOD$_{ITNs}$ parameter could therefore provide a measure of ITN efficacy at the individual level. An individual biomarker would also be relevant at the large-scale operational studies or surveillance in the field, e.g. in National Malaria Control Programs (NMCP). In addition, the high sensitivity and specificity of the gSG6-P1 Ab response make it ideal for the evaluation of low-level ex-

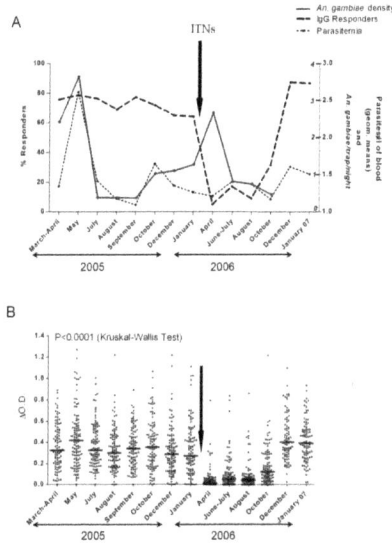

Figure 14. IgG Ab responses to gSG6-P1 before and after ITN use [30]. The percentage (%) of anti-gSG6-P1 IgG im-mune responders (thick-dotted line) in the "immunological" sub-population (n=105), before (2005) and after (2006 and January 2007) the installation of ITNs (A). These results are presented together with the intensity of *P. falciparum* infection (mean parasitaemia – fine-dotted line) measured in the same population and the mean of number of *An. gambiae* (solid line) in the studied area (A). Entomological data were not available in December 2006 and January 2007 (the last two months of the study). Arrows indicate the installation of Insecticide Treated Nets (ITNs) in February 2006. Individual anti-gSG6-P1 IgG levels (ΔOD) are presented before (2005) and after (2006) the installation of ITNs (B). Bars indicate the median value for each studied month. Statistically significant differences between months are indicated.

posure to *Anopheles bites* [27, 28], even when exposure or transmission is curtailed by NMCP efforts. Taken together, the estimation of human IgG responses to *Anopheles* gSG6-P1 could provide a reliable indicator for evaluating the efficacy of ITN-based strategies against malar-ia vectors, at individual and population levels, even after vector control generating particu-lar low exposure/transmission contexts. This salivary biomarker is a relevant tool for the evaluation of short-term efficacy as well as longer-term monitoring of malaria VCMs.

Evaluation of effectiveness of diverse vector control measures

A recent cross-sectional study conducted from October to December 2008 on 2,774 residents (children and adults) of 45 districts of urban Dakar (Senegal) has validated IgG responses to gSG6-P1 as an epidemiological indicator evaluating the effectiveness of a range of VCMs. Indeed, in this area, IgG levels to gSG6-P1 as well as the use of diverse malaria VCMs (ITNs, mosquito coils, spray bombs, ventilation and/or incense) highly varied between districts [124]. This difference of use suggests some socio-economical and cultural discrepancies between householders as described in large cities of Ivory Coast [132] and Tanzania [123]. At the district level, specific IgG levels significantly decreased with VCM use in children as well as in adults.

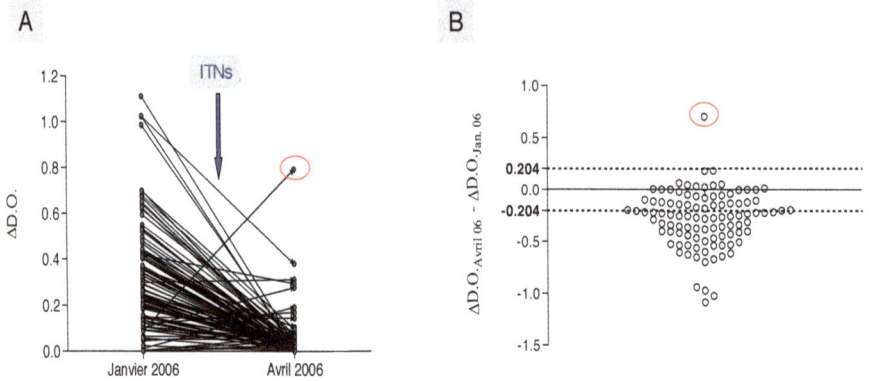

Figure 15. IgG response to gSG6-P1 as biomarker for short-term ITN efficacy. Changes in individual IgG levels (ΔOD) are presented between "just before" (January 2006) and "just after" (April 2006) ITN introduction (n=105; children and adults) (A). The arrow indicates the installation of Insecticide Treated Nets (ITNs) in February 2006. Individual IgG level changes from January (before) to April are presented (B) by individual ΔOD_{ITNs} value ($\Delta OD_{ITNs} = \Delta OD_{April06} - \Delta OD_{January06}$). The threshold of specific IgG responders (TR=0.204) is indicated (dotted line). Significant positive (ΔOD>0.204) or negative (ΔOD<−0.204) changes are therefore individually presented.

Among used VCM, ITNs, the 1st chosen preventive method (43.35% rate of use), by reducing drastically the human-*Anopheles* contact level and specific IgG levels in children as well as in adults, were by far the most efficient whatever age, period of sampling or the exposure level to mosquito bites. Spray bombs were secondarily associated to a decrease of specific IgG level, due certainly to their power and fast knock-down action. But, their effects can be limited by the non-persistence of used products and some socio-economic considerations [133]. In addition, they only have been recently adopted and are more expensive in the majority of sub-Saharan Africa cities [133], explaining their less frequent use (9.57% rate of use) in the Dakar area. The non-effect of mosquito coil use is surprising, regardless to their well-adoption by residents (36.68% of rate of use), but it can be explained by their power deterrent effect which tends to push *Anopheles* vectors outside where they can remain active [133]. However, the protection ensured by ITN use seemed to be insufficient because anti-gSG6-P1 IgG levels in ITN users were specifically high in some periods of fairly high exposure to *Anopheles* bites. Changes in *An. arabiensis* behaviour, the major malaria vector in the area, can also explain this lack of protection. It can bite outside the rooms/ habitations with a maximal activity around 10.00 pm, when people are not in bed and ITNs not hanged [123]. Therefore, ITNs must be associated to a complementary VCM for an effective protection against *Anopheles* bites.

Taken together, these results suggest that the assessment of human IgG responses to *Anopheles* gSG6-P1 salivary peptide can provide a reliable evaluation of the effectiveness of malaria vector control in urban settings of Dakar whatever the age, sex, level of exposure to bites or period of malaria transmission. Therefore, this salivary biomarker can be used to compare the effectiveness of different anti-malaria vector strategies in order to identify the most suitable for a given area.

Comparing effectiveness of combined or not vector control measures

In parallel to an entomological and parasitological evaluation, IgG responses to gSG6-P1 were also used to assess, in a randomized controlled trial in 28 villages in southern Benin, four malaria vector control interventions: Long-Lasting Insecticide-treated Net (LLIN) targeted coverage to pregnant women and children younger than 6 years (TLLIN, reference group), LLIN universal coverage of all sleeping units (ULLIN), TLLIN plus full coverage of carbamate-indoor residual spraying (IRS) applied every 8 months (TLLIN+IRS), and ULLIN plus full coverage of carbamate-treated plastic sheeting (CTPS) lined up to the upper part of the household walls (ULLIN+CTPS). Results from this study have shown that specific IgG levels were similar in the 4 groups before intervention and only significantly lower in the ULLIN group compared to the others after intervention. In contrast to immunological data, clinical incidence density of malaria, the prevalence and parasite density of asymptomatic infections, and the density and aggressiveness of *Anopheles* mosquitoes, were not significantly different between the four groups before as well as after interventions [134]. These findings mean that LLIN used along by all the population of a given area may be more suitable in reducing the contact between human populations and the *Anopheles* vectors, even if any effect on malaria morbidity, infection, and transmission was not observed. Therefore, combining anti-vector tools do not undeniably reduce individual exposure to malaria vectors, even if significant effect on reducing more rapidly malaria transmission and burden has been reported [135]. These findings confirm that anti-vector saliva Ab response as a biomarker of exposure is also important for NMCPs and should help the design of more cost-effective strategies for malaria control and elimination.

3.4.4. Importance to develop a specific biomarker of infecting Anopheles bites

Recent data have shown that the use of the gSG6-P1 biomarker for the assessment of the differential risk of the disease transmission may have some limitations in high exposure areas (Drame *et al.*, submitted). Indeed, the gSG6-P1 assesses the exposure level to both infective and not infective *Anopheles* bites. In malaria hyperendemic areas, resident people are highly exposed to mainly not infective bites and present almost all Ab specific to gSG6-P1 levels relatively high. Therefore it should be relevant to develop a biomarker of exposure specific to infective bites in order to assess the human risk of malaria transmission in such contexts. Such epidemiological parameter would be important to define in the context of malaria control. The transmission depends on the density of competent *Anopheles*, of their *Plasmodium* infective rate and of the intensity of human-vector contact. In addition, current methods to measure the intensity of malaria transmission show several limitations, especially in low transmission areas. The EIR (entomological inoculation rate) is a commonly used metric rate that estimates the number of bites by infectious mosquitoes per person per unit time. It is the product of the "human biting rate" – the number of bites per person per day by vector mosquitoes – and the fraction of vector mosquitoes that are infectious (the "sporozoite rate"). The classical method to estimate the density of sporozoites in mosquitoes is the dissection of salivary glands and the sporozoites counting under microscope. But in area of low exposure and because few mosquitoes are infected, many mosquitoes must be caught and dissected. The salivary glands dissection is a tedious technique which required well trained and studious personnel. More-over this technique cannot differentiate *Plasmodium* species. Another technique named CSP-ELISA detects the CSP (Circumsporozoite protein) parasite surface protein and is generally done on head/thorax of mosquitoes. However the CSP protein is expressed at the oocyst stage, consequently the CSP can be detected in the mosquito before the sporozoites have reached the salivary glands (until 2-3 days) [136, 137]. Therefore, this method induced a bias with an overestimation of sporozoites index [138, 139]. Other traditional epidemiological estimates mainly based on parasitological tests are very sensitive and specific allowing the determination of parasite species, but the examination of finger prick and thick blood smear is also labour intensive and time-consuming requiring well trained staff for a reliable examination [140]. To improve the measure of transmission, antibody responses against parasite proteins (CSP, AMA1, MSP1, MSP3, etc...) could be used but several studies have highlighted limits of this approach. Actually, people exposed to malaria can be seropositive during several months [141, 142], even after transmission has stopped [141] or in the context of low transmission [143]. So by using this method we are not able to distinguish old and new infection which is particularly important in the context of evaluation of the effectiveness of vector control program. Consid-ering these limits, these serological parameters seem inappropriate to assess the malaria exposure at the individual level. Some proteomic and transcriptomic studies highlighted that the composition of *Anopheles* salivary glands could be modified with the presence of *Plasmo-dium* parasite [15, 144, 145]. Therefore, the development of a biomarker specific of infective bites based on the analysis of antibody response against salivary proteins should represent an alternative method to assess the parasite transmission to the human.

The principle of biomarker of infective bites is based on the use of immunogenic salivary protein like marker of transmission. The expression of some salivary proteins could be induced or regulated when the salivary glands are infected. Therefore, if one of such protein presents also immunogenic properties, we can probably use the specific immune response to this protein like a marker of transmission in human. Such a biomarker will be also particularly relevant in the context of re-emergence after malaria transmission reduction or in area of low exposure. This tool will allow focusing the intervention (vector control strategies and drugs distribution) on the most exposed and the most susceptible population.

4. Conclusions

In the present chapter, we have described the development of a biomarker (the *An. gambiae* gSG6-P1 peptide) of *Anopheles* mosquito bites by using an original approach coupling bioinformatic tools and immuno-epidemiological assays. Then, measurements of IgG level specific to gSG6-P1 at individual as well as population level, represent a tool/biomarker for accurately evaluate the level of human exposure to *Anopheles* bites and the risk of malaria in all age-classes of populations (newborns, infants, children, adults) living in various settings (very-low, low, moderate, and high malaria transmission areas) of rural, semi-urban and urban regions of Senegal, Angola and Benin. In the majority of these areas, this biomarker appeared to be promising and complementary to classical entomological methods, because it can give a reliable evaluation of the individual contact with anthropophilic *Anopheles* even if exposure to bites is low/very low (urban area). Therefore, such biomarker would be particularly relevant in places where malaria transmission is low, e.g. in foci of urban, high-altitude or seasonal malaria, and in travelers in endemic areas. This chapter has also shown that the availability of such a biomarker could allow the evaluation of the exposure to the main *P. falciparum* vectors (*An. gambiae s.s.*, *An. arabiensis*, *An. funestus*, *An. melas*) in Africa where different species of malaria vector co-inhabit. One direct application of such a gSG6 peptide marker of exposure could be in the elaboration of maps representing the risk of exposure to *Anopheles* bites. It could represent a geographic indicator of the risks of malaria transmission and thus a useful tool for predicting malaria morbidity risk as previously described. Furthermore, it represents a powerful and reliable tool for the evaluation of the effectiveness of vector control strategies. Such an indicator could also represent an alternative to classical entomological-parasitological monitoring methods for measuring and following the effectiveness of vector control strategies used by the National Malaria Control Programmes in various settings across Africa. Finally, this biomarker approach could be similarly applied to vector-control strategies for other mosquito-borne diseases such as emergent or re-emergent arbovirus diseases and trypanosomiasis.

Author details

Papa M. Drame[1*], Anne Poinsignon[1], Alexandra Marie[1], Herbert Noukpo[2], Souleymane Doucoure[1], Sylvie Cornelie[1,2] and Franck Remoue[1,2]

*Address all correspondence to: drpapamak@gmail.com

1 Universités Montpellier 1 et 2, Institut de Recherche pour le Développement (IRD), Montpellier, France

2 Universités Montpellier 1 et 2, Centre de Recherche Entomologique de Cotonou (CREC), Cotonou, Bénin

References

[1] Gubler DJ. Resurgent vector-borne diseases as a global health problem. Emerg Infect Dis 1998;4:442-50.

[2] WHO. 2011. In: Organization WH, ed. Geneva: World Health Organization, World Malaria Report 2011.

[3] Guerra CA, Gikandi PW, Tatem AJ, et al. The limits and intensity of *Plasmodium falciparum* transmission: implications for malaria control and elimination worldwide. PLoS Med 2008;5:e38.

[4]   Hay SI, Guerra CA, Gething PW, et al. A world malaria map: *Plasmodium falciparum* endemicity in 2007. PLoS Med 2009;6:e1000048.

[5]   WHO. Global Malaria Action Plan World Health Organization. Geneva, Switzerland: World Health Organization, 2009.

[6]   The MalERA Consultative group on Monitoring EaS. A research agenda for malaria eradication: monitoring, evaluation, and surveillance. PLoS Med. 2011;8:e1000400.

[7]   Beier JC, Killeen GF and Githure JI. Short report: entomologic inoculation rates and *Plasmodium falciparum* malaria prevalence in Africa. Am J Trop Med Hyg 1999;61:109-13.

[8]   Drakeley CJ, Corran PH, Coleman PG, et al. Estimating medium- and long-term trends in malaria transmission by using serological markers of malaria exposure. Proc Natl Acad Sci U S A 2005;102:5108-13.

[9]   Hay SI, Rogers DJ, Toomer JF and Snow RW. Annual *Plasmodium falciparum* entomological inoculation rates (EIR) across Africa: literature survey, Internet access and review. Trans R Soc Trop Med Hyg 2000;94:113-27.

[10] Smith DL, Dushoff J, Snow RW and Hay SI. The entomological inoculation rate and *Plasmodium falciparum* infection in African children. Nature 2005;438:492-5.

[11] Clements AP, Ferry JG. Cloning, nucleotide sequence, and transcriptional analyses of the gene encoding a ferredoxin from *Methanosarcina thermophila*. J Bacteriol 1992;174:5244-50.

[12] Vanderberg JP, Frevert U. Intravital microscopy demonstrating antibody-mediated immobilisation of *Plasmodium berghei* sporozoites injected into skin by mosquitoes. Int J Parasitol 2004;34:991-6.

[13] Champagne DE. Antihemostatic strategies of blood-feeding arthropods. Curr Drug Targets Cardiovasc Haematol Disord 2004;4:375-96.

[14] Champagne DE. Antihemostatic molecules from saliva of blood-feeding arthropods. Pathophysiol Haemost Thromb 2005;34:221-7.

[15] Choumet V, Carmi-Leroy A, Laurent C, et al. The salivary glands and saliva of *Anopheles gambiae* as an essential step in the *Plasmodium* life cycle: a global proteomic study. Proteomics 2007;7:3384-94.

[16] Ribeiro JM, Francischetti IM. Role of arthropod saliva in blood feeding: sialome and post-sialome perspectives. Annu Rev Entomol 2003;48:73-88.

[17] Peng Z, Simons FE. Mosquito allergy: immune mechanisms and recombinant salivary allergens. Int Arch Allergy Immunol 2004;133:198-209.

[18] Donovan MJ, Messmore AS, Scrafford DA, Sacks DL, Kamhawi S and McDowell MA. Uninfected mosquito bites confer protection against infection with malaria parasites. Infect Immun 2007;75:2523-30.

[19] Schneider BS, Mathieu C, Peronet R and Mecheri S. *Anopheles stephensi* saliva enhances progression of cerebral malaria in a murine model. Vector Borne Zoonotic Dis 2011;11:423-32

[20] Andrade BB, Rocha BC, Reis-Filho A, et al. Anti-*Anopheles darlingi* saliva antibodies as marker of *Plasmodium vivax* infection and clinical immunity in the Brazilian Amazon. Malar J 2009;8:121.

[21] Orlandi-Pradines E, Almeras L, Denis de Senneville L, et al. Antibody response against saliva antigens of *Anopheles gambiae* and *Aedes aegypti* in travellers in tropical Africa. Microbes Infect 2007;9:1454-62.

[22] Remoue F, Cisse B, Ba F, et al. Evaluation of the antibody response to *Anopheles* salivary antigens as a potential marker of risk of malaria. Trans R Soc Trop Med Hyg 2006;100:363-70

[23] Waitayakul A, Somsri S, Sattabongkot J, Looareesuwan S, Cui L and Udomsangpetch R. Natural human humoral response to salivary gland proteins of *Anopheles* mosquitoes in Thailand. Acta Trop 2006;98:66-73.

[24] Schneider BS, Higgs S. The enhancement of arbovirus transmission and disease by mosquito saliva is associated with modulation of the host immune response. Trans R Soc Trop Med Hyg 2008;102:400-8.

[25] Londono-Renteria BL, Eisele TP, Keating J, James MA and Wesson DM. Antibody response against *Anopheles albimanus* (Diptera: Culicidae) salivary protein as a measure of mosquito bite exposure in Haiti. J Med Entomol 2010;47:1156-63.

[26] Poinsignon A, Cornelie S, Mestres-Simon M, et al. Novel peptide marker corresponding to salivary protein gSG6 potentially identifies exposure to *Anopheles* bites. PLoS One 2008;3:e2472

[27] Drame PM, Machault V, Diallo A, et al. IgG responses to the gSG6-P1 salivary peptide for evaluating human exposure to *Anopheles* bites in urban areas of Dakar region, Senegal. Malar J 2012;11:72.

[28] Poinsignon A, Cornelie S, Ba F, et al. Human IgG response to a salivary peptide, gSG6-P1, as a new immuno-epidemiological tool for evaluating low-level exposure to *Anopheles* bites. Malar J 2009;8:198.

[29] Poinsignon A, Samb B, Doucoure S, et al. First attempt to validate the gSG6-P1 salivary peptide as an immuno-epidemiological tool for evaluating human exposure to *Anopheles funestus* bites. Trop Med Int Health 2010;15:1198-203.

[30] Drame PM, Poinsignon A, Besnard P, et al. Human antibody responses to the *Anopheles* salivary gSG6-P1 peptide: a novel tool for evaluating the efficacy of ITNs in malaria vector control. PLoS One 2010;5:e15596.

[31] Odegaard F. How many species of arthropods? Erwin's estimate revised. Biological Journal of the Linnean Society 2000;71:583-597.

[32] Ribeiro JM. Blood-feeding arthropods: live syringes or invertebrate pharmacologists? Infect Agents Dis 1995;4:143-52.

[33] Foster WA. Mosquito sugar feeding and reproductive energetics. Annu Rev Entomol 1995;40:443-74.

[34] Ribeiro JM. Role of saliva in blood-feeding by arthropods. Annu Rev Entomol 1987;32:463-78.

[35] Francischetti IM, Sa-Nunes A, Mans BJ, Santos IM and Ribeiro JM. The role of saliva in tick feeding. Front Biosci 2009;14:2051-88.

[36] Ribeiro JM, Rossignol PA and Spielman A. Role of mosquito saliva in blood vessel location. J Exp Biol 1984;108:1-7.

[37] Champagne DE. The role of salivary vasodilators in bloodfeeding and parasite transmission. Parasitol Today 1994;10:430-3.

[38] Stark KR, James AA. Salivary gland anticoagulants in culicine and anopheline mosquitoes (Diptera:Culicidae). J Med Entomol 1996;33:645-50.

[39] Francischetti IM. Platelet aggregation inhibitors from hematophagous animals. Toxicon 2010;56:1130-44.

[40] Lombardo F, Di Cristina M, Spanos L, Louis C, Coluzzi M and Arca B. Promoter sequences of the putative *Anopheles gambiae* apyrase confer salivary gland expression in *Drosophila melanogaster*. J Biol Chem 2000;275:23861-8.

[41] Arca B, Lombardo F, Capurro M, et al. Salivary gland-specific gene expression in the malaria vector *Anopheles gambiae*. Parassitologia 1999;41:483-7.

[42] Arca B, Lombardo F, de Lara Capurro M, et al. Trapping cDNAs encoding secreted proteins from the salivary glands of the malaria vector *Anopheles gambiae*. Proc Natl Acad Sci U S A 1999;96:1516-21.

[43] Calvo E, Andersen J, Francischetti IM, et al. The transcriptome of adult female *Anopheles darlingi* salivary glands. Insect Mol Biol 2004;13:73-88.

[44] Calvo E, Mans BJ, Andersen JF and Ribeiro JM. Function and evolution of a mosquito salivary protein family. J Biol Chem 2006;281:1935-42.

[45] Yoshida S, Sudo T, Niimi M, et al. Inhibition of collagen-induced platelet aggregation by anopheline antiplatelet protein, a saliva protein from a malaria vector mosquito. Blood 2008;111:2007-14.

[46] Francischetti IM, Valenzuela JG and Ribeiro JM. Anophelin: kinetics and mechanism of thrombin inhibition. Biochemistry 1999;38:16678-85.

[47] Isawa H, Yuda M, Orito Y and Chinzei Y. A mosquito salivary protein inhibits activation of the plasma contact system by binding to factor XII and high molecular weight kininogen. J Biol Chem 2002;277:27651-8.

[48] Champagne DE, Ribeiro JM. Sialokinin I and II: vasodilatory tachykinins from the yellow fever mosquito *Aedes aegypti*. Proc Natl Acad Sci U S A 1994;91:138-42.

[49] Ribeiro JM. Characterization of a vasodilator from the salivary glands of the yellow fever mosquito *Aedes aegypti*. J Exp Biol 1992;165:61-71.

[50] Ribeiro JM, Valenzuela JG. Purification and cloning of the salivary peroxidase/catechol oxidase of the mosquito *Anopheles albimanus*. J Exp Biol 1999;202:809-16.

[51] Fontaine A, Pascual A, Diouf I, et al. Mosquito salivary gland protein preservation in the field for immunological and biochemical analysis. Parasit Vectors 2011;4:33.

[52] Wikel SK. Immune responses to arthropods and their products. Annu Rev Entomol 1982;27:21-48.

[53] Konik P, Slavikova V, Salat J, Reznickova J, Dvoroznakova E and Kopecky J. Antitumour necrosis factor-alpha activity in *Ixodes ricinus* saliva. Parasite Immunol 2006;28:649-56.

[54] Titus RG, Bishop JV and Mejia JS. The immunomodulatory factors of arthropod saliva and the potential for these factors to serve as vaccine targets to prevent pathogen transmission. Parasite Immunol 2006;28:131-41.

[55] Andrade BB, Barral-Netto M. Biomarkers for susceptibility to infection and disease severity in human malaria. Mem Inst Oswaldo Cruz 2011;106 Suppl 1:70-8.

[56] Peng Z, Estelle F and Simons R. Mosquito allergy and mosquito salivary allergens. Protein Pept Lett 2007;14:975-81.

[57] Poole S, Lorenzetti BB, Cunha JM, Cunha FQ and Ferreira SH. Bradykinin B1 and B2 receptors, tumour necrosis factor alpha and inflammatory hyperalgesia. Br J Pharmacol 1999;126:649-56.

[58] Demeure CE, Brahimi K, Hacini F, et al. *Anopheles* mosquito bites activate cutaneous mast cells leading to a local inflammatory response and lymph node hyperplasia. J Immunol 2005;174:3932-40

[59] Billingsley PF, Baird J, Mitchell JA and Drakeley C. Immune interactions between mosquitoes and their hosts. Parasite Immunol 2006;28:143-53.

[60] Depinay N, Hacini F, Beghdadi W, Peronet R and Mecheri S. Mast cell-dependent down-regulation of antigen-specific immune responses by mosquito bites. J Immunol 2006;176:4141-6.

[61] Gillespie RD, Mbow ML and Titus RG. The immunomodulatory factors of blood-feeding arthropod saliva. Parasite Immunol 2000;22:319-31.

[62] Edwards JF, Higgs S and Beaty BJ. Mosquito feeding-induced enhancement of Cache Valley Virus (Bunyaviridae) infection in mice. J Med Entomol 1998;35:261-5.

[63] Schneider BS, Soong L, Girard YA, Campbell G, Mason P and Higgs S. Potentiation of West Nile encephalitis by mosquito feeding. Viral Immunol 2006;19:74-82.

[64] Schneider BS, Soong L, Zeidner NS and Higgs S. *Aedes aegypti* salivary gland extracts modulate anti-viral and TH1/TH2 cytokine responses to sindbis virus infection. Viral Immunol 2004;17:565-73.

[65] Esmon CT. Interactions between the innate immune and blood coagulation systems. Trends Immunol 2004;25:536-42.

[66] Bissonnette EY, Rossignol PA and Befus AD. Extracts of mosquito salivary gland inhibit tumour necrosis factor alpha release from mast cells. Parasite Immunol 1993;15:27-33.

[67] Rocha AC, Braga EM, Araujo MS, Franklin BS and Pimenta PF. Effect of the *Aedes fluviatilis* saliva on the development of *Plasmodium gallinaceum* infection in *Gallus (gallus) domesticus*. Mem Inst Oswaldo Cruz 2004;99:709-15.

[68] Thomson SA, Sherritt MA, Medveczky J, et al. Delivery of multiple CD8 cytotoxic T cell epitopes by DNA vaccination. J Immunol 1998;160:1717-23.

[69] Ader DB, Celluzzi C, Bisbing J, et al. Modulation of dengue virus infection of dendritic cells by *Aedes aegypti* saliva. Viral Immunol 2004;17:252-65.

[70] Remoue F, Alix E, Cornelie S, et al. IgE and IgG4 antibody responses to *Aedes* saliva in African children. Acta Trop 2007;104:108-15.

[71] Ramasamy MS, Srikrishnaraj KA, Wijekoone S, Jesuthasan LS and Ramasamy R. Host immunity to mosquitoes: effect of antimosquito antibodies on *Anopheles tessellatus* and *Culex quinquefasciatus* (Diptera: Culicidae). J Med Entomol 1992;29:934-8.

[72] Siden-Kiamos I, Louis C. Interactions between malaria parasites and their mosquito hosts in the midgut. Insect Biochem Mol Biol 2004;34:679-85.

[73] Suneja A, Gulia M and Gakhar SK. Blocking of malaria parasite development in mosquito and fecundity reduction by midgut antibodies in *Anopheles stephensi* (Diptera: Culicidae). Arch Insect Biochem Physiol 2003;52:63-70.

[74] Gomes R, Teixeira C, Teixeira MJ, et al. Immunity to a salivary protein of a sand fly vector protects against the fatal outcome of visceral leishmaniasis in a hamster model. Proc Natl Acad Sci U S A 2008;105:7845-50.

[75] Brennan JD, Kent M, Dhar R, Fujioka H and Kumar N. *Anopheles gambiae* salivary gland proteins as putative targets for blocking transmission of malaria parasites. Proc Natl Acad Sci U S A 2000;97:13859-64.

[76] Ramamoorthi N, Narasimhan S, Pal U, et al. The Lyme disease agent exploits a tick protein to infect the mammalian host. Nature 2005;436:573-7.

[77] Dai J, Wang P, Adusumilli S, et al. Antibodies against a tick protein, Salp15, protect mice from the Lyme disease agent. Cell Host Microbe 2009;6:482-92.

[78] Peng Z, Beckett AN, Engler RJ, Hoffman DR, Ott NL and Simons FE. Immune responses to mosquito saliva in 14 individuals with acute systemic allergic reactions to mosquito bites. J Allergy Clin Immunol 2004;114:1189-94.

[79] Peng Z, Ho MK, Li C and Simons FE. Evidence for natural desensitization to mosquito salivary allergens: mosquito saliva specific IgE and IgG levels in children. Ann Allergy Asthma Immunol 2004;93:553-6.

[80] Schwartz BS, Ford DP, Childs JE, Rothman N and Thomas RJ. Anti-tick saliva antibody: a biologic marker of tick exposure that is a risk factor for Lyme disease seropositivity. Am J Epidemiol 1991;134:86-95.

[81] Schwartz BS, Ribeiro JM and Goldstein MD. Anti-tick antibodies: an epidemiologic tool in Lyme disease research. Am J Epidemiol 1990;132:58-66.

[82] Barral A, Honda E, Caldas A, et al. Human immune response to sand fly salivary gland antigens: a useful epidemiological marker? Am J Trop Med Hyg 2000;62:740-5.

[83] Nascimento RJ, Santana JM, Lozzi SP, Araujo CN and Teixeira AR. Human IgG1 and IgG4: the main antibodies against *Triatoma infestans* (Hemiptera: Reduviidae) salivary gland proteins. Am J Trop Med Hyg 2001;65:219-26.

[84] Drame PM, Poinsignon A, Besnard P, et al. Human antibody response to *Anopheles gambiae* saliva: an immuno-epidemiological biomarker to evaluate the efficacy of insecticide-treated nets in malaria vector control. Am J Trop Med Hyg 2010;83:115-21.

[85] Brosseau L, Drame PM, Besnard P, et al. Human antibody response to *Anopheles* saliva for comparing the efficacy of three malaria vector control methods in Balombo, Angola. PLoS One 2012;7:e44189.

[86] Ribeiro JM. A catalogue of *Anopheles gambiae* transcripts significantly more or less expressed following a blood meal. Insect Biochem Mol Biol 2003;33:865-82.

[87] Lombardo F, Lanfrancotti A, Mestres-Simon M, Rizzo C, Coluzzi M and Arca B. At the interface between parasite and host: the salivary glands of the African malaria vector *Anopheles gambiae*. Parassitologia 2006;48:573-80.

[88] Valenzuela JG. High-throughput approaches to study salivary proteins and genes from vectors of disease. Insect Biochem Mol Biol 2002;32:1199-209

[89] Charlab R, Valenzuela JG, Rowton ED and Ribeiro JM. Toward an understanding of the biochemical and pharmacological complexity of the saliva of a hematophagous sand fly *Lutzomyia longipalpis*. Proc Natl Acad Sci U S A 1999;96:15155-60

[90] Holt RA, Subramanian GM, Halpern A, et al. The genome sequence of the malaria mosquito *Anopheles gambiae*. Science 2002;298:129-49

[91] Wang Z, Gerstein M and Snyder M. RNA-Seq: a revolutionary tool for transcriptomics. Nat Rev Genet 2009;10:57-63

[92] Jariyapan N, Roytrakul S, Paemanee A, et al. Proteomic analysis of salivary glands of female *Anopheles barbirostris* species A2 (Diptera: Culicidae) by two-dimensional gel electrophoresis and mass spectrometry. Parasitol Res 2012. 111(3), 1239-49.

[93] Valenzuela JG, Belkaid Y, Garfield MK, et al. Toward a defined anti-*Leishmania* vaccine targeting vector antigens: characterization of a protective salivary protein. J Exp Med 2001;194:331-42

[94] Arca B, Lombardo F, Valenzuela JG, et al. An updated catalogue of salivary gland transcripts in the adult female mosquito, *Anopheles gambiae*. J Exp Biol 2005;208:3971-86

[95] Calvo E, Dao A, Pham VM and Ribeiro JM. An insight into the sialome of *Anopheles funestus* reveals an emerging pattern in anopheline salivary protein families. Insect Biochem Mol Biol 2007;37:164-75

[96] Das S, Radtke A, Choi YJ, Mendes AM, Valenzuela JG and Dimopoulos G. Transcriptomic and functional analysis of the *Anopheles gambiae* salivary gland in relation to blood feeding. BMC Genomics 2010;11:566.

[97] Jariyapan N, Baimai V, Poovorawan Y, et al. Analysis of female salivary gland proteins of the *Anopheles barbirostris* complex (Diptera: Culicidae) in Thailand. Parasitol Res 2010;107:509-16.

[98] Jariyapan N, Choochote W, Jitpakdi A, et al. Salivary gland proteins of the human malaria vector, *Anopheles dirus* B (Diptera: Culicidae). Rev Inst Med Trop Sao Paulo 2007;49:5-10.

[99] Lombardo F, Ronca R, Rizzo C, et al. The *Anopheles gambiae* salivary protein gSG6: an anopheline-specific protein with a blood-feeding role. Insect Biochem Mol Biol 2009;39:457-66.

[100] Valenzuela JG, Francischetti IM, Pham VM, Garfield MK and Ribeiro JM. Exploring the salivary gland transcriptome and proteome of the *Anopheles stephensi* mosquito. Insect Biochem Mol Biol 2003;33:717-32.

[101] Calvo E, Pham VM, Marinotti O, Andersen JF and Ribeiro JM. The salivary gland transcriptome of the neotropical malaria vector *Anopheles darlingi* reveals accelerated evolution of genes relevant to hematophagy. BMC Genomics 2009;10:57.

[102] Francischetti IM, Valenzuela JG, Pham VM, Garfield MK and Ribeiro JM. Toward a catalog for the transcripts and proteins (sialome) from the salivary gland of the malaria vector *Anopheles gambiae*. J Exp Biol 2002;205:2429-51.

[103] Li S, Kwon J and Aksoy S. Characterization of genes expressed in the salivary glands of the tsetse fly, *Glossina morsitans morsitans*. Insect Mol Biol 2001;10:69-76.

[104] Arca B, Lombardo F, Lanfrancotti A, et al. A cluster of four D7-related genes is expressed in the salivary glands of the African malaria vector *Anopheles gambiae*. Insect Mol Biol 2002;11:47-55.

[105] Valenzuela JG, Charlab R, Gonzalez EC, et al. The D7 family of salivary proteins in blood sucking Diptera. Insect Mol Biol 2002;11:149-55.

[106] Simons FE, Peng Z. Mosquito allergy: recombinant mosquito salivary antigens for new diagnostic tests. Int Arch Allergy Immunol 2001;124:403-5.

[107] Jariyapan N, Choochote W, Jitpakdi A, et al. A glycine- and glutamate-rich protein is female salivary gland-specific and abundant in the malaria vector *Anopheles dirus* B (*Diptera: Culicidae*). J Med Entomol 2006;43:867-74.

[108] Ribeiro JM, Arca B, Lombardo F, et al. An annotated catalogue of salivary gland transcripts in the adult female mosquito, *Aedes aegypti*. BMC Genomics 2007;8:6.

[109] Lanfrancotti A, Lombardo F, Santolamazza F, et al. Novel cDNAs encoding salivary proteins from the malaria vector *Anopheles gambiae*. FEBS Lett 2002;517:67-71.

[110] Neira Oviedo M, Ribeiro JM, Heyland A, VanEkeris L, Moroz T and Linser PJ. The salivary transcriptome of *Anopheles gambiae* (Diptera: Culicidae) larvae: A microarray-based analysis. Insect Biochem Mol Biol 2009;39:382-94.

[111] Okulate MA, Kalume DE, Reddy R, et al. Identification and molecular characterization of a novel protein Saglin as a target of monoclonal antibodies affecting salivary gland infectivity of *Plasmodium* sporozoites. Insect Mol Biol 2007;16:711-22.

[112] Shen Z, Jacobs-Lorena M. A type I peritrophic matrix protein from the malaria vector *Anopheles gambiae* binds to chitin. Cloning, expression, and characterization. J Biol Chem 1998;273:17665-70.

[113] Calvo E, Pham VM, Lombardo F, Arca B and Ribeiro JM. The sialotranscriptome of adult male *Anopheles gambiae* mosquitoes. Insect Biochem Mol Biol 2006;36:570-5.

[114] Isawa H, Orito Y, Iwanaga S, et al. Identification and characterization of a new kallikrein-kinin system inhibitor from the salivary glands of the malaria vector mosquito *Anopheles stephensi*. Insect Biochem Mol Biol 2007;37:466-77.

[115] Arca B, Lombardo F, Francischetti IM, et al. An insight into the sialome of the adult female mosquito *Aedes albopictus*. Insect Biochem Mol Biol 2007;37:107-27.

[116] Ribeiro JM, Charlab R, Pham VM, Garfield M and Valenzuela JG. An insight into the salivary transcriptome and proteome of the adult female mosquito *Culex pipiens quinquefasciatus*. Insect Biochem Mol Biol 2004;34:543-63.

[117] Cornelie S, Remoue F, Doucoure S, et al. An insight into immunogenic salivary proteins of *Anopheles gambiae* in African children. Malar J 2007;6:75.

[118] Rizzo C, Ronca R, Fiorentino G, et al. Humoral response to the *Anopheles gambiae* salivary protein gSG6: a serological indicator of exposure to Afrotropical malaria vectors. PLoS One 2011;6:e17980.

[119] Rizzo C, Ronca R, Fiorentino G, et al. Wide cross-reactivity between *Anopheles gambiae* and *Anopheles funestus* SG6 salivary proteins supports exploitation of gSG6 as a marker of human exposure to major malaria vectors in tropical Africa. Malar J 2011;10:206.

[120] Larru B, Molyneux E, Ter Kuile FO, Taylor T, Molyneux M and Terlouw DJ. Malaria in infants below six months of age: retrospective surveillance of hospital admission records in Blantyre, Malawi. Malar J 2009;8:310.

[121] Rogier C. [Childhood malaria in endemic areas: epidemiology, acquired immunity and control strategies]. Med Trop (Mars) 2003;63:449-64.

[122] Carnevale P, Frezil JL, Bosseno MF, Le Pont F and Lancien J. [The aggressiveness of *Anopheles gambiae* A in relation to the age and sex of the human subjects]. Bull World Health Organ 1978;56:147-54.

[123] Geissbuhler Y, Chaki P, Emidi B, et al. Interdependence of domestic malaria prevention measures and mosquito-human interactions in urban Dar es Salaam, Tanzania. Malar J 2007;6:126.

[124] Drame PM, Diallo A, Poinsignon A, et al. Evaluation of the effectiveness of malaria vector control measures in urban settings of Dakar by a specific *Anopheles* salivary biomarker. PLoS One (2013). In press.

[125] Palmeira P, Quinello C, Silveira-Lessa AL, Zago CA and Carneiro-Sampaio M. IgG placental transfer in healthy and pathological pregnancies. Clin Dev Immunol 2012;2012:985646.

[126] Kinyanjui SM, Bull P, Newbold CI and Marsh K. Kinetics of antibody responses to *Plasmodium falciparum*-infected erythrocyte variant surface antigens. J Infect Dis 2003;187:667-74.

[127] Gadiaga L, Machault V, Pages F, et al. Conditions of malaria transmission in Dakar from 2007 to 2010. Malar J 2011;10:312.

[128] Machault V, Gadiaga L, Vignolles C, et al. Highly focused anopheline breeding sites and malaria transmission in Dakar. Malar J 2009;8:138.

[129] Kalluri S, Gilruth P, Rogers D and Szczur M. Surveillance of arthropod vector-borne infectious diseases using remote sensing techniques: a review. PLoS Pathog 2007;3:1361-71.

[130] Smith T, Killeen G, Lengeler C and Tanner M. Relationships between the outcome of *Plasmodium falciparum* infection and the intensity of transmission in Africa. Am J Trop Med Hyg 2004;71:80-6.

[131] Corran P, Coleman P, Riley E and Drakeley C. Serology: a robust indicator of malaria transmission intensity? Trends Parasitol 2007;23:575-82

[132] Doannio JM, Doudou DT, Konan LY, et al. [Influence of social perceptions and practices on the use of bednets in the malaria control programme in Ivory Coast (West Africa)]. Med Trop (Mars) 2006;66:45-52.

[133] Pages F, Orlandi-Pradines E and Corbel V. [Vectors of malaria: biology, diversity, prevention, and individual protection]. Med Mal Infect 2007;37:153-61.

[134] Corbel V, Akogbeto M, Damien GB, et al. Combination of malaria vector control interventions in pyrethroid resistance area in Benin: a cluster randomised controlled trial. Lancet Infect Dis 2012;12:617-26.

[135] Okumu FO, Moore SJ. Combining indoor residual spraying and insecticide-treated nets for malaria control in Africa: a review of possible outcomes and an outline of suggestions for the future. Malar J 2011;10:208.

[136] Beier JC. Malaria parasite development in mosquitoes. Annu Rev Entomol 1998;43:519-43.

[137] Lombardi S, Esposito F, Zavala F, et al. Detection and anatomical localization of *Plasmodium falciparum* circumsporozoite protein and sporozoites in the Afrotropical malaria vector *Anopheles gambiae* s.l. Am J Trop Med Hyg 1987;37:491-4.

[138] Burkot TR, Williams JL and Schneider I. Identification of *Plasmodium falciparum*-infected mosquitoes by a double antibody enzyme-linked immunosorbent assay. Am J Trop Med Hyg 1984;33:783-8.

[139] Fontenille D, Meunier JY, Nkondjio CA and Tchuinkam T. Use of circumsporozoite protein enzyme-linked immunosorbent assay compared with microscopic examination of salivary glands for calculation of malaria infectivity rates in mosquitoes (Diptera: Culicidae) from Cameroon. J Med Entomol 2001;38:451-4.

[140] Siala E, Ben Abdallah R, Bouratbine A, Aoun K. Current biological diagnosis of malaria. Revue Tunisienne d'Infectiologie 2010;4:5-9.

[141] Druilhe P, Pradier O, Marc JP, Miltgen F, Mazier D and Parent G. Levels of antibodies to *Plasmodium falciparum* sporozoite surface antigens reflect malaria transmission rates and are persistent in the absence of reinfection. Infect Immun 1986;53:393-7.

[142] Greenhouse B, Ho B, Hubbard A, et al. Antibodies to *Plasmodium falciparum* antigens predict a higher risk of malaria but protection from symptoms once parasitemic. J Infect Dis 2011;204:19-26.

[143] Clark EH, Silva CJ, Weiss GE, et al. *Plasmodium falciparum* malaria in the Peruvian Amazon, a region of low transmission, is associated with immunologic memory. Infect Immun 2012;80:1583-92.

[144] Dixit R, Sharma A, Mourya DT, Kamaraju R, Patole MS and Shouche YS. Salivary gland transcriptome analysis during *Plasmodium* infection in malaria vector *Anopheles stephensi*. Int J Infect Dis 2009;13:636-46.

[145] Rosinski-Chupin I, Briolay J, Brouilly P, et al. SAGE analysis of mosquito salivary gland transcriptomes during *Plasmodium* invasion. Cell Microbiol 2007;9:708-24.

Chapter 10

Transgenic Mosquitoes for Malaria Control: From the Bench to the Public Opinion Survey

Christophe Boëte and Uli Beisel

Additional information is available at the end of the chapter

1. Introduction

The recent field releases of genetically modified mosquitoes in inter alia The Cayman Islands, Malaysia and Brazil have been the source of intense debate in the specialized press [1, 2] as well as in the non-specialized mass media. For the first time in history (to our knowledge), transgenic *Aedes aegypti* were released in the Cayman Islands in 2010 by a private company, Oxitec, in collaboration with the local Mosquito Research and Control Unit (MRCU) [3]. The releases were followed by other releases in Malaysia in 2010/11 and then in Brazil in 2011 [4]. While the releases in Malaysia and Brazil were publicised beforehand, the releases in The Cayman Islands were only announced publicly one year after the fact [1, 5]. This lack of transparency, not to say the secrecy, in the way the first trial was conducted is without much doubt the major reason for the controversy that emerged. Brushing aside years of discussion in the scientific world and a shared recognition of the importance to consider ethical, legal and social issues this first trial could be read as a fait-accompli: the cage of transgenic mosquitoes has now been opened [6]. Oxitec faced harsh criticism for these releases, both within the scientific community, as well as from non-governmental organisations, such as GeneWatch that accused the company of acting like "a last bastion of colonialism". A vector-borne diseases method for control has rarely been the subject of such discussion not even concerning its potential efficacy at reducing the burden associated with a vector-borne disease.

Focusing on malaria control, this chapter reviews the major technological milestones associated with this technique from its roots to its most recent development. Key-points in the understanding of mosquito ecology are going to be presented, as well as their use in models whose major aim is to determine the validity of the transgenic approach and to help designing successful strategies for disease control.

Furthermore, the ethical and social points related to both field trials and wide-scale releases aiming at modifying mosquito populations (and thus controlling vector-borne diseases) are going to be discussed as well as the question of public engagement and the role scientists might play in fostering debate and public deliberation. While large part of the laboratory research is done in the Global North, most of the vector-borne diseases are endemic in the Global South. We suggest that the geopolitics related to the genetically modified (GM) mosquitoes as well as the specificity of Southern contexts needs to be considered when discussing the application of this technology.

2. Why acting on the vector population: How efficient are transgenic methods for malaria control?

When discussing the epidemiology of malaria the gold standard is the description of the R_0 [7-9]. Focusing on the vector compartment suggests that the spread of malaria can be curved either by reducing the mosquito population or by decreasing their vectorial capacity. In other words, one either aims to decrease the number of mosquitoes or to make them less efficient in transmitting the parasites. These two strategies can both be addressed by vector control including through a transgenic approach: population reduction or population replacement. However, when looking closely at R_0 one can notice that the parameters that are affected by those strategies are not the most likely ones to curve transmission efficiently. The mortality of mosquitoes (μ) and their biting rate (a) are indeed affecting R_0 in an exponential and in a quadratic manner respectively. In this respect, they are the parameters whose modifications affect R_0 and consequently the human prevalence mostly (see Box 1). This means that modifying a linear parameter is less likely to lead to a drastic change in malaria epidemiology. For example halving the vector population density (m) is going to reduce R_0 by two but because of the non-linear relationship between R_0 and the human prevalence (y) the decrease of the latter one is not going to be affected in such a manner especially in a context of high transmission.

3. Technology: What has lead to GM mosquitoes for malaria control?

The roots of the technology can be traced back to the early 80's/90's when the knowledge gained in genetics in *Drosophila* research sparked the development of new tools in the fight of vector-borne diseases. The plan was straightforward with three milestones to be achieved in a decade: i) the stable transformation of *Anopheles* mosquitoes by 2000 ii) the engineering of a mosquito unable to carry malaria parasites by 2005 and iii) the development of controlled experiments to understand how to drive this genotype of interest into wild populations by 2010 [10].

Regarding malaria most recent research has concentrated on the development of an *Anopheles* strain that has the ability to interrupt transmission through the synthesis and production of molecules able to block the development of the parasite. A few years ago, the SM1 peptide was shown to reduce malaria oocysts number by about 80% [11]. More recently, it was

$$R_0 = \frac{ma^2 b_1 b_2 e^{-\mu T}}{r\mu} \qquad \text{(equation 1)}$$

m : Number of mosquitoes per host.
a : Biting rate of mosquitoes on their host.
μ : Mortality of adult mosquitoes
T : Incubation time of the the parasite in the mosquito vector
r : Recovery rate of humans
b1 : Infectiousness of hosts to mosquitoes.
b2 : Susceptibility of humans

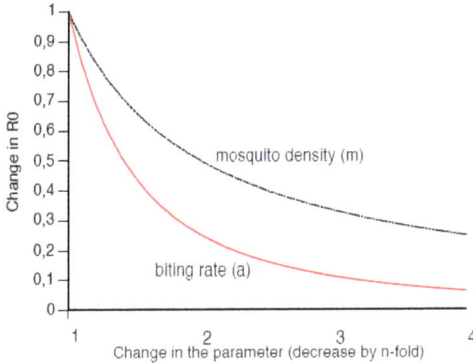

Evaluating the impact of several parameters on R0 permits to determine that a decrease in the biting rate is affecting R0 in a greater manner than a change of the same magnitude in mosquito density. The biting rate (a) appears indeed quadratically whereas the mosquito density (m) is a linear factor in equation 1.

$$y = \frac{R_0 - 1}{R_0 + \dfrac{a}{\mu}} \qquad \text{(equation 2)}$$

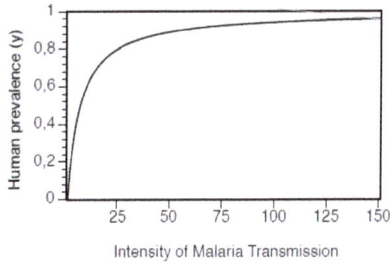

Box 1. The Ross-MacDonald model permits to describe R0 which is the number of secondary case arising from a single one in an otherwise uninfected population (Macdonald 1957; Koella, 1991). It permits to determine the relative importance of the different parameters implicated in the transmission of malaria (equation 1). From the R0 value, a simple expression permits to determine the prevalence in the human population (equation 2). As seen on the graph above, only a large decrease in the intensity of transmission (estimated by R0) can affect significantly the human prevalence (y).

synthesised from a transgenic entomopathogenic fungi [12], this later one is by-itself (in its natural version) already considered as a potentially interesting method to develop [13-15]. Other potential solutions currently developed rely on single-chain antibodies [16-18]. Using the φC31 integration system for the first time in *An. stephensi* it is now possible to insert the transgene of interest in a permanent manner at chromosomal 'docking' site using site-specific recombination and to have a tissue- and sex-specific expression. The authors have then shown that the prevalence and number of oocysts decreased when the transgenic mosquitoes were challenged with *Plasmodium falciparum* [17]. If technology has been able to determine how the insertion of a transgene can be made to change a vector to a quasi non-vector, the next question to answer concerns the spread of this construction in natural populations of mosquitoes.

4. Mosquito ecology: First hurdle at the door of the Lab

When the ecological and evolutionary issues related to the potential use and impact of *Plasmodium*-resistant transgenic mosquitoes started to be discussed about a decade ago [19, 20], most studies aimed at providing information on the fitness of genetically-modified mosquitoes were based on the use of natural mosquito immune responses as a model system. This was mainly driven by the fact that using the natural immune system of mosquitoes in a transgenic approach was considered of some potential interest [21], and also because the only fully effective system against malaria parasite was the melanization response (also known as melanotic encapsulation) in selected lines of mosquitoes [22]. The mechanism leading to the death of the parasite because of melanization remains unclear. It seems that death can occur because of starvation (by isolation from the hemolymph) as well as because of the cytotoxic function of melanin [21, 23]. The melanization response was then considered as a model of what could happen with an artificial peptide mimicking an immune response and thus aiming at reducing the number of parasites in the mosquito.

Before considering the cost associated with resistance that could impair the spread of resistance in mosquito populations, it is important to notice that the sole insertion of an exogenous gene (not even conferring any anti-parasitic advantage) leads to a drastic decrease in *Anopheles stephensi* fitness [24]. However, recent work with site-specific insertion seems to bring a less negative outcome in term of fitness [18]. This even seems to be the case when all different groups including the control group (called wild) derive from a lab colony and the fitness reduction due to the colonisation process is probably significant. Concerning the cost of resistance, mosquitoes are no exception and reduced fitness associated with the absence of parasite can be observed. Thus, several studies have measured the associated cost in *Anopheles stephensi* carrying a transgene conferring resistance again the rodent malaria parasite *P. gallinaceum*. Regardless if resistance was provided by the expression of SM1 (termed for salivary gland- and midgut binding peptide 1) [25] or the phospholipase A2 gene (PLA2) [26], a fitness cost was associated with it. Even in conditions where harbouring an allele conferred an advantage i.e. when mosquitoes were fed on *Plasmodium*-infected blood, the SM1 transgene could not reach fixation revealing that the benefit of resistance was counterbalanced by the cost of resistance in the transgenic homozygotes [27]. In any case the construction needs to follow a couple of requirements for the promoter and the gene of interest for the method to have some chances of success [28]. The gene of interest needs to express in a temporal manner i.e. after a blood-meal is taken, but also only in the tissues where it could efficiently impact the parasite life cycle, such as the midgut epithelium and the salivary glands.

Recent work on GM mosquitoes have also been done with *Aedes* that are not resistant towards a pathogen but that are carrying a gene that makes nearly all their offspring non-viable in a natural environment [29-31]. To date such a strategy has not been developed for the *Anopheles* genus.

For the strategy considering the replacement of malaria vector by their modified non-vector version, this question of a cost associated with resistance leads necessarily to the idea of the need to use a driving system in order to favour the spread of resistance in natural populations of mosquitoes.

5. Driving an allele of interest in natural populations of mosquitoes

The idea of using a gene drive to affect the epidemiology of vector-borne diseases is not a recent idea as the use of chromosomal translocation to reduce mosquito populations was already proposed in 1940 by Serebrovskii [32]. It was revived later with the idea to use those translocations to drive alleles conferring refractoriness in mosquito populations [33].

Thus the spread of refractoriness in mosquito populations could be facilitated if the allele, conferring resistance but also associated with a cost, was linked with an element whose spread is not Mendelian. One of the techniques for which various models provide information is the use of transposable elements. A tandem made of a transposon and an allele of interest can spread easily and fixation can be reached [34, 35], even if the cost of resistance is particularly high [36].

Using intracellular bacteria associated with cytoplasmic incompatibility, such as *Wolbachia*, is also an idea that has been explored. Modifying them so that they could harbour the allele of interest would permit, at least in theory, to favour the spread of the allele of interest [37, 38]. There is no natural infection of *Anopheles* by *Wolbachia* but work is in progress trialling infections of *Anopheles gambiae* cells by *Wolbachia pipientis* (strains wRi and wAlbB) in the lab [39]. However, up to now no such sustainable transformation has been done [40].

Other constructions that would favour the spread of resistance have also been considered [41, 42]. Among them the use of HEG (Homing Endonuclease Genes) has been the centre of a lot of attention in the last years [43-45]. Apart from those systems another approach relies on the use of pairs of unlinked lethal genes. In this case, each gene is associated with the repressor of the lethality of the other one and this system is called engineered underdominance [46]. With respect to those methods a number of recent papers have been focusing on theoretical work aiming at spreading an allele conferring resistance as well as containing it. If the aim of a GM approach is to favour the spread of an allele conferring resistance it is also important to consider that self-limitation could be a real advantage to avoid the establishment of the transgene in non-target populations. Such an approach has been studied in theoretical analysis with the *Inverse Medea* gene drive system [47] and with the *Semele* one [48].

If the speed at which the construction of interest can spread in mosquito populations is a major issue, authors have also shown that in the case of the use of transposable elements one of the problems is the stability of the system with the probability of disruption [49].

However, if the spread of an allele conferring resistance is a target that can be reached, the real aim should be a strong decrease in the prevalence of the disease or even its elimination. Two models merging population genetics and epidemiology have pointed out the major importance of the efficacy of resistance [36, 50]. They have shown that a significant reduction in malaria prevalence can only be obtained if the efficacy is close to 1 especially when a release of resistant mosquitoes is done in high transmission areas.

If recent work claims that the engineered-mosquito do not suffer too much from carrying a resistant allele [17], this remain only valid under lab conditions where environmental conditions remain fairly stable and usually favourable. It is interesting to note that the survival of the mosquitoes in Isaacs et al. study reaches about 35 to 40 days which is probably far more that what happens under natural conditions.

As shown with natural immune responses, environmental conditions experienced at the larval or at the adult stage can greatly affect the host-parasite interactions and thus the outcome of an infection [51]. A reduction of 75% on food availability at the larval stage in lines selected for refractoriness [22] leads to a decrease in the proportion of the mosquitoes able to melanize half of the surface of a foreign body (a Sephadex bead) of more than 50% of it [52]. Even more worryingly, a recent paper [53] revealed the complex effects of temperature on both the cellular and humoral immune responses on the malaria vector *Anopheles stephensi*. What is highly interesting in this study is that not only temperature can affect immune responses but also that different immune responses are affected in different manners by temperature. The authors have studied the melanization response, the phagocytosis (a cellular immune response that lead to the destruction of small organisms or apoptotic cells) and the defensin (an antimicrobial peptide) expression. The three of them are higher at 18°C while the expression of Nitric Oxide Synthase (active against a large number of pathogens [54]) peaks at 30°C and the one of cecropin (an antimicrobial peptide) seems to be temperature-independent. Concerning melanization it is important to note that if the melanization rate is higher at 18°C, the percentage of melanised beads -introduced inside the mosquito to measure its immunocompetence- (at least partly) was higher when the temperature increased (fig. 1).

This result highlights the difficulties to define what is an optimal temperature for the melanization response especially as it is also involved in developmental processes. The complexity of the immune function appears also with cecropin expression that despite being independent from temperature was affected by the administration of an injury or the injection of heat-killed *E. coli*. Other works have also revealed that the immune function is affected in a complex manner by a variety of environmental parameters such as the density of conspecifics or the quality of food resources [55]. Apart from showing the need to better understand the impact of the complex interactions between temperature and other variables on the vector competence, this work also highlights the crucial importance to take them into account when determining the potential outcome of the interactions between the natural immune function, the allele conferring resistance in a GM mosquito and finally the resulting vectorial competence under a large variety of ecological conditions.

What appears to be clear is that the expression of genes involved in the anti-parasitic response are not only influenced by the sole host-parasite interactions but that the environment is a

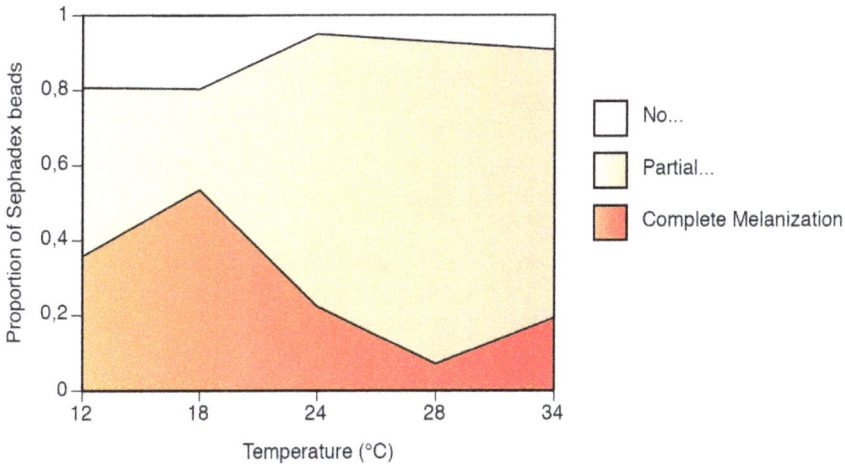

Figure 1. Influence of the temperature on the melanization response of Sephadex beads in the malaria vector Anopheles stephensi. The melanization of beads was measured 24h after the injection. The proportion of completely melanized beads was the highest at 18°C whereas the higher proportion of beads being at least partially melanized occurs at higher temperatures (modified after Murdock et al. 2012)[53].

crucial factor be it the abiotic conditions, such as temperature and its daily variations, or biotic factors, such as parasites encountered at the larval or adult stage [56, 57].

On the side of the parasite it would be naïve not to consider an evolutionary response in the face of selective pressure represented by any (natural or artificial) resistance. The quick selection of resistance against artemisinin in South-East Asia in the last years [58] and the evidence of its genetic basis [59] suggests that it is reasonable to envision the selection of parasite strains able to overcome any engineered resistance mechanism. Using transgenic *Plasmodium*-resistant mosquitoes can be considered equivalent to artificially increasing the investment of the mosquito in an immune response. Referring to some theoretical work [60] this is assumed to be followed by an increase in the parasite investment to avoid resistance. In the long term this would lead to a decrease in the effectiveness of the programme aiming at decreasing malaria prevalence or the need to 'play evolution' by monitoring the parasite population and releasing transgenic mosquitoes for which resistance could be modified as in an arm race with parasite evasion.

What is then important is to determine the longer-term of such a strategy regarding parasite virulence. Some answers have already been provided by theoretical work concerning the impact on parasite virulence to humans and mosquitoes in the case of dengue [61]. The authors examined four distinct situations: blocking transmission, decreasing mosquito biting rate, increasing mosquito background mortality or increasing the mortality due to infection; if all of them are associated with a benefit in terms of disease incidence, only the ones affecting mosquito mortality seem to pose the smallest risk in term of virulence to humans. It is important to note the scarcity of studies aiming at providing empirical data on this topic even if experimental evolution with mosquitoes and parasite can provide interesting results in a reasonable number of generations [62]. This lack of data not only concerns dengue but also malaria as has already been discussed in a paper on possible outcomes of the use of transgenic *Plasmodium*-resistant mosquitoes [63].

6. Vector control: To be or not to be transgenic-based

As mentioned earlier one of the major points to consider with transgenic mosquitoes used for malaria control are the ethical and societal issues and public acceptance of this high-tech method. Even though the importance of societal acceptance of GM mosquitoes has been recognised for a decade [64], studies on acceptability remain scarce. One first study conducted in Mali mapped out several crucial aspects of potential acceptance or rejection of GM mosquitoes [65]. While Marshall reports that his interviewees were generally "pragmatic" about the technology, acceptance was dependent on several conditions.

If people were supportive of a release of transgenic mosquitoes for malaria control, they first wanted to see evidence of safety for human health and the environment prior to releases. In addition, proof of efficacy of the technology in reducing malaria prevalence was requested. Lastly people declared that they would prefer the trial to be done outside of their village and when comparing GM crops and GM mosquitoes, people were more sceptical of the latter. Even if this not a rejection of the idea of using a GM technology for health purpose, it is important to note that a population, even if at risk of contracting malaria, remains cautious about the idea of using such a technology. This should remind us how, in the 70's, a decade-long programme conducted by the WHO in India utilising the sterile insect technique (SIT) ended in a chaotic way after the publication of inaccurate information in the Indian press [66].

Secondly, the question of regulation has recently been highlighted as crucial [5, 67]. Because the social and environmental implications of GM mosquitoes are significant and potentially irreversible, and as the regulatory attention that GMOs have received in Europe suggests broad-based trials and releases require robust legislation and international agreements. These regulations are still under development, and it is important to note that at the time of the first releases in The Cayman Islands international guidance on open field releases of GM mosquitoes was still in preparation [67, 68]. While the existing Cartagena Protocol on Biosafety is considered to be applicable to GM crops, it is in need of specific amendments in order to work for GM mosquitoes [69].

Furthermore, in terms of regulation one has to distinguish between two different types of GM mosquitoes. While regulation and tracking might be possible for genetically sterilised mosquitoes as they are self-limiting in their spread, tracking and containment of GM mosquitoes with self-spreading genetics, i.e. fertile mosquitoes that block disease transmission, is considered almost impossible, or at the very least extremely difficult [70, 71]. This distinguishes GM mosquitoes from earlier GM technologies, such as for the modification of crops. GM and non-GM crops can be separated from each other and marked by labels on GM products, it can thus be seen as a technology of choice. However, the accuracy of this argument is only limited. As for instance Lezaun has shown, bees have proven to be effective agents of cross-pollination between GM and non-GM crops, thus subverting regulations that aim to keep GM and non-GM crops separate [72]. GM insects, however, are markedly different. The elusiveness of mosquitoes will likely be a major impediment to tracking, containment and comprehensive regulation, as for instance the spread of *Aedes albopictus* and herewith the increased risk of arboviral transmission in new locations across the world has shown, mosquitoes are hard to contain. This renders GM mosquitoes as a no-choice technology – once released, GM mosquitoes will stay in our environments.

A second major issue in terms of the social and ethical implications of GM mosquitoes is the question by whom and how they are produced and implemented. GM modification of insects is an expensive high-tech intervention and research so far has mainly been located in resource rich laboratories in the Global North, rather than in disease-endemic developing countries [73]. This enrols the technology thoroughly into discussions about technology transfer and development initiatives from North to South, and sits uncomfortably with the West's history in colonial exploitation and tropical medicine. Aside from this imbalance in bio-capital and agenda setting, GM mosquitoes are as much a product of the biotech industry as they are tools for public or global health. Are GM mosquitoes currently seen as a public good or a commercial product? While most of the research and development of GM mosquitoes has so far been funded by public institutions –both national research foundations -such as the US National Science Foundation- and philanthropic organisations -such as the Bill and Melinda Gates Foundation and the Wellcome Trust, the mosquitoes that have been released were part of a commercial project. The emerging GM mosquito industry has caught the interest of private biotech firms. The first company to produce and market GM mosquitoes is Oxford Insect Technologies (Oxitec), founded by a group of entomologists as a spin-off company of Oxford University. The company is a for-profit-enterprise, so far has mainly been funded by public entities and venture capitalists, and is one of the main drivers of high-end developments in the field. As discussed in the introduction, Oxitec was the first to release sterile GM mosquitoes into the wild in the field trials in The Cayman Islands. A fundamental issue that is raised through the dominance of Oxitec in the field is the tension between GM mosquitoes as a public health tool and a commercial product [74-76]. While GM mosquitoes in malaria control would be used as a tool of disease control and to foster public health, companies like Oxitec follow different aims – they have to become profitable and eventually make profits with their GM entities. This tension brings another social issue of GM mosquitoes to the forefront, namely the question of how one conducts field trials with GM mosquitoes in an ethical way?

As we alluded to in the introduction, the first releases in The Cayman Islands were conducted in a rather secretive fashion. Oxitec only published the news about the release with a one-year delay [1], leading to accusations that the releases were deliberately done in secret [75, 76]. Oxitec stated the trials were prepared and conducted in close cooperation with local Mosquito Control and Research Unit, had conformed to the British Overseas Territory's biosafety rules, and that information had been sent to local newspapers preceding the trials. However, many locals claimed they were not informed and no risk assessment documents were made available to the public on the internet. The only risk assessment document that can be found was published by the UK parliament in 2011, over one year after the releases started [5]. The Cayman Island releases have triggered fears for entomologists working on GM mosquitoes that such secretive trials might lead to a public backlash and undermine their own extensive efforts at public engagement, some scientists for instance claimed they have spent years preparing a study site through "extensive dialogues with citizen groups, regulators, academics and farmers"[1].

GeneWatch argued that Oxitec purposefully bypassed existing international GM regulations (developed mainly for GM crops), because Cayman Islands does not have biosafety laws and is not a signatory to the Cartagena Protocol on Biosafety or the Aarhus Convention (even though since the UK is a signatory to the protocol, Oxitec had a duty to report the export of GM eggs to UK government). As a result GeneWatch reads Oxitec's actions as colonialist tactics: "the British scientific establishment is acting like the last bastion of colonialism, using an Overseas Territory as a private lab" [76].

All in all, this raises the question what ethically and socially responsible research on GM mosquitoes means? Here, the ability of researchers and stakeholders to communicate with each other is key for meaningful public engagement. In this respect, a recent survey has focused on the willingness of scientists to have interactions with a non-scientific audience [77]. One of the main findings of the survey indicates that more than 90% of scientists working on GM mosquitoes are agreeable to interactions with the public on their research. However, communication might not be enough and real discussion might not be easy between researchers and a non-scientific audience. This has been underlined by the reluctance of a fraction of the research community to have their research project evaluated by a non-scientific public [77]. Thus, while a significant proportion of researchers are ready to interact with a non-scientific audience, they seem to be less likely to accept an evaluation and a prior-agreement of a research proposal by the general public, interestingly especially researchers from the Global North are hesitant. On the other hand, many scientists in malarious countries do welcome exchanges with publics and are more willing to negotiate their research project with members of the disease-endemic communities.

In summary, the GM mosquito technology in malaria control raises a set of challenging questions. Challenges from a biological and ecological perspective are interlinked with questions about democratic decision-making, local acceptance and international regulation of these emerging entities. Such a potentially controversial technology cannot afford to skip these debates and time is ripe to focus on the ethical and sociological aspects governing the potential use of GM mosquitoes. Furthermore, it is crucial that the development of transgenic methods does not lead to a decrease in funding of classical, accepted and efficient vector control methods – indeed, they should be favoured and enhanced to continue curbing the malaria burden today.

Acknowledgements

Thanks to Sylvie Manguin for the kind invitation to write this chapter. Thanks to Courtney C Murdock for providing necessary data and to Silke Fuchs for a preprint. We are also grateful to Luisa Reis de Castro and Guy Reeves for helpful comments on a previous version of this paper. Both authors wish also to thank the Institut des Sciences de la Communication, CNRS (France) for financial support.

Author details

Christophe Boëte[1*] and Uli Beisel[2]

*Address all correspondence to: cboete@gmail.com

1 UMR 190 "Emergence des Pathologies Virales", Aix Marseille Université IRD (Institut de Recherche pour le Développement) EHESP (Ecole des Hautes Etudes en Santé Publique), France

2 Lancaster Environment Centre, Lancaster University, Lancaster LA1 4YQ, UK

References

[1] Enserink M. Science and society. GM mosquito trial alarms opponents, strains ties in Gates-funded project. Science 2010;330:1030-1031.

[2] Subbaraman N. Science snipes at Oxitec transgenic-mosquito trial. Nature Biotechnology 2011;29:9-11.

[3] Harris AF, Nimmo D, McKemey AR, Kelly N, Scaife S, Donnelly CA, et al. Field performance of engineered male mosquitoes. Nature Biotechnology 2011;29:1034-1037.

[4] Harris AF, McKemey AR, Nimmo D, Curtis Z, Black I, Morgan SA, et al. Successful suppression of a field mosquito population by sustained release of engineered male mosquitoes. Nature Biotechnology 2012;30:828-830.

[5] Reeves RG, Denton JA, Santucci F, Bryk J, Reed FA. Scientific standards and the regulation of genetically modified insects. PLoS Neglected Tropical Diseases 2012;6:e1502. doi: 10.1371/journal.pntd.0001502

[6] Boëte C. Moustiques Transgéniques: La cage est ouverte. Les blogs du Diplo (http://blog.mondediplo.net/2011-02-10-Moustiques-transgeniques-la-cage-est-ouverte) (accessed 20 February 2013).

[7] Koella JC. On the use of mathematical models of malaria transmission. Acta Tropica 1991;49:1-25.

[8] Smith DL, Battle KE, Hay SI, Barker CM, Scott TW, McKenzie FE. Ross, Macdonald, and a theory for the dynamics and control of mosquito-transmitted pathogens. PLoS Pathogens 2012;8:e1002588. doi: 10.1371/journal.ppat.1002588.

[9] Smith DL, McKenzie FE, Snow RW, Hay SI. Revisiting the basic reproductive number for malaria and its implications for malaria control. PLoS Biology2007;5:e42. doi: 10.1371/journal.pbio.0050042.

[10] World Health Organization. Prospects for malaria control by genetic manipulation of its vectors TDR/BCV/ MAL-ENT/91.3. Geneva; 1991.

[11] Ito J, Ghosh A, Moreira LA, Wimmer EA, Jacobs-Lorena M. Transgenic anopheline mosquitoes impaired in transmission of a malaria parasite. Nature 2002;417:452-455.

[12] Fang W, Vega-Rodriguez J, Ghosh AK, Jacobs-Lorena M, Kang A, St Leger RJ. Development of transgenic fungi that kill human malaria parasites in mosquitoes. Science 2011;331:1074-1077.

[13] Scholte EJ, Knols BG, Takken W. Infection of the malaria mosquito *Anopheles gambiae* with the entomopathogenic fungus *Metarhizium anisopliae* reduces blood feeding and fecundity. Journal of Invertebrate Pathology 2006;91:43-49.

[14] Scholte EJ, Ng'habi K, Kihonda J, Takken W, Paaijmans K, Abdulla S, et al. An entomopathogenic fungus for control of adult African malaria mosquitoes. Science 2005;308:1641-1642.

[15] Scholte EJ, Njiru BN, Smallegange RC, Takken W, Knols BG. Infection of malaria (*Anopheles gambiae* s.s.) and filariasis (*Culex quinquefasciatus*) vectors with the entomopathogenic fungus *Metarhizium anisopliae*. Malaria Journal 2003;2:29. doi: 10.1186/1475-2875-2-29

[16] de Lara Capurro M, Coleman J, Beerntsen BT, Myles KM, Olson KE, Rocha E, et al. Virus-expressed, recombinant single-chain antibody blocks sporozoite infection of salivary glands in *Plasmodium gallinaceum*-infected *Aedes aegypti*. American Journal of Tropical Medicine and Hygiene 2000;62:427-433.

[17] Isaacs AT, Jasinskiene N, Tretiakov M, Thiery I, Zettor A, Bourgouin C, et al. Transgenic *Anopheles stephensi* coexpressing single-chain antibodies resist *Plasmodium falciparum* development. Proceedings of the National Academy of Sciences U S A 2012;109:E1922-1930.

[18] Isaacs AT, Li F, Jasinskiene N, Chen X, Nirmala X, Marinotti O, et al. Engineered resistance to *Plasmodium falciparum* development in transgenic *Anopheles stephensi*. PLoS Pathogens 2011;7:e1002017. doi:10.1371/journal.ppat.1002017

[19] Boëte C, Koella JC. Evolutionary ideas about genetically manipulated mosquitoes and malaria control. Trends in Parasitology 2003;19:32-38.

[20] Scott TW, Takken W, Knols BG, Boëte C. The ecology of genetically modified mosquitoes. Science 2002;298:117-119.

[21] Christensen BM, Li J, Chen CC, Nappi AJ. Melanization immune responses in mosquito vectors. Trends in Parasitology 2005;21:192-199.

[22] Collins FH, Sakai RK, Vernick KD, Paskewitz S, Seeley DC, Miller LH, et al. Genetic selection of a *Plasmodium*-refractory strain of the malaria vector *Anopheles gambiae*. Science 1986;234:607-610.

[23] Nappi AJ, Christensen BM. Melanogenesis and associated cytotoxic reactions: applications to insect innate immunity. Insect Biochemistry and Molecular Biology 2005;35:443-459.

[24] Catteruccia F, Godfray HC, Crisanti A. Impact of genetic manipulation on the fitness of *Anopheles stephensi* mosquitoes. Science 2003;299:1225-1227.

[25] Marrelli MT, Li CY, Rasgon JL, Jacobs-Lorena M. Transgenic malaria-resistant mosquitoes have a fitness advantage when feeding on *Plasmodium*-infected blood. Proceedings of the National Academy of Sciences U S A 2007;104:5580-5583.

[26] Moreira LA, Wang J, Collins FH, Jacobs-Lorena M. Fitness of anopheline mosquitoes expressing transgenes that inhibit *Plasmodium* development. Genetics 2004;166:1337-1341.

[27] Lambrechts L, Koella JC, Boëte C. Can transgenic mosquitoes afford the fitness cost? Trends in Parasitology 2008;24:4-7.

[28] Fuchs S, Nolan T, Crisanti A. Mosquito transgenic technologies to reduce *Plasmodium* transmission. Methods in Molecular Biology 2013;923:601-622.

[29] Bargielowski I, Nimmo D, Alphey L, Koella JC. Comparison of life history characteristics of the genetically modified OX513A line and a wild type strain of *Aedes aegypti*. PLoS One 2011 6(6): e20699. doi:10.1371/journal.pone.0020699

[30] Bargielowski I, Kaufmann C, Alphey L, Reiter P, Koella J. Flight Performance and Teneral Energy Reserves of Two Genetically-Modified and One Wild-Type Strain of the Yellow Fever Mosquito *Aedes aegypti*. Vector Borne Zoonotic Diseases 2012.

[31] Bargielowski I, Alphey L, Koella JC. Cost of mating and insemination capacity of a genetically modified mosquito *Aedes aegypti* OX513A compared to its wild type counterpart. PLoS One 2011 6(10) :e26086. doi:10.1371/journal.pone.0026086

[32] Serebrovskii AS. On the possibility of a new method for the control of insect pests. (In Russian). Zoologichesky Zhurnal 1940;19:618-630.

[33] Curtis CF. Possible use of translocations to fix desirable genes in insect pest populations. Nature 1968;218:368-369.

[34] Kiszewski AE, Spielman A. Spatially explicit model of transposon-based genetic drive mechanisms for displacing fluctuating populations of anopheline vector mosquitoes. Journal of Medical Entomology 1998;35:584-590.

[35] Ribeiro JM, Kidwell MG. Transposable elements as population drive mechanisms: specification of critical parameter values. Journal of Medical Entomology 1994;31:10-16.

[36] Boëte C, Koella JC. A theoretical approach to predicting the success of genetic manipulation of malaria mosquitoes in malaria control. Malaria Journal 2002;1:3. doi: 10.1186/1475-2875-1-3

[37] Curtis CF, Sinkins SP. *Wolbachia* as a possible means of driving genes into populations. Parasitology 1998;116 Suppl:S111-115.

[38] Rasgon JL, Scott TW. Impact of population age structure on *Wolbachia* transgene driver efficacy: ecologically complex factors and release of genetically modified mosquitoes. Insect Biochemistry and Molecular Biology 2004;34:707-713.

[39] Rasgon JL, Ren X, Petridis M. Can *Anopheles gambiae* be infected with *Wolbachia pipientis*? Insights from an in vitro system. Applied and Environmental Microbiology 2006;72:7718-7722.

[40] Hughes GL, Koga R, Xue P, Fukatsu T, Rasgon JL. *Wolbachia* infections are virulent and inhibit the human malaria parasite *Plasmodium falciparum* in *Anopheles gambiae*. PLoS Pathogens 2011 7(5): e1002043. doi:10.1371/journal.ppat.1002043

[41] Sinkins SP, Gould F. Gene drive systems for insect disease vectors. Nature Reviews Genetics 2006;7:427-435.

[42] Hay BA, Chen CH, Ward CM, Huang H, Su JT, Guo M. Engineering the genomes of wild insect populations: challenges, and opportunities provided by synthetic *Medea* selfish genetic elements. Journal of Insect Physiology 2010;56:1402-1413.

[43] Burt A. Site-specific selfish genes as tools for the control and genetic engineering of natural populations. Proceedings of the Royal Society B: Biological Sciences 2003;270:921-928.

[44] Deredec A, Godfray HC, Burt A. Requirements for effective malaria control with homing endonuclease genes. Proceedings of the National Academy of Sciences U S A 2011;108:E874-880.

[45] Windbichler N, Menichelli M, Papathanos PA, Thyme SB, Li H, Ulge UY, et al. A synthetic homing endonuclease-based gene drive system in the human malaria mosquito. Nature 2011;473:212-215.

[46] Davis S, Bax N, Grewe P. Engineered underdominance allows efficient and economical introgression of traits into pest populations. Journal of Theoretical Biology 2001;212:83-98.

[47] Marshall JM, Hay BA. Inverse *Medea* as a novel gene drive system for local population replacement: a theoretical analysis. Journal of Heredity 2011;102:336-341.

[48] Marshall JM, Pittman GW, Buchman AB, Hay BA. *Semele*: a killer-male, rescue-female system for suppression and replacement of insect disease vector populations. Genetics 2011;187:535-551.

[49] Curtis CF, Coleman P, Kelly DW, Campbell-Lendrum DH. Advantages and Limitations of Transgenic Vector Control: Sterile Males versus Gene Drivers. In: Boëte C. (ed.). Genetically Modified Mosquitoes for Malaria Control. Georgetown, TX, USA: Landes Biosciences - Eurekah 2006. p60-78.

[50] Koella JC, Zaghloul L. Using evolutionary costs to enhance the efficacy of malaria control via genetically manipulated mosquitoes. Parasitology 2008;135:1489-1496.

[51] Lambrechts L, Chavatte JM, Snounou G, Koella JC. Environmental influence on the genetic basis of mosquito resistance to malaria parasites. Proceedings of the Royal Society B: Biological Sciences 2006;273:1501-1506.

[52] Suwanchaichinda C, Paskewitz SM. Effects of larval nutrition, adult body size, and adult temperature on the ability of *Anopheles gambiae* (Diptera: Culicidae) to melanize Sephadex beads. Journal of Medical Entomology 1998;35:157-161.

[53] Murdock CC, Paaijmans KP, Bell AS, King JG, Hillyer JF, Read AF, et al. Complex effects of temperature on mosquito immune function. Proceedings of the Royal Society B: Biological Sciences 2012;279:3357-3366.

[54] Rivero A. Nitric oxide: an antiparasitic molecule of invertebrates. Trends in Parasitology 2006;22:219-225.

[55] Triggs A, Knell RJ. Interactions between environmental variables determine immunity in the Indian meal moth *Plodia interpunctella*. Journal of Animal Ecology 2012;81:386-394.

[56] Boëte C. *Anopheles* mosquitoes: not just flying malaria vectors... especially in the field. Trends in Parasitology 2009;25:53-55.

[57] Aliota MT, Chen CC, Dagoro H, Fuchs JF, Christensen BM. Filarial worms reduce *Plasmodium* infectivity in mosquitoes. PLoS Neglected Tropical Diseases 2011;5:e963.

[58] Dondorp AM, Nosten F, Yi P, Das D, Phyo AP, Tarning J, et al. Artemisinin resistance in *Plasmodium falciparum* malaria. New England Journal of Medicine 2009;361:455-467.

[59] Anderson TJ, Nair S, Nkhoma S, Williams JT, Imwong M, Yi P, et al. High heritability of malaria parasite clearance rate indicates a genetic basis for artemisinin resistance in western Cambodia. Journal of Infectious Diseases 2010;201:1326-1330.

[60] Koella JC, Boëte C. A model for the coevolution of immunity and immune evasion in vector-borne diseases with implications for the epidemiology of malaria. The American Naturalist 2003;161:698-707.

[61] Medlock J, Luz PM, Struchiner CJ, Galvani AP. The impact of transgenic mosquitoes on dengue virulence to humans and mosquitoes. The American Naturalist 2009;174:565-577.

[62] Legros M, Koella JC. Experimental evolution of specialization by a microsporidian parasite. BMC Evolutionary Biology 2010;10:159.

[63] Ferguson HM, Gandon S, Mackinnon MJ, Read AF. Malaria parasite virulence in mosquitoes and its implications for the introduction of Efficacy of GMM malaria Control Programs. In: Boëte C. (ed.). Genetically Modified Mosquitoes for Malaria Control. Georgetown, TX, USA: Landes Biosciences - Eurekah 2006. p103-116.

[64] Touré YT, Oduola AMJ, Sommerfeld J, Morel CM. Biosafety and risk assessment in the use of genetically modified mosquiotes for disease control. In: Takken W, Scott TW, editors. Ecological Aspects for Application of Genetically Modified Mosquitoes. Wageningen: Kluwer Academic Publishers; 2003.

[65] Marshall JM, Toure MB, Traore MM, Famenini S, Taylor CE. Perspectives of people in Mali toward genetically-modified mosquitoes for malaria control. Malaria Journal 2010;9:128. doi:10.1186/1475-2875-9-128.

[66] Anonymous Oh New Delhi, Oh Geneva. Nature 1975;256:355-357.

[67] Mumford JD. Science, regulation, and precedent for genetically modified insects. PLoS Neglected Tropical Diseases 2012 6(1): e1504. doi:10.1371/journal.pntd.0001504

[68] World Health Organization. Progress and prospects for the use of genetically modified mosquitoes to inhibit disease transmission. Geneva; 2009.

[69] Marshall JM. The Cartagena Protocol and genetically modified mosquitoes. Nature Biotechnology 2010;28:896-897.

[70] Angulo E, Gilna B. International law should govern release of GM mosquitoes. Nature 2008;454:158.

[71] Angulo E, Gilna B. When biotech crosses borders. Nature Biotechnology 2008;26:277-282.

[72] Lezaun J. Bees, beekeepers, and bureaucrats: parasitism and the politics of transgenic lifeEnvironment and Planning D: Society and Space 2011;29(4):738-756.

[73] Mshinda H, Killeen GF, Mukabana WR, Mathenge EM, Mboera LE, Knols BG. Development of genetically modified mosquitoes in Africa. The Lancet Infectious diseases 2004;4:264-265.

[74] Beisel U, Boëte C. The Flying Public Health Tool: Genetically Modified mosquitoes in malaria control. Science as Culture 2013 22(1).

[75] Genewatch UK Oxitec's genetically-modified mosquitoes: in the public interest? http://tinyurl.com/by8vsvd (accessed 20 February 2013)

[76] Genewatch UK British Overseas Territory used as private lab for GM mosquito company. 2010. http://www.genewatch.org/uploads/f03c6d66a9b354535738483c1c3d49e4/Oxitecbrief_fin.pdf (accessed 20 February 2013)

[77] Boëte C. Scientists and public involvement: a consultation on the relation between malaria, vector control and transgenic mosquitoes. Transactions of the Royal Society of Tropical Medicine and Hygiene 2011;105:704-710.

Permissions

The contributors of this book come from diverse backgrounds, making this book a truly international effort. This book will bring forth new frontiers with its revolutionizing research information and detailed analysis of the nascent developments around the world.

We would like to thank Sylvie Manguin and Prof. Jean Mouchet, for lending their expertise to make the book truly unique. They have played a crucial role in the development of this book. Without their invaluable contribution this book wouldn't have been possible. They have made vital efforts to compile up to date information on the varied aspects of this subject to make this book a valuable addition to the collection of many professionals and students.

This book was conceptualized with the vision of imparting up-to-date information and advanced data in this field. To ensure the same, a matchless editorial board was set up. Every individual on the board went through rigorous rounds of assessment to prove their worth. After which they invested a large part of their time researching and compiling the most relevant data for our readers. Conferences and sessions were held from time to time between the editorial board and the contributing authors to present the data in the most comprehensible form. The editorial team has worked tirelessly to provide valuable and valid information to help people across the globe.

Every chapter published in this book has been scrutinized by our experts. Their significance has been extensively debated. The topics covered herein carry significant findings which will fuel the growth of the discipline. They may even be implemented as practical applications or may be referred to as a beginning point for another development. Chapters in this book were first published by InTech; hereby published with permission under the Creative Commons Attribution License or equivalent.

The editorial board has been involved in producing this book since its inception. They have spent rigorous hours researching and exploring the diverse topics which have resulted in the successful publishing of this book. They have passed on their knowledge of decades through this book. To expedite this challenging task, the publisher supported the team at every step. A small team of assistant editors was also appointed to further simplify the editing procedure and attain best results for the readers.

Our editorial team has been hand-picked from every corner of the world. Their multi-ethnicity adds dynamic inputs to the discussions which result in innovative outcomes. These outcomes are then further discussed with the researchers and contributors who give their valuable feedback and opinion regarding the same. The feedback is then collaborated with the researches and they are edited in a comprehensive manner to aid the understanding of the subject.

Apart from the editorial board, the designing team has also invested a significant amount of their time in understanding the subject and creating the most relevant covers. They scrutinized every image to scout for the most suitable representation of the subject and create an appropriate cover for the book.

The publishing team has been involved in this book since its early stages. They were actively engaged in every process, be it collecting the data, connecting with the contributors or procuring relevant information. The team has been an ardent support to the editorial, designing and production team. Their endless efforts to recruit the best for this project, has resulted in the accomplishment of this book. They are a veteran in the field of academics and their pool of knowledge is as vast as their experience in printing. Their expertise and guidance has proved useful at every step. Their uncompromising quality standards have made this book an exceptional effort. Their encouragement from time to time has been an inspiration for everyone.

The publisher and the editorial board hope that this book will prove to be a valuable piece of knowledge for researchers, students, practitioners and scholars across the globe.

List of Contributors

Indra Vythilingam
Parasitology Department, Faculty of Medicine, University of Malaya, Kuala Lumpur, Malaysia Formerly WHO Malaria Scientist, World Health Organization, Philippines

Jeffery Hii
Taman Damai, Jalan Fung Yei Ting, Kota Kinabalu, Sabah, Malaysia Formerly WHO Malaria Scientist, World Health Organization, Philippines

Mathilde Gendrin and George K. Christophides
Department of Life Sciences, Imperial College London, UK

Chloé Lahondère and Claudio R. Lazzari
Institut de Recherche sur la Biologie de l'Insecte, UMR CNRS - Université François Rabelais, Tours, France

Sylvie Manguin
Institut de Recherche pour le Développement (IRD), Faculté de Pharmacie, Montpellier, France

Chung Thuy Ngo
Institut de Recherche pour le Développement (IRD), Faculté de Pharmacie, Montpellier, France National Institute of Veterinary Research, Ha Noi, Vietnam

Krajana Tainchum, Waraporn Juntarajumnong and Theeraphap Chareonviriyaphap
Department of Entomology, Faculty of Agriculture, Kasetsart University, Bangkok, Thailand

Anne-Laure Michon and Estelle Jumas-Bilak
University Montpellier, Equipe Pathogènes et Environnements, Faculté de Pharmacie, Montpellier, France

Vincent Corbel
Institut de Recherche pour le Développement, Maladies Infectieuses et Vecteurs, Ecologie, Génétique, Evolution et Contrôle (IRD 224-CNRS 5290 UM1-UM2), Benin Department of Entomology, Kasetsart University, Bangkok, Thailand

Raphael N'Guessan
London School of Hygiene & Tropical Medicine, London, UK Centre de Recherches Entomologiques de Cotonou, Cotonou, Benin

Lies Durnez
Department of Biomedical Sciences, Institute of Tropical Medicine, Antwerp, Belgium

sMarc Coosemans
Department of Biomedical Sciences, Institute of Tropical Medicine, Antwerp, Belgium
Department of Biomedical Sciences, Faculty of Pharmaceutical, Veterinary and Biomedical
Sciences, University of Antwerp, Antwerpen (Wilrijk), Belgium

Claire Duchet
Entente InterDépartementale de Démoustication du Littoral Méditerranéen, Montpellier,
France Community Ecology Laboratory, Institute of Evolution and Department of
Evolutionary & Environmental Biology, University of Haifa, Israel

Richard Allan
The MENTOR Initiative, Crawley, UK

Pierre Carnevale
Portiragnes, France

Donald R. Roberts
Uniformed Services University of the Health Sciences, Bethesda, MD, USA Retired,
Professor Emeritus, Clifton Forge, VA, USA

Kimberly Hess
Africa Fighting Malaria, Washington, DC, USA

Papa M. Drame, Souleymane Doucoure, Anne Poinsignon and Alexandra Marie
Universités Montpellier 1 et 2, Institut de Recherche pour le Développement (IRD),
Montpellier, France

Sylvie Cornelie and Franck Remoue
Universités Montpellier 1 et 2, Institut de Recherche pour le Développement (IRD),
Montpellier, France Universités Montpellier 1 et 2, Centre de Recherche Entomologique
de Cotonou (CREC), Cotonou, Bénin

Herbert Noukpo
Universités Montpellier 1 et 2, Centre de Recherche Entomologique de Cotonou (CREC),
Cotonou, Bénin

Christophe Boëte
UMR 190 "Emergence des Pathologies Virales", Aix Marseille Université IRD (Institut de
Recherche pour le Développement) EHESP (Ecole des Hautes Etudes en Santé Publique),
France

Uli Beisel
Lancaster Environment Centre, Lancaster University, Lancaster LA1 4YQ, UK

www.ingramcontent.com/pod-product-compliance
Lightning Source LLC
Chambersburg PA
CBHW070727190326
41458CB00004B/1074